Assessment of Preclinical Organ Damage in Hypertension

Enrico Agabiti Rosei • Giuseppe Mancia
Editors

Assessment of Preclinical Organ Damage in Hypertension

Springer

Editors
Enrico Agabiti Rosei
Department of Clinical
and Experimental Sciences
University of Brescia
Brescia
Italy

Giuseppe Mancia
IRCCS Istituto Auxologico Italiano
University of Milano-Bicocca
Milano
Italy

This book is endorsed by the European Society of Hypertension

ISBN 978-3-319-15602-6 ISBN 978-3-319-15603-3 (eBook)
DOI 10.1007/978-3-319-15603-3

Library of Congress Control Number: 2015940816

Springer Cham Heidelberg New York Dordrecht London

Printed on acid-free paper

Springer International Publishing AG Switzerland is part of Springer Science+Business Media (www.springer.com)

Foreword

Primary prevention of cardiovascular events and complications in the modern management of hypertension requires precise methods of assessment of preclinical organ damage. This excellent book provides a comprehensive know-how for all clinical practitioners involved in the management of patients with hypertension.

There is an excellent coverage of traditional and modern techniques, with all aspects of cardiac, arterial, renal and brain damage evaluation described and illustrated in detail. This book will facilitate practical management of hypertensive patients according to the current guidelines. It will also allow us to be ready for the future guidelines and recommendations through critical and detailed assessment of new methods and techniques, which are not yet in routine clinical use. One could ask an important question regarding genomics and other "omics", which are not covered in the text. We are aware that there is a large genetic component (30–50 %) in individuals' predisposition to hypertension, but further work is necessary to justify large-scale genetic screening for very early prediction of hypertension and cardiovascular disease risk. I believe that the next edition of this book will be able to discuss precision medicine strategies as they develop and mature.

In the meantime, the book *Assessment of Preclinical Organ Damage in Hypertension* will be used by specialist centres and primary care physicians now, and for many years to come, to answer practical questions on management of hypertension.

Anna F. Dominiczak, MD, FRCP
University of Glasgow, Glasgow, UK

Contents

Part I

Heart

Evaluation of Cardiac Damage in Hypertension: Electrocardiography

1

Anders M. Greve, Peter M. Okin, Michael Hecht Olsen, and Kristian Wachtell

1.1 Pathophysiology of Cardiac Target-Organ Damage

In the pressure-loaded heart, changes in cardiac structure and function, such as left ventricular (LV) hypertrophy, initially occur as adaptive responses to reduce wall stress and maintain cardiac output. However, depending on a combination of known and lesser understood factors, e.g., antihypertensive therapy, genes, and age, the heart will at a varying pace transition towards increasing cardiac fibrosis, LV dilation, pump failure, and ultimately death [1]. Importantly, substantial evidence has documented that early identification and therapy aimed at preventing or reversing subclinical cardiac target-organ damage is associated with improved outcomes in

A.M. Greve, MD, PhD (✉)
Department of Medicine, Glostrup University Hospital,
Glostrup, Copenhagen 2600, Denmark
e-mail: Greve_anders@outlook.com

P.M. Okin, MD
Division of Cardiology, Department of Medicine, Weill Cornell Medical College,
525 East 68th Street, New York, NY 10065, USA
e-mail: pokin@med.cornell.edu

M.H. Olsen, MD, PhD, DMSc
The Cardiovascular and Metabolic Preventive Clinic, Department of Endocrinology, Centre for Individualized Medicine in Arterial Diseases (CIMA), Odense University Hospital,
Sønder Boulevard 29, Odense 5000, Denmark
e-mail: mho@dadlnet.dk

K. Wachtell, MD, PhD, DMSc
Department of Medicine, Glostrup University Hospital,
Glostrup, Copenhagen 2600, Denmark

Division of Cardiology, Department of Medicine, Weill Cornell Medical College,
525 East 68th Street, New York, NY 10065, USA

Department of Cardiology, Örebro University Hospital, Örebro, Sweden

E. Agabiti Rosei, G. Mancia (eds.), *Assessment of Preclinical Organ Damage in Hypertension*, DOI 10.1007/978-3-319-15603-3_1

hypertension [2]. In current practice, the treating physician is well equipped to detect and monitor temporal changes in subclinical cardiac target-organ damage. The purpose of this chapter is to give an introduction to the usefulness of electrocardiography in evaluating patients with hypertension. The first subchapter presents a brief overview of the electrocardiogram in order for the main attention to be focused on the clinical evidence pertaining to its use in assessing cardiac target-organ damage.

1.2 The Electrocardiogram

In spite of its centenarian status, the electrocardiogram remains one of the most ubiquitous tools in modern cardiology (>150,000,000 performed per year in the USA and the European Union). Its advantages are clear: it is widely available, can be interpreted without expert knowledge, and provides prognostic information at low cost in patients with and without established cardiovascular disease [3]. The basis for electrocardiography is the sequential depolarization of the heart, which under physiologic conditions initiates in the sinoatrial node to move through the cardiac conductive system and reach the ventricular cardiomyocytes via the Purkinje fibers. The surface electrocardiographic signal is by definition positive if the vector of electrical current points towards the electrode and negative if the net flux directs away from the electrode. Today's standard is to use 10 electrodes to construct 12 different leads. Each lead views the depolarization and repolarization of atrial (P-wave) and ventricular (QRS-complex) cardiomyocytes from a different angle and under many circumstances allows for prediction of the anatomic localization underlying the observed electrocardiographic findings. By principle, cardiac cellular hypertrophy or a lean body stature will tend to increase QRS voltage amplitude [4]. Conversely, a loss of cardiac cells, due to, for example, cardiac fibrosis, or an increased distance from heart to the electrode, e.g., obesity or a posterior shift of cardiac positioning within the thorax, will attenuate electrocardiographic voltage [5]. Placement of the surface electrodes therefore also influences voltage-sensitive criteria for LV hypertrophy [6]. QRS duration reflects the time it takes for the initial depolarization of the LV. The latter is an integrated function of cardiac size and the speed with which the electrical pulse is propagated through the heart. Longer QRS duration may therefore be associated with intrinsic myocardial cell damage or slowing of propagation in specialized conduction tissue, perhaps due to aging in itself [7, 8]. The mechanisms underlying ST-segment deviation and T-wave inversion, although not fully understood, appear to involve a repolarization disparity between the endo- and epicardial layer induced by the effects of impaired myocardial blood flow [9]. The consequent ST/T abnormalities are not specific for underlying pathology, as they could equally reflect insufficient blood flow due to epicardial disease or an oxygen supply–demand mismatch in patients with concentric LV hypertrophy and normal coronary arteries [10, 11]. Of note, unlike ST elevation and transmural ischemia, ST depression and most instances of T-wave inversion do not localize the anatomic region with insufficient subendocardial blood flow [12]. The following subchapters highlight the clinical correlates of specific electrocardiographic findings in patients with hypertension.

1.3 Electrocardiographic Left Ventricular Hypertrophy

The most common criteria for assessing electrocardiographic LV hypertrophy are listed in Table 1.1 [13]. In general, the presence of electrocardiographic LV hypertrophy is regarded as highly predictive of anatomic LV hypertrophy (specificity 85–90 %), whereas the absence of electrocardiographic LV hypertrophy is considered less useful for ruling out cardiac hypertrophy (sensitivity less than 50 %) [13, 14]. As noted earlier, the latter may in part relate to the confounding effects of race, age, gender, and obesity on the diagnostic accuracy of the various electrocardiographic criteria [15–17]. In spite of its modest sensitivity, numerous studies have related electrocardiographic indices of cardiac hypertrophy to increased cardiovascular event rates in patients with hypertension [18]. It is therefore very important for the clinician to be familiar with the evidence linking electrocardiographic LV hypertrophy to target-organ damage and an independent increase in the risk of adverse outcomes including stroke, heart failure, myocardial infarction, and sudden cardiac death [19, 20]. Of equal importance is the fact that regression of electrocardiographic LV hypertrophy during antihypertensive treatment is associated with improved outcomes independent of changes in blood pressure per se [21, 22]. This suggests that LV hypertrophy is a more sensitive marker of cellular damage than brachial blood pressure. A mechanism may be that LV hypertrophy is closely associated with increased renin-angiotensin system activity and development of cardiac fibrosis (Fig. 1.1) [23, 24]. In conclusion, there is low to moderate agreement between the electrocardiographic LV hypertrophy and anatomic LV mass as determined by echocardiogram or magnetic resonance imaging (MRI) in patients with hypertension. However, strong evidence links LV hypertrophy on the electrocardiogram to risk of adverse outcomes in the same patient population. The beneficial effect of electrocardiographic LV hypertrophy regression during antihypertensive treatment suggests that electrocardiographic LV hypertrophy is a potential therapeutic target in hypertension.

1.4 Electrocardiographic ST/T Abnormalities

Electrocardiographic repolarization abnormalities are often observed in conjunction with electrocardiographic LV hypertrophy. It has been documented that adding electrocardiographic repolarization patterns to electrocardiographic voltage and QRS duration may improve the diagnostic accuracy for detection of anatomic LV hypertrophy [13]. Specifically, the additional presence of LV repolarization abnormalities is believed to be a marker of severe concentric LV hypertrophy [25, 26]. In turn, this may partly explain why the electrocardiographic "strain" pattern of lateral ST depression and T-wave inversion has emerged as an independent risk attribute

Table 1.1 Electrocardiographic criteria for assessing left ventricular hypertrophy

	Amplitude	First author of study	Year of study publication
Limb lead voltage			
(R I–S I)+(S III–R III)	>16 mm	Lewis	1914
R I+S III	>25 mm	Gubner	1943
R I	>15 mm	Gubner	1943
R aVL	>11 mm	Sokolow	1949
R aVF	>20 mm	Goldberger	1949
Q or S aVR	>19 mm	Schack	1950
R+S in any limb lead	>19 mm	Romhilt	1968
Precordial lead voltage			
S V_1	>23 mm	Wilson	1944
S V_2	>25 mm	Mazzoleni	1964
S V_1+R V_5	>35 mm	Sokolow	1949
S V_2+R $V_{5,6}$	>45 mm	Romhilt	1969
S $V_{1,2}$+R $V_{5,6}$	>35 mm	Murphy	1984
S $V_{1,2}$+R V_6	>40 mm	Grant	1957
R+S any precordial lead	>35 mm	Grant	1957
R V_5: R V_6	>1.0	Holt	1962
R, any precordial lead	>26 mm	McPhie	1958
S V_2+R $V_{4,5}$	>45 mm	Wolff	1956
R V_5	>33 mm	Wilson	1944
R V_6	>25 mm	Wilson	1944
Combinations of limb and precordial voltage			
RS aVF+V_2+V_6 (>30 years)	>59 mm	Manning	1964
RS aVF+V_2+V_6 (<30 years)	>93 mm	Manning	1964
S V_3+R aVL (men)	>28 mm	Casale	1985
S V_3+R aVL (women)	>20 mm	Casale	1985
Total 12-lead voltage	>175 mm	Siegel	1982
Combinations of voltage and non-voltage			
Voltage-STT-LAA-axis-QRS duration	Point score	Romhilt	1968
(R aVL+S V_3)×QRS duration	>2,436 mm/s	Molloy	1992
Total 12-lead voltage×QRS duration	>1,742 mm/s	Molloy	1992
Criteria for use with left anterior fascicular block			
S V_1+R V_5+S V_5	>25	Bozzi	1976
S $V_{1,2}$+R V_6+S V_6	>25	Bozzi	1976
S III+max R/S any lead (men)	>30	Gertsch	1988
S III+max R/S any lead (women)	>28	Gertsch	1988

Table 1.1 (continued)

	Amplitude	First author of study	Year of study publication
Criteria for use with right bundle-branch block			
Max R/S precordial lead (with LAD)	>29 mm	Vandenberg	1991
S V_1	>2 mm	Vandenberg	1991
R $V_{5,6}$	>15 mm	Vandenberg	1991
S III + max R/S precordial (with LAD)	>40 mm	Vandenberg	1991
R I	>11 mm	Vandenberg	1991

Reproduced with permission from [13]
Amplitudes are given in millimeters, where 1 mm = 0.1 mV
LAD left axis deviation

even when adjusting for the presence of electrocardiographic voltage criteria for LV hypertrophy [27–29]. In the losartan intervention for endpoint reduction (LIFE) study, new development of electrocardiographic strain was a strong predictor of adverse outcome in the setting of electrocardiographic LV hypertrophy regression [30].In conclusion, electrocardiographic strain patterns refine cardiovascular risk prediction and may improve detection of anatomic LV hypertrophy when combined with electrocardiographic LV hypertrophy. The mechanisms underlying regression and development of electrocardiographic strain, at baseline and during antihypertensive therapy, require further study to fully unveil its prognostic potential.

1.5 QRS Duration

Longer QRS duration is an independent predictor of increased sudden cardiac death in patients with hypertension [31]. Moreover, longitudinal changes in QRS duration during follow-up in hypertensive patients are closely related to risk of incident heart failure [32]. It is less evident if QRS duration should be considered a separate risk marker as compared to electrocardiographic voltage in itself. This is further complicated by the fact that some electrocardiographic criteria for LV hypertrophy include QRS duration in their calculation, whereas others rely entirely on electrocardiographic voltage. Clearly, electrocardiographic voltage and QRS duration will be differently affected by confounding factors such as obesity and age-related calcification of conduction tissue [33]. From a pathophysiological standpoint, there may also be important differences between QRS duration and voltage, as only viable cardiomyocytes can produce electrocardiographic voltage. Conversely, longer QRS duration is in itself associated with cardiac fibrosis and LV dilatation, both of which are regarded as hallmarks of end-stage LV failure [34]. Thus, while greater QRS voltage mirrors hypertrophy of viable cardiomyocytes, longer QRS duration may reflect greater cellular hypertrophy or delayed cardiac activation due to regional or more widespread cardiac

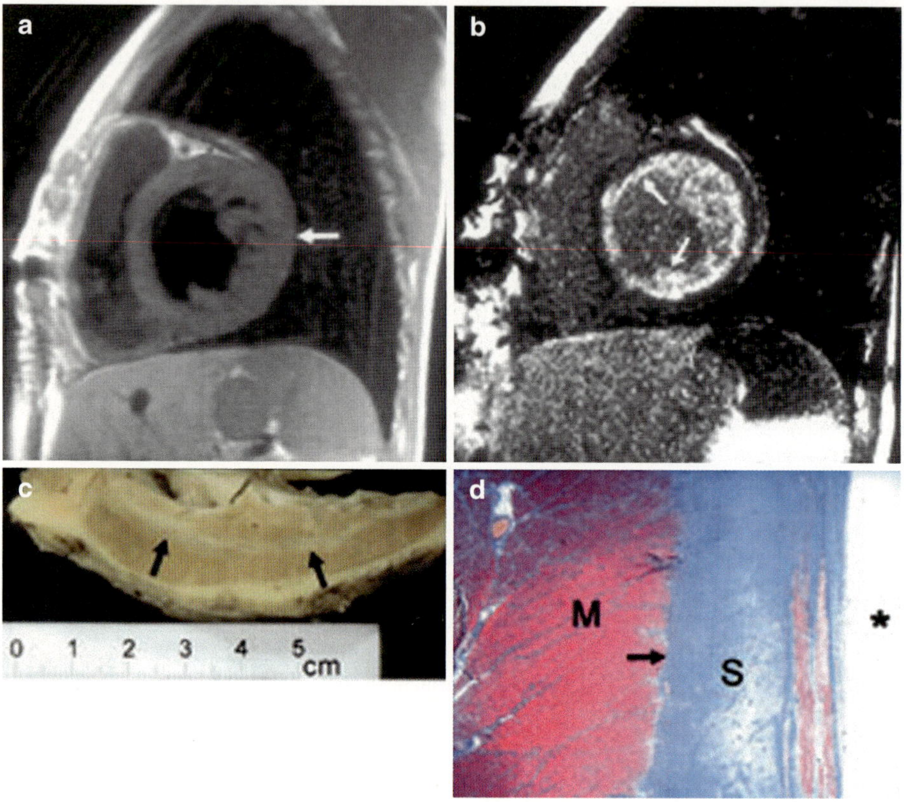

Fig. 1.1 (**a**) Short-axis T1-weighted image of the mid-left ventricle demonstrating left ventricular hypertrophy with normal myocardial signal (*arrow*). (**b**) Corresponding midventricular MRI image with delayed gadolinium enhancement shows extensive subendocardial enhancement consistent with diffuse fibrosis (*arrows*). (**c**) Gross examination of the explanted left ventricle fixed in formalin shows extensive subendocardial fibrosis. Note the sharp demarcation from normal tan-colored myocardium (*arrows*). (**d**) Masson's trichrome stain confirms extensive subendocardial fibrosis (*S*), *stained blue* with this stain (*arrow*) and sharply demarcated from normal myocardium (*M*), *staining red* (original magnification, ×40). *Asterisk* denotes endocardial surface (Reproduced with permission from Salvia et al. [23])

fibrosis, which may (reactive interstitial fibrosis) or may not be reversible (replacement fibrosis) [35]. Worsening fibrosis in the setting of increasing LV hypertrophy may in part explain why electrocardiographic voltage is not linearly related to cardiac mass and suggests that the current clinical standard of dichotomizing electrocardiographic criteria for LV hypertrophy may in itself lead to poor diagnostic performance of the electrocardiogram [5]. In conclusion, QRS duration is an independent predictor of heart failure and sudden cardiac death in hypertensive patients. QRS duration and QRS voltage may reflect different stages or components of cardiac maladaptations to increased LV afterload. Further studies are needed to elucidate the differential implications of longer QRS duration as compared increased QRS voltage.

1.6 Atrial Fibrillation

Atrial fibrillation is an independent predictor of adverse outcomes including stroke, heart failure, and cardiovascular mortality in hypertensive patients [36]. There is mounting evidence to indicate that new-onset atrial fibrillation should be regarded as target-organ damage [37]. One potential mechanism may involve increased LV pressures that translate to a dilatation of the thin-walled left atria, thereby increasing risk of atrial arrhythmia [38]. As such, regression of electrocardiographic indices of LV hypertrophy is associated with a reduced incidence of new-onset atrial fibrillation [39]. Importantly, it has been well documented that prevention of new-onset atrial fibrillation is associated with less fewer clinical endpoints, including stroke and sudden cardiac death [40, 41]. In conclusion, atrial fibrillation is a well-established marker of cardiovascular risk in hypertensive patients. Preexisting atrial fibrillation might relate to different factors than hypertension. However, there is now clear evidence to suggest that new-onset atrial fibrillation during follow-up of hypertensive patients is a sign of target-organ damage, which should elicit more aggressive lowering of blood pressure and risk factors to prevent catastrophic events like stroke and sudden cardiac death.

1.7 Electrocardiography vs. Echocardiography and Magnetic Resonance Imaging

Historically, the electrocardiogram has been used to detect cardiac arrhythmias and as a surrogate marker of anatomic LV hypertrophy. Based on the published evidence, sensitivity of LV hypertrophy on the electrocardiogram is too low to serve as a discriminatory marker of anatomic LV hypertrophy in patients with hypertension. The next question then becomes, is the electrocardiogram therefore a rudimentary tool that will eventually be phased out as echocardiography and cardiac MRI becomes more routine and cost is driven down. So far, the answer to that question seems to be both yes and no. Favoring a continued important role of electrocardiography in hypertension is the fact that several studies have now shown that electrocardiographic LV hypertrophy and anatomic LV hypertrophy, as determined by echocardiography or MRI, are separately predictive of adverse cardiovascular outcomes [37, 42]. It has therefore been proposed that anatomical and electrical hypertrophy might reflect different aspects of cardiac maladaptations to increased LV afterload [43]. Novel cardiac MRI measures, such as extracellular volume mapping and pixel-wise quantification of myocardial blood flow, are likely to provide further insight into the mechanisms underlying electrocardiographic abnormalities in the hypertensive heart [44]. On the other hand, there is now sufficient evidence to conclude that electrocardiogram is not useful tool to screen for anatomic LV hypertrophy and that many electrocardiographic changes overlap with changes in cardiac structure and function that are not specific to cardiac organ damage induced by hypertension. Thus, the electrocardiogram cannot stand alone in cardiovascular risk stratification of hypertensive patients, but it can provide low-cost and very valuable prognostic information when ordered and interpreted in light of its strengths and limitations. There is no randomized comparison of antihypertensive management with and without guidance from the electrocardiographic findings. Thus, until new evidence becomes available, the clinician must rely on observational evidence as presented in this chapter.

References

1. Hein S, Arnon E, Kostin S, et al. Progression from compensated hypertrophy to failure in the pressure-overloaded human heart: structural deterioration and compensatory mechanisms. Circulation. 2003;107:984–91.
2. Agabiti-Rosei E, Muiesan ML, Salvetti M. Evaluation of subclinical target organ damage for risk assessment and treatment in the hypertensive patients: left ventricular hypertrophy. J Am Soc Nephrol. 2006;17:S104–8.
3. Kannel WB. Prevalence and natural history of electrocardiographic left ventricular hypertrophy. Am J Med. 1983;75:4–11.
4. Sokolow M, Lyon TP. The ventricular complex in left ventricular hypertrophy as obtained by unipolar precordial and limb leads. Am Heart J. 1949;37:161–86.
5. Roberts WC, Filardo G, Ko JM, et al. Comparison of total 12-lead QRS voltage in a variety of cardiac conditions and its usefulness in predicting increased cardiac mass. Am J Cardiol. 2013;112:904–9.
6. Angeli F, Verdecchia P, Angeli E, et al. Day-to-day variability of electrocardiographic diagnosis of left ventricular hypertrophy in hypertensive patients. Influence of electrode placement. J Cardiovasc Med (Hagerstown). 2006;7:812–6.
7. Dhingra R, Ho NB, Benjamin EJ, et al. Cross-sectional relations of electrocardiographic QRS duration to left ventricular dimensions: the Framingham Heart Study. J Am Coll Cardiol. 2005;45:685–9.
8. Wiegerinck RF, Verkerk AO, Belterman CN, et al. Larger cell size in rabbits with heart failure increases myocardial conduction velocity and QRS duration. Circulation. 2006;113:806–13.
9. Johnson NP, Gould KL. Physiological basis for angina and ST-segment change PET-verified thresholds of quantitative stress myocardial perfusion and coronary flow reserve. JACC Cardiovasc Imaging. 2011;4:990–8.
10. Cabrera E, Monroy JR. Systolic and diastolic loading of the heart. II. Electrocardiographic data. Am Heart J. 1952;43:669–86.
11. Pichard AD, Gorlin R, Smith H, Ambrose J, Meller J. Coronary flow studies in patients with left ventricular hypertrophy of the hypertensive type. Evidence for an impaired coronary vascular reserve. Am J Cardiol. 1981;47:547–54.
12. Li D, Li CY, Yong AC, Kilpatrick D. Source of electrocardiographic ST changes in subendocardial ischemia. Circ Res. 1998;82:957–70.
13. Hancock EW, Deal BJ, Mirvis DM, et al. AHA/ACCF/HRS recommendations for the standardization and interpretation of the electrocardiogram: part V: electrocardiogram changes associated with cardiac chamber hypertrophy: a scientific statement from the American Heart Association Electrocardiography and Arrhythmias Committee, Council on Clinical Cardiology; the American College of Cardiology Foundation; and the Heart Rhythm Society. Endorsed by the International Society for Computerized Electrocardiology. J Am Coll Cardiol. 2009;53:992–1002.
14. Pewsner D, Juni P, Egger M, Battaglia M, Sundstrom J, Bachmann LM. Accuracy of electrocardiography in diagnosis of left ventricular hypertrophy in arterial hypertension: systematic review. BMJ. 2007;335:711.
15. Alfakih K, Walters K, Jones T, Ridgway J, Hall AS, Sivananthan M. New gender-specific partition values for ECG criteria of left ventricular hypertrophy: recalibration against cardiac MRI. Hypertension. 2004;44:175–9.

16. Okin PM, Devereux RB, Jern S, Kjeldsen SE, Julius S, Dahlof B. Baseline characteristics in relation to electrocardiographic left ventricular hypertrophy in hypertensive patients: the Losartan intervention for endpoint reduction (LIFE) in hypertension study. The Life Study Investigators. Hypertension. 2000;36:766–73.
17. Angeli F, Verdecchia P, Iacobellis G, Reboldi G. Usefulness of QRS voltage correction by body mass index to improve electrocardiographic detection of left ventricular hypertrophy in patients with systemic hypertension. Am J Cardiol. 2014;114(3):427–32.
18. Ang D, Lang C. The prognostic value of the ECG in hypertension: where are we now? J Hum Hypertens. 2008;22:460–7.
19. Verdecchia P, Porcellati C, Reboldi G, et al. Left ventricular hypertrophy as an independent predictor of acute cerebrovascular events in essential hypertension. Circulation. 2001;104:2039–44.
20. Schillaci G, Battista F, Pucci G. A review of the role of electrocardiography in the diagnosis of left ventricular hypertrophy in hypertension. J Electrocardiol. 2012;45:617–23.
21. Okin PM, Devereux RB, Jern S, et al. Regression of electrocardiographic left ventricular hypertrophy during antihypertensive treatment and the prediction of major cardiovascular events. JAMA. 2004;292:2343–9.
22. Wachtell K, Okin PM, Olsen MH, et al. Regression of electrocardiographic left ventricular hypertrophy during antihypertensive therapy and reduction in sudden cardiac death: the LIFE Study. Circulation. 2007;116:700–5.
23. La Salvia EA, Gilkeson RC, Dahms BB, Siwik E. Delayed contrast enhancement magnetic resonance imaging in congenital aortic stenosis. Pediatr Cardiol. 2006;27:388–90.
24. Muiesan ML. Left ventricular hypertrophy: a new approach for fibrosis inhibition. J Hypertens. 2002;20:611–3.
25. Buchner S, Debl K, Haimerl J, et al. Electrocardiographic diagnosis of left ventricular hypertrophy in aortic valve disease: evaluation of ECG criteria by cardiovascular magnetic resonance. J Cardiovasc Magn Reson. 2009;11:18.
26. Okin PM, Devereux RB, Nieminen MS, et al. Relationship of the electrocardiographic strain pattern to left ventricular structure and function in hypertensive patients: the LIFE study. Losartan Intervention For End point. J Am Coll Cardiol. 2001;38:514–20.
27. Okin PM, Devereux RB, Nieminen MS, et al. Electrocardiographic strain pattern and prediction of cardiovascular morbidity and mortality in hypertensive patients. Hypertension. 2004;44:48–54.
28. Verdecchia P, Reboldi G, Angeli F, et al. Prognostic value of serial electrocardiographic voltage and repolarization changes in essential hypertension: the HEART Survey study. Am J Hypertens. 2007;20:997–1004.
29. Schillaci G, Pirro M, Pasqualini L, et al. Prognostic significance of isolated, non-specific left ventricular repolarization abnormalities in hypertension. J Hypertens. 2004;22:407–14.
30. Okin PM, Oikarinen L, Viitasalo M, et al. Prognostic value of changes in the electrocardiographic strain pattern during antihypertensive treatment: the Losartan Intervention for End-Point Reduction in Hypertension Study (LIFE). Circulation. 2009;119:1883–91.
31. Morin DP, Oikarinen L, Viitasalo M, et al. QRS duration predicts sudden cardiac death in hypertensive patients undergoing intensive medical therapy: the LIFE study. Eur Heart J. 2009;30:2908–14.
32. Okin PM, Devereux RB, Kjeldsen SE, Edelman JM, Dahlof B. Incidence of heart failure in relation to QRS duration during antihypertensive therapy: the LIFE study. J Hypertens. 2009;27:2271–7.
33. Lenegre J. Etiology and pathology of bilateral bundle branch block in relation to complete heart block. Prog Cardiovasc Dis. 1964;6:409–44.
34. Drazner MH. The progression of hypertensive heart disease. Circulation. 2011;123:327–34.
35. Mewton N, Liu CY, Croisille P, Bluemke D, Lima JA. Assessment of myocardial fibrosis with cardiovascular magnetic resonance. J Am Coll Cardiol. 2011;57:891–903.
36. Wachtell K, Hornestam B, Lehto M, et al. Cardiovascular morbidity and mortality in hypertensive patients with a history of atrial fibrillation: the Losartan Intervention For End Point Reduction in Hypertension (LIFE) study. J Am Coll Cardiol. 2005;45:705–11.

37. Chrispin J, Jain A, Soliman EZ, et al. Association of electrocardiographic and imaging surrogates of left ventricular hypertrophy with incident atrial fibrillation: MESA (Multi-Ethnic Study of Atherosclerosis). J Am Coll Cardiol. 2014;63:2007–13.
38. Wachtell K, Devereux RB, Lyle PA, Okin PM, Gerdts E. The left atrium, atrial fibrillation, and the risk of stroke in hypertensive patients with left ventricular hypertrophy. Ther Adv Cardiovasc Dis. 2008;2:507–13.
39. Okin PM, Wachtell K, Devereux RB, et al. Regression of electrocardiographic left ventricular hypertrophy and decreased incidence of new-onset atrial fibrillation in patients with hypertension. JAMA. 2006;296:1242–8.
40. Wachtell K, Lehto M, Gerdts E, et al. Angiotensin II receptor blockade reduces new-onset atrial fibrillation and subsequent stroke compared to atenolol: the Losartan Intervention For End Point Reduction in Hypertension (LIFE) study. J Am Coll Cardiol. 2005;45:712–9.
41. Okin PM, Bang CN, Wachtell K, et al. Relationship of sudden cardiac death to new-onset atrial fibrillation in hypertensive patients with left ventricular hypertrophy. Circ Arrhythm Electrophysiol. 2013;6:243–51.
42. Sundstrom J, Lind L, Arnlov J, Zethelius B, Andren B, Lithell HO. Echocardiographic and electrocardiographic diagnoses of left ventricular hypertrophy predict mortality independently of each other in a population of elderly men. Circulation. 2001;103:2346–51.
43. Bacharova L, Szathmary V, Kovalcik M, Mateasik A. Effect of changes in left ventricular anatomy and conduction velocity on the QRS voltage and morphology in left ventricular hypertrophy: a model study. J Electrocardiol. 2010;43:200–8.
44. Ann Noninvasive Electrocardiol. 2014;19(6):524–33. doi: 10.1111/anec.12223. Epub 2014 Nov 4.

Evaluation of Cardiac Damage in Hypertension: Echocardiography

2

Enrico Agabiti Rosei and Maria Lorenza Muiesan

2.1 How to Assess

The presence of cardiac target organ damage, and in particular of left ventricular hypertrophy (LVH), has prognostic relevance and may influence the choice of treatment options.

The recent guidelines of the European Society of Hypertension (ESH) and of the European Society of Cardiology (ESC) [1] include echocardiography among the recommended techniques to be considered in hypertensive patients.

Echocardiography is a relatively easy method, is repeatable, is specific, and is a more sensitive measure of LVH than electrocardiography. It is more expensive than electrocardiography but may provide additional information on the anatomy and function of the heart and valves and can be performed before starting antihypertensive therapy but also during treatment (Table 2.1).

2.1.1 Cardiac Structure

In hypertensive patients, the main goal of echocardiography is the detection of LVH, and to this regard, the calculation of left ventricular mass (LVM) is mandatory. Hypertrophy cannot be defined according to wall thickness only, and wall thickness alone is not predictive of cardiovascular risk [3, 4].

Both mono-dimensional (M-mode) and two-dimensional (2D) echocardiography have been used in the measurement of LVM and have been anatomically validated [5, 6].

E. Agabiti Rosei, MD (✉) • M.L. Muiesan
Department of Clinical and Experimental Sciences, Clinica Medica, University of Brescia, Piazzale Spedali Civili 1, Brescia 25121, Italy
e-mail: enrico.agabitirosei@unibs.it; marialorenza.muiesan@unibs.it

E. Agabiti Rosei, G. Mancia (eds.), *Assessment of Preclinical Organ Damage in Hypertension*, DOI 10.1007/978-3-319-15603-3_2

Table 2.1 Parameters to be included in the echocardiographic report

LV mass indexed to BSA, $g/m^2 < 96$ in women,< 116 in men (when BMI 30 kg/m^2)
LV mass indexed to height 2.7, g/m 2.7 < 45 in women,<49 in men (when BMI > 30 kg/m^2)
LV relative wall thickness (RWT) < 0.43
Transmitral flow
Peak *E* velocity, cm/s
Peak *A* velocity, cm/s
E/A ratio, under quiet breathing and if necessary during Valsalva maneuver
E wave deceleration time, ms
LV isovolumic relaxation time, ms
Tissue Doppler imaging
e′ septal, cm/s ≥ 8
e′ lateral, cm/s ≥ 10
E/e′ ratio (septal and lateral averaged) < 13
LV ejection fraction, % > 55
Left atrial diameter, cm < 3.9 in women,<4.1 in men
Left atrial volume indexed to BSA, $ml/m^2 < 34$ (ESH ESC) (mild, EAE, ASE < 29)
Aortic diameter at the sinuses of Valsalva, indexed to BSA, $cm/m^2 < 2.1$

Normality reference values are derived from the ASE committee recommendations [2] and ESH/ESC guidelines [1], with permission

BSA body surface area, *BMI* body mass index, *RWT* relative wall thickness, *LA* left atrium, *ESH/ESC* European Society Hypertension/European Society Cardiology, *ASE* American Society Echocardiography

Linear measurements of interventricular septum wall thickness (IVST), as well as of left ventricular internal diameter (LVID) and posterior wall thickness (PWT), should be obtained with the beam perpendicular to the minor axis at the mitral valve leaflet tips, in the left parasternal acoustic window, at end diastole, from 2D-targeted M-mode, or directly from 2D images. Calculation of LVM is based on a mathematical formula assuming a prolate ellipsoid shape for the LV (LVM = 0.8 × (1.04 [(LVIDD + PWTD + IVSTD)3 − (LVIDD)3]) + 0.6 g, where LVIDD is left ventricle internal dimension in diastole, PWTD is posterior wall thickness in diastole, and IVSTD is intraventricular septal thickness in diastole [2].

LVM normalization for an anthropometric measure, such as height or body surface area, is needed to identify LVH. Weight and height should be measured simultaneously to the echocardiographic examination, avoiding the use of patients self-reported data, that is a source of potential error in the indexation of LVM and finally in the risk stratification [7]. The indexation of LVM to body surface area underestimates the prevalence of LVH and the LVH attributable risk in populations with overweight or obese subjects [8]. In these patients indexation of LVM for height (height to the allometric power of 1.7 or 2.7) can be considered. Indexation by height 2.7 was derived from a cohort of Caucasian children and adults, and indexation by height 1.7 was derived from a study including 1,035 Chinese and Caucasian adults [9, 10]. Recent data from the Echocardiographic Normal Ranges Meta-Analysis of the Left heart (EchoNoRMAL) project suggest that different allometric power for BSA and height should be applied according to gender and ethnic group [11].

The evaluation of geometric adaptation of the left ventricle to the increased hemodynamic load implies the calculation of the relative wall thickness (RWT or wall to radius ratio, i.e., the ratio between LV end-diastolic wall thicknesses and diameter) and may significantly differ among hypertensive patients [12]. A cutoff value of 0.42 permits categorization of an increase in left ventricular mass as either concentric (RWT = or > 0.42) or eccentric (RWT < 0.42) hypertrophy and also allows the identification of concentric remodeling, defined as a normal left ventricular mass with increased RWT > 0.42 [1].

These different LV geometric patterns are associated with different hemodynamic characteristics, and peripheral resistances are greater in patients with concentric geometry, while cardiac index is increased in those with eccentric hypertrophy [13]. In addition concentric remodeling, eccentric and concentric hypertrophy all predict an increased incidence of cardiovascular disease, but concentric hypertrophy has consistently been shown to be the condition that most markedly increases the risk, even in very high-risk patients [14–16]. Very recently, a new reclassification of LVH, based on LVM, relative wall thickness, and LV dilatation, has been proposed in hypertensive patients [17]. The subclassification of hypertensive patients with eccentric LVH into groups with normal or increased LV chamber volume revealed that the latter, but not the former, predicted increased risk for all-cause and cardiovascular mortality and cardiovascular events. In contrast, the subclassification of patients with concentric LVH into groups with normal or increased LV chamber volume revealed the association of both dilated and non-dilated concentric LVH with poor outcome. The low-risk group of patients with relatively mild LVH, no concentric geometry, or dilatation among patients with eccentric LVH had a similar risk of all-cause mortality or cardiovascular events as patients with normal LVM. The verification of the enhanced prognostic power of the 4-group classification of LVH in other populations is needed before recommending that this more refined approach replaces the established classification of LVH into eccentric and concentric subgroups.

Evaluating LVM increase by taking into account gender and cardiac loading conditions has been proposed in order to discriminate the amount of LVM adequate to compensate the hemodynamic load (adequate or appropriate) from the amount in excess to loading conditions (and therefore inappropriate or not compensatory) [18]. LVM is inappropriate when the value of LVM measured in a single subject exceeds the amount needed to adapt to the stroke work for that given gender and body size.

Technical variability represents a potential limitation of echocardiographic measurement of LVM. An assessment of LVM reproducibility has shown that LVM changes of 10–15 % may have biological significance in individual patients [19]. When changes in LVM inappropriateness are evaluated, changes of 15–25 % may reflect true changes [20]. Real-time 3D echocardiography permits a more reliable measurement of LVM, and its accuracy has been shown to compare favorably with that of cardiac magnetic resonance imaging [21]. Despite the relationship between LVM and incidence of cardiovascular events is continuous [22], several criteria for the diagnosis of echocardiographic LVH have been proposed. These criteria are based on the distribution of LVM index in general population samples (average LVM value plus one standard deviation in apparently healthy population-based samples) or on the association between increased values of LVM and occurrence of cardiovascular events in longitudinal studies. The presence of echocardiographic LVH is associated with an incidence of cardiovascular events equal or greater than 20 % in 10 years [23].

The American Society of Echocardiography and the European Association of Echocardiography (EAE/ASE) have published ranges for several echocardiographic parameters derived from a population of about 500 multiethnic, normotensive, and normal weight subjects, and the Pamela study has provided new reference limits in an Italian population [2, 24]. A revision of previous diagnostic criteria will probably come from new ethnic and gender-specific group reference values from the Echocardiographic Normal Ranges Meta-Analysis of the Left heart (EchoNoRMAL) project [11].

2.1.2 LV Diastolic Function

In hypertensive patients diastolic dysfunction is characterized by alterations of LV relaxation and filling that may precede abnormalities of systolic function [25]; these abnormalities should be interpreted according to the presence of LVH or concentric geometry in order to give a correct interpretation of LV diastolic function and filling pressure parameters. In fact, in patients with LV hypertrophy or concentric remodeling, LV relaxation is usually slowed, with a decrease in early diastolic filling; in the presence of normal left atrial pressure, a greater proportion of LV filling is shifted from early to late diastole after atrial contraction. Therefore, the presence of a predominant early filling in these patients should suggest the presence of increased LV filling pressures [2, 26].

An improvement in the study of LV diastolic function has been provided by the assessment of Doppler transmitral flow velocities and by pulsed Doppler tissue imaging (DTI). LA size is a further parameter to be assessed in the evaluation of diastolic function [27].

The influence of factors such as age, gender, body mass index, heart rate, and blood pressure on Doppler flow velocities has been extensively evaluated. Normal values for Doppler parameters according to age groups have been assessed in a relatively small sample of 117 subjects [28].

The analysis of myocardial velocities at the mitral annulus may reveal an increase in left ventricular filling pressure; in respect to Doppler transmitral flow velocities,

DTI velocities show no "pseudonormalization" pattern [29, 30]. The average value of DTI velocities at the septal and lateral sides of the mitral annulus should be used for the assessment of global LV diastolic function. The *E*/*e*′ ratio represents a reliable estimate of LV filling pressures, and different cutoff values have been proposed for the definition of normal or progressively higher LV filling pressure. *E*/*e*′ ratio > 13 indicates a severe increase in LV filling pressure. In the Anglo-Scandinavian Cardiac Outcomes Trial (ASCOT) echocardiographic sub-study, *E*/*e*′ ratio was the strongest predictor of first cardiac events, independent of LVM and geometry [31]. The combination of transmitral flow velocities, mitral annulus DTI velocities, and left atrial volume should be used for diastolic dysfunction diagnosis and stratification [26]. The grading suggested by the EAE/ASE recommendations is an important predictor of all-cause mortality, as shown in the Olmsted County epidemiological study.

An accurate measurement of left atrial (LA) size should be an integral part of the standard echocardiogram in hypertensive patients. LA enlargement may reflect the increase in left ventricular filling pressure; in patients with preserved systolic function, it may be a marker of diastolic dysfunction and is predictive of an increased risk of atrial fibrillation, stroke, heart failure, and mortality. This has been shown by the measurement of LA anteroposterior linear dimension by M-mode from the parasternal long axis view and by the more accurate evaluation of LA volume from 2D images. The measurement of LA volume is recommended both in clinical practice and in research studies, and most guidelines recommend the biplane area-length method. The recent 2013 ESH/ESC guidelines for the management of arterial hypertension and the EAE/ASE guidelines recommend a cutoff value of > 34 ml/m^2 for left atrial enlargement [1].

Compared to the conventional two-dimensional approach, 3D echocardiography appears superior in the assessment of LA volume; at present, however, this application is limited to research studies. The same consideration applies to several other parameters of left atrial function, based on 2D or 3D measures, conventional and tissue Doppler, or strain rate imaging [32, 33].

2.1.3 LV Systolic Function

LV dysfunction includes segmental and global alterations of LV that may differently affect pump function and prognosis. In uncomplicated hypertensive patients, LV shortening fraction (FS) and ejection fraction (EF) express endocardial fiber shortening and are usually preserved or even "supernormal," mainly in the presence of concentric geometry [2]. However, midwall myocardial fibers contribute to a greater extent than subendocardial fibers to LV ejection, and the difference between the conventional and midwall indexes of LV systolic function is more evident in the presence of a concentric LV geometry; therefore, in the presence of a concentric LV geometry, LV midwall fractional shortening is considered a more appropriate index of LV systolic function than conventional FS [34–36].

LVEF, derived from two-dimensional calculation of the LV end-diastolic volume (EDV) and the LV end-systolic volume (ESV) according to the modified Simpson method (average of apical four and two chamber views), is the most sensitive index of systolic ventricular function with a high prognostic value. LVEF values >55 % define a normal systolic function, while a slight or moderate reduction in systolic function is present when EF values are between 45 % and 55 % and between 35 % and 45 %, respectively; values below 35 % identify patients with severe LV systolic dysfunction.

In the absence of major structural abnormalities, a single-plane measurement of the LV area is obtained from the apical four-chamber window. The longitudinal myocardial systolic velocity (Sm), measured by TDI at the mitral annulus level, has been proposed as a reliable and accurate index of myocardial fiber performance, independent of LV preload and afterload. In normal conditions, its value is higher than 8 cm/s and in severe pathological conditions is less than 5 cm/s [26].

More recently a 3D probe (multiplane) has become available and allows the calculation of LV volumes by the Simpson triplane method [32, 37]. The accuracy of 3D echocardiographic in the measurement of LV volumes has been confirmed by the comparison with magnetic resonance imaging [38]. Speckle-tracking echocardiography, a technique based on the analysis of interference patterns and natural acoustic reflections generated by tissue motion which are ultimately resolved into angle-independent 2D and 3D strain-based sequences, may reveal early subclinical abnormalities in regional systolic and diastolic LV myocardial function in hypertension and can also be used to evaluate left atrial mechanics [39, 40].

2.1.4 Aortic Root

Finally, the measurement of the aortic size provides useful information in hypertensive patients undergoing echocardiography. As hypertension exerts a relevant effect on aortic size, an enlarged aorta has been associated with adverse cardiovascular outcomes and mortality.

Most guidelines currently underline the importance of including measurements at the aortic valve annulus (i.e., the hinge point of aortic leaflets) and at the sino-tubular junction in addition to the standard approach of measurement of aorta diameter at the sinuses of Valsalva from the 2D view in order to obtain the largest diameter. Furthermore, the subcostal approach allows in a large majority of patients the evaluation of the abdominal aorta, and these measurements are therefore recommended in clinical practice. Indexation for BSA is recommended for clinical purposes, a prognostically validated upper normal threshold for the diameter at the Valsalva sinus is 2.1 cm/m^2, and nomograms taking into account the age of patients are also available. In obese or overweight patients, indexation to body height should be considered [41].

2.2 Prevalence

Prevalence of left ventricular hypertrophy (LVH) in patients with hypertension mostly derives from population-based studies and selected hypertensive cohorts, with a quite large range according to demographic characteristics of subjects and to cutoff criteria used for the diagnosis. This variability is also potentiated by the different criteria used in different studies to calculate LVH. Cuspidi et al. have analyzed the available studies in 2012 and found that LVH prevalence consistently varied among studies from 9 % to 77 %, being lowest in population-based studies (<10 %) and highest in high-risk hypertensive patients (58–77 %) [42].

In a multicenter Italian study conducted in several hypertension specialist outpatient clinic, the prevalence of LVH was 60 % according to sex-specific criteria of LVM indexed by height to the 2.7 power and 37 % according to sex-specific criteria for LVM indexed by BSA [7].

2.3 Change with Treatment

Antihypertensive treatment is associated with a significant reduction in LVM. The magnitude of the decrease is related to the baseline LVM; according to variability in LVM measurements, only changes >10–15 % can be considered of biological relevance. The correlation between changes of LVM and changes in clinic BP is modest and increases when 24 h BP is considered [43].

Among all classes of antihypertensive drugs, ACE inhibitors, angiotensin receptor blockers, and calcium antagonists seem to be more effective as compared with beta-blockers [44]. It should kept in mind, however, that in most studies patients were receiving a combination of drugs (usually with a diuretic) and not monotherapy. Therefore, the efficacy of antihypertensive treatment in inducing adequate and long-term blood pressure control seems more important than the choice of a specific class.

A normalization of LVM is more difficult and cannot be always reached in women [25], obese or diabetic patients [45], elderly subjects with isolated systolic hypertension [46], or patients with coronary artery disease, despite adequate treatment. A normalization of LV geometry is also possible, and in the LIFE study, a conversion of concentric to eccentric LVH was reported in 34 % of subjects, whereas only 3 % of patients with eccentric LVH transitioned to concentric LVH [47]. In the ASCOT study, a modest change in LVM and persistence of elevated relative wall thickness were observed from the first to the third year of therapy [48].

Several studies have also noted an improvement of midwall FS [49] and of diastolic function parameters in response to antihypertensive therapy. However, two studies have recently shown no favorable changes in diastolic filling or E/e' ratio, despite adequate BP control; in these studies, however, a limited, despite statistically significant, decrease of LVM and no change in RWT were noted.

It is possible that the partial dissociation between structural and functional changes during antihypertensive treatment may reflect, at least in part, the effect of treatment on several factors influencing diastolic function, including heart rate, humoral changes, and extracellular matrix composition.

The deposition of perivascular and interstitial fibrosis has been noninvasively evaluated by some ultrasound methods, showing that drugs interfering with the renin-angiotensin-aldosterone system may be particularly effective in inducing changes that might reflect a decrease of myocardial tissue collagen content. Cardiac magnetic resonance may provide accurate and noninvasive assessment of regional myocardial fibrosis using late gadolinium enhancement, while diffuse interstitial myocardial fibrosis is accurately assessed with post-contrast T1 mapping [38]. In the future this technique will allow the assessment of the effects of different drugs on interstitial fibrosis in hypertensive patients.

2.4 Prognostic Value of Change

In hypertensive patients LVH may predict the occurrence of cardiovascular events, including myocardial infarction, stroke sudden death, and heart failure [50]. The incidence of atrial fibrillation and of renal events, such as creatinine doubling, estimated glomerular filtration rate<30 ml/min/1.73 m^2, or the need for end-stage renal disease, are higher in the presence of LVH [51].

Changes of LVM index during treatment, and not only the baseline value of LVM, may have prognostic relevance. In the prospective randomized clinical study Losartan Intervention For Endpoint reduction in hypertension (LIFE), it was shown that in patients with electrocardiographic LVH, the absence of LVH during treatment was associated with a lower incidence of cardiovascular events, while the opposite was true for patients with no regression of LVH induced by long-term antihypertensive therapy [52]. Several other studies have confirmed the results of the LIFE study; these studies were performed in cohorts of hypertensive patients with different demographic and clinical characteristics, with and without LVH at baseline, treated according to the decision of their general practitioner (Fig. 2.1) [50, 53, 54]. In addition a different statistical approach, evaluating the change of the echocardiographic LVM from baseline to follow-up and not the "in-treatment" value, was used.

Regression of LVH may have a prognostic significance independently of blood pressure values, even when measured by 24 h BP. Changes in LVM and in renal function may independently predict the occurrence of cardiovascular events [55].

Study name	Statistics for each study					Events/Total		
	Odds ratio	Lower limit	Upper limit	Z-Value	p-Value	LVH absence or regression	LVH persistence or development	Total
Muiesan, 1995	0.136	0.052	0.355	−4.074	0.000	8/110	15/41	23/151
Verdecchia, 1998	0.448	0.215	0.934	−2.142	0.032	15/285	16/145	31/430
Cipriano, 2001	0.219	0.098	0.487	−3.722	0.000	8/218	32/216	40/434
Koren, 2002	0.376	0.162	0.873	−2.278	0.023	17/130	12/42	29/172
Muiesan, 2007	0.200	0.118	0.342	−5.907	0.000	31/321	40/115	71/436
Pierdomenico, 2008	0.150	0.080	0.281	−5.899	0.000	15/245	44/145	59/390
Gosse, 2012	0.282	0.162	0.490	−4.483	0.000	19/202	63/234	82/436
	0.236	0.182	0.305	−11.039	0.000	113/1511	222/938	335/2449

Odds ratio and 95 % CI

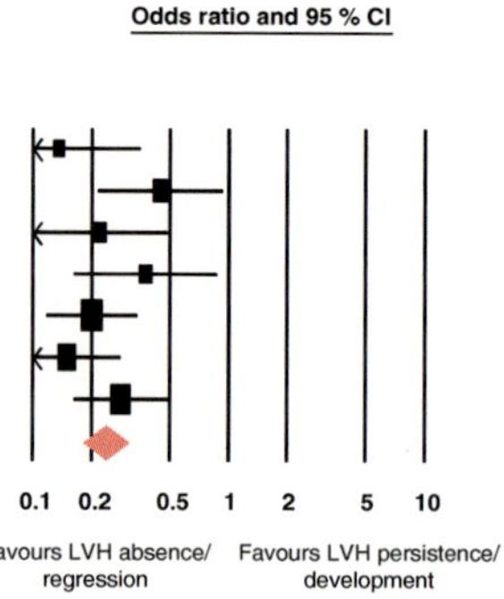

Fig. 2.1 Update of studies evaluating the occurrence of CV events in hypertensive patients according to changes in LV mass

During antihypertensive treatment, the modifications of LV geometry, of left atrial size, of midwall fractional shortening, and of diastolic dysfunction parameters have been also shown to be associated with the incidence of cardiovascular events, independently of LVM change [14, 27, 56].

Therefore, although it must not be considered an absolute indication, in a patient with LVH at baseline, it is recommended to repeat an echocardiogram after 12 months of treatment, for the great amount of given information [1]. During this time interval, it is greatest the probability that the degree of anatomic and/or functional changes indicate a real biological modification.

References

1. Mancia G, Fagard R, Narkiewicz K, Redon J, Zanchetti A, Bohm M, et al. 2013 ESH/ESC guidelines for the management of arterial hypertension: the task force for the management of arterial hypertension of the European Society of Hypertension (ESH) and of the European Society of Cardiology (ESC). J Hypertens. 2013;31(7):1281–357.
2. Lang RM, Bierig M, Devereux RB, Flachskampf FA, Foster E, Pellikka PA, et al. Recommendations for chamber quantification: a report from the American Society of Echocardiography's Guidelines and Standards Committee and the Chamber Quantification Writing Group, developed in conjunction with the European Association of Echocardiography, a branch of the European Society of Cardiology. J Am Soc Echocardiogr. 2005;18(12):1440–63.
3. Leibowitz D, Planer D, Ben-Ibgi F, Rott D, Weiss AT, Bursztyn M. Measurement of wall thickness alone does not accurately assess the presence of left ventricular hypertrophy. Clin Exp Hypertens. 2007;29(2):119–25.
4. Barbieri A, Bursi F, Mantovani F, Valenti C, Quaglia M, Berti E, et al. Left ventricular hypertrophy reclassification and death: application of the Recommendation of the American Society of Echocardiography/European Association of Echocardiography. Eur Heart J Cardiovasc Imaging. 2012;13(1):109–17.
5. Devereux RB, Alonso DR, Lutas EM, Gottlieb GJ, Campo E, Sachs I, et al. Echocardiographic assessment of left ventricular hypertrophy: comparison to necropsy findings. Am J Cardiol. 1986;57(6):450–8.
6. Reichek N, Devereux RB. Left ventricular hypertrophy: relationship of anatomic, echocardiographic and electrocardiographic findings. Circulation. 1981;63(6):1391–8.
7. Cuspidi C, Negri F, Giudici V, Muiesan ML, Grandi AM, Ganau A, et al. Self-reported weight and height: implications for left ventricular hypertrophy detection. An Italian multi-center study. Clin Exp Hypertens. 2011;33(3):192–201.
8. Gosse P, Jullien V, Jarnier P, Lemetayer P, Clementy J. Echocardiographic definition of left ventricular hypertrophy in the hypertensive: which method of indexation of left ventricular mass? J Hum Hypertens. 1999;13(8):505–9.
9. de Simone G, Daniels SR, Devereux RB, Meyer RA, Roman MJ, de Divitiis O, et al. Left ventricular mass and body size in normotensive children and adults: assessment of allometric relations and impact of overweight. J Am Coll Cardiol. 1992;20(5):1251–60.
10. Chirinos JA, Segers P, De Buyzere ML, Kronmal RA, Raja MW, De BD, et al. Left ventricular mass: allometric scaling, normative values, effect of obesity, and prognostic performance. Hypertension. 2010;56(1):91–8.
11. Poppe KK, Doughty RN, Whalley GA. Redefining normal reference ranges for echocardiography: a major new individual person data meta-analysis. Eur Heart J Cardiovasc Imaging. 2013;14(4):347–8.
12. Ganau A, Devereux RB, Roman MJ, de Simone G, Pickering TG, Saba PS, et al. Patterns of left ventricular hypertrophy and geometric remodeling in essential hypertension. J Am Coll Cardiol. 1992;19(7):1550–8.

13. Linzbach AJ. Heart failure from the point of view of quantitative anatomy. Am J Cardiol. 1960;5:370–82.
14. Muiesan ML, Salvetti M, Monteduro C, Bonzi B, Paini A, Viola S, et al. Left ventricular concentric geometry during treatment adversely affects cardiovascular prognosis in hypertensive patients. Hypertension. 2004;43(4):731–8.
15. Verdecchia P, Schillaci G, Borgioni C, Ciucci A, Battistelli M, Bartoccini C, et al. Adverse prognostic significance of concentric remodeling of the left ventricle in hypertensive patients with normal left ventricular mass. J Am Coll Cardiol. 1995;25(4):871–8.
16. Cuspidi C, Giudici V, Meani S, Negri F, Sala C, Zanchetti A, et al. Extracardiac organ damage in essential hypertensives with left ventricular concentric remodelling. J Hum Hypertens. 2009;19.
17. Bang CN, Gerdts E, Aurigemma GP, Boman K, de Simone G, Dahlof B, et al. Four-group classification of left ventricular hypertrophy based on ventricular concentricity and dilatation identifies a low-risk subset of eccentric hypertrophy in hypertensive patients. Circ Cardiovasc Imaging. 2014;7(3):422–9.
18. de Simone G, Palmieri V, Koren MJ, Mensah GA, Roman MJ, Devereux RB. Prognostic implications of the compensatory nature of left ventricular mass in arterial hypertension. J Hypertens. 2001;19(1):119–25.
19. de Simone G, Muiesan ML, Ganau A, Longhini C, Verdecchia P, Palmieri V, et al. Reliability and limitations of echocardiographic measurement of left ventricular mass for risk stratification and follow-up in single patients: the RES trial. Working Group on Heart and Hypertension of the Italian Society of Hypertension. Reliability of M-mode Echocardiographic Studies. J Hypertens. 1999;17(12 Pt 2):1955–63.
20. Muiesan ML, de Simone G, Ganau A, Longhini C, Verdecchia P, Mancia G, et al. Inappropriate left ventricular mass: reliability and limitations of echocardiographic measurement for risk stratification and follow-up in single patients. J Hypertens. 2006;24(11):2293–8.
21. Kusunose K, Kwon DH, Motoki H, Flamm SD, Marwick TH. Comparison of three-dimensional echocardiographic findings to those of magnetic resonance imaging for determination of left ventricular mass in patients with ischemic and non-ischemic cardiomyopathy. Am J Cardiol. 2013;112(4):604–11.
22. Schillaci G, Verdecchia P, Porcellati C, Cuccurullo O, Cosco C, Perticone F. Continuous relation between left ventricular mass and cardiovascular risk in essential hypertension. Hypertension. 2000;35(2):580–6.
23. Yasuno S, Ueshima K, Oba K, Fujimoto A, Ogihara T, Saruta T, et al. Clinical significance of left ventricular hypertrophy and changes in left ventricular mass in high-risk hypertensive patients: a subanalysis of the Candesartan Antihypertensive Survival Evaluation in Japan trial. J Hypertens. 2009;27(8):1705–12.
24. Cuspidi C, Facchetti R, Sala C, Bombelli M, Negri F, Carugo S, et al. Normal values of left-ventricular mass: echocardiographic findings from the PAMELA study. J Hypertens. 2012;30(5):997–1003.
25. Perlini S, Chung ES, Aurigemma GP, Meyer TE. Alterations in early filling dynamics predict the progression of compensated pressure overload hypertrophy to heart failure better than abnormalities in midwall systolic shortening. Clin Exp Hypertens. 2013;35(6):401–11.
26. Mor-Avi V, Lang RM, Badano LP, Belohlavek M, Cardim NM, Derumeaux G, et al. Current and evolving echocardiographic techniques for the quantitative evaluation of cardiac mechanics: ASE/EAE consensus statement on methodology and indications endorsed by the Japanese Society of Echocardiography. J Am Soc Echocardiogr. 2011;24(3):277–313.
27. Kurt M, Wang J, Torre-Amione G, Nagueh SF. Left atrial function in diastolic heart failure. Circ Cardiovasc Imaging. 2009;2(1):10–5.
28. Klein AL, Burstow DJ, Tajik AJ, Zachariah PK, Bailey KR, Seward JB. Effects of age on left ventricular dimensions and filling dynamics in 117 normal persons. Mayo Clin Proc. 1994;69(3):212–24.
29. Nagueh SF. Echocardiographic assessment of left ventricular relaxation and cardiac filling pressures. Curr Heart Fail Rep. 2009;6(3):154–9.

30. Wang J, Nagueh SF. Echocardiographic assessment of left ventricular filling pressures. Heart Fail Clin. 2008;4(1):57–70.
31. Sharp AS, Tapp RJ, Thom SA, Francis DP, Hughes AD, Stanton AV, et al. Tissue Doppler E/E′ ratio is a powerful predictor of primary cardiac events in a hypertensive population: an ASCOT substudy. Eur Heart J. 2010;31(6):747–52.
32. Jenkins C, Chan J, Hanekom L, Marwick TH. Accuracy and feasibility of online 3-dimensional echocardiography for measurement of left ventricular parameters. J Am Soc Echocardiogr. 2006;19(9):1119–28.
33. Marwick TH. Application of 3D echocardiography to everyday practice: development of normal ranges is step 1. JACC Cardiovasc Imaging. 2012;5(12):1198–200.
34. Vinch CS, Aurigemma GP, Simon HU, Hill JC, Tighe DA, Meyer TE. Analysis of left ventricular systolic function using midwall mechanics in patients >60 years of age with hypertensive heart disease and heart failure. Am J Cardiol. 2005;96(9):1299–303.
35. de Simone G, Devereux RB, Roman MJ, Ganau A, Saba PS, Alderman MH, et al. Assessment of left ventricular function by the midwall fractional shortening/end-systolic stress relation in human hypertension. J Am Coll Cardiol. 1994;23(6):1444–5.
36. Bella JN, Devereux RB. Left ventricular midwall function in systemic hypertension. Cardiologia. 1998;43(5):465–8.
37. Jenkins C, Bricknell K, Hanekom L, Marwick TH. Reproducibility and accuracy of echocardiographic measurements of left ventricular parameters using real-time three-dimensional echocardiography. J Am Coll Cardiol. 2004;44(4):878–86.
38. Maceira AM, Mohiaddin RH. Cardiovascular magnetic resonance in systemic hypertension 2. J Cardiovasc Magn Reson. 2012;14:28.
39. Celic V, Tadic M, Suzic-Lazic J, Andric A, Majstorovic A, Ivanovic B, et al. Two- and three-dimensional speckle tracking analysis of the relation between myocardial deformation and functional capacity in patients with systemic hypertension. Am J Cardiol. 2014;113(5):832–9.
40. Wang J, Khoury DS, Yue Y, Torre-Amione G, Nagueh SF. Left ventricular untwisting rate by speckle tracking echocardiography. Circulation. 2007;116(22):2580–6.
41. Sahn DJ, DeMaria A, Kisslo J, Weyman A. Recommendations regarding quantitation in M-mode echocardiography: results of a survey of echocardiographic measurements. Circulation. 1978;58(6):1072–83.
42. Cuspidi C, Sala C, Negri F, Mancia G, Morganti A. Prevalence of left-ventricular hypertrophy in hypertension: an updated review of echocardiographic studies. J Hum Hypertens. 2012;26(6):343–9.
43. Mancia G, Zanchetti A, Agabiti-Rosei E, Benemio G, De Cesaris R, Fogari R, et al. Ambulatory blood pressure is superior to clinic blood pressure in predicting treatment-induced regression of left ventricular hypertrophy. SAMPLE Study Group Study on Ambulatory Monitoring of Blood Pressure and Lisinopril Evaluation. Circulation. 1997;95(6):1464–70.
44. Fagard RH, Celis H, Thijs L, Wouters S. Regression of left ventricular mass by antihypertensive treatment: a meta-analysis of randomized comparative studies. Hypertension. 2009;54(5):1084–91.
45. de Simone G, Devereux RB, Izzo R, Girfoglio D, Lee ET, Howard BV, et al. Lack of reduction of left ventricular mass in treated hypertension: the strong heart study. J Am Heart Assoc. 2013;2(3):e000144.
46. Mancusi C, Gerdts E, de Simone G, Abdelhai YM, Lonnebakken MT, Boman K, et al. Impact of isolated systolic hypertension on normalization of left ventricular structure during antihypertensive treatment (the LIFE study). Blood Press. 2014;23(4):206–12.
47. Wachtell K, Dahlof B, Rokkedal J, Papademetriou V, Nieminen MS, Smith G, et al. Change of left ventricular geometric pattern after 1 year of antihypertensive treatment: the Losartan Intervention For Endpoint reduction in hypertension (LIFE) study. Am Heart J. 2002;144(6):1057–64.
48. Barron AJ, Hughes AD, Sharp A, Baksi AJ, Surendran P, Jabbour RJ, et al. Long-term antihypertensive treatment fails to improve E/e′ despite regression of left ventricular mass: an Anglo-Scandinavian cardiac outcomes trial substudy. Hypertension. 2014;63(2):252–8.

49. Perlini S, Muiesan ML, Cuspidi C, Sampieri L, Trimarco B, Aurigemma GP, et al. Midwall mechanics are improved after regression of hypertensive left ventricular hypertrophy and normalization of chamber geometry. Circulation. 2001;103(5):678–83.
50. Verdecchia P, Angeli F, Borgioni C, Gattobigio R, de Simone G, Devereux RB, et al. Changes in cardiovascular risk by reduction of left ventricular mass in hypertension: a meta-analysis. Am J Hypertens. 2003;16(11 Pt 1):895–9.
51. Tsioufis C, Kokkinos P, Macmanus C, Thomopoulos C, Faselis C, Doumas M, et al. Left ventricular hypertrophy as a determinant of renal outcome in patients with high cardiovascular risk. J Hypertens. 2010;28(11):2299–308.
52. Devereux RB, Wachtell K, Gerdts E, Boman K, Nieminen MS, Papademetriou V, et al. Prognostic significance of left ventricular mass change during treatment of hypertension. JAMA. 2004;292(19):2350–6.
53. Muiesan ML, Salvetti M, Rizzoni D, Castellano M, Donato F, Agabiti-Rosei E. Association of change in left ventricular mass with prognosis during long-term antihypertensive treatment. J Hypertens. 1995;13(10):1091–5.
54. Gosse P, Cremer A, Vircoulon M, Coulon P, Jan E, Papaioannou G, et al. Prognostic value of the extent of left ventricular hypertrophy and its evolution in the hypertensive patient. J Hypertens. 2012;30(12):2403–9.
55. Salvetti M, Muiesan ML, Paini A, Monteduro C, Agabiti-Rosei C, Aggiusti C, et al. Left ventricular hypertrophy and renal dysfunction during antihypertensive treatment adversely affect cardiovascular prognosis in hypertensive patients. J Hypertens. 2012;30(2):411–20.
56. Wachtell K, Gerdts E, Palmieri V, Olsen MH, Nieminen MS, Papademetriou V, et al. In-treatment midwall and endocardial fractional shortening predict cardiovascular outcome in hypertensive patients with preserved baseline systolic ventricular function: the Losartan Intervention For Endpoint reduction study. J Hypertens. 2010;28(7):1541–6.

3 Modern Diagnostic Approach for the Assessment of Cardiac Damage in Hypertension: 3D, CT and MRI

Athanasios J. Manolis, Eftichia Chamodraka, and Ioanna Zacharopoulou

3.1 Three-Dimensional Echocardiography in Hypertension

Hypertension (HTN) is a leading cause of cardiovascular morbidity and mortality. Asymptomatic organ disease (OD) is crucial in determining the cardiovascular (CV) risk of hypertensive individuals, and the significance of OD in determining calculation of overall risk depends on how carefully the damage is assessed, based on available facilities.

Echocardiography represents a significant clinical tool in determining cardiac structural and functional changes. Although it has some technical limitations, it represent the gold standard in the assessment of cardiac function and structure. Hypertension is associated with alterations in cardiac structure and function such as left ventricular hypertrophy as well as alterations in left ventricular filling and relaxation [1, 2]. Left ventricular hypertrophy (LVH) can predict CV mortality independently of SCORE stratification, and this obviates the need of using echocardiographic assessment of hypertensive patients in daily clinical practice [3–5].

3.1.1 Left Ventricular Systolic Function

A sine qua non in the assessment of left ventricular function is the estimation of left ventricular ejection fraction (LVEF). Traditional measurement of LVEF by two-dimensional (2D) echocardiography using Simpson's biplane technique relies on optimal visualization of the endocardial border. Additional limitations of 2D imaging include:

- The 'missing third dimension' that has been considered the main source of the relatively wide interobserver variability of 2D diameters and volumes

A.J. Manolis (✉) • E. Chamodraka • I. Zacharopoulou
Cardiology Department, Asklepeion Hospital, Athens, Greece
e-mail: ajmanol@otenet.gr

E. Agabiti Rosei, G. Mancia (eds.), *Assessment of Preclinical Organ Damage in Hypertension*, DOI 10.1007/978-3-319-15603-3_3

- The need for 'foreshortened' views of the ventricle, in order to improve endocardial visualization particularly of the apical-lateral segments of the left ventricle resulting in less accurate and reproducible model-based measurements

Three-dimensional (3D) technology permits frame-by-frame detection of the endocardial surface from real-time 3D datasets. Most studies that have directly compared the accuracy of 3D measurements of left ventricular (LV) volumes and LVEF have demonstrated the superiority of the 3D technique in comparison to 2D. This superiority was demonstrated in both accuracy and reproducibility when compared against independent reference techniques, such as radionuclide ventriculography or cardiovascular magnetic resonance [6, 7].

Recently, real-time full-volume three-dimensional transthoracic echocardiography (3D RT-VTTE) has used a fully automated endocardial contouring algorithm to identify and automatically correct the contours to obtain accurate LV volumes in both patients with sinus rhythm and atrial fibrillation (Fig. 3.1). This fully automated technique, which decreases the time required to obtain measurements, showed results which correlated well with CMR measurements of LV end-diastolic volume, LV end-systolic volume and LVEF (r-values greater than 0.9) [8].

Importantly, reference values for 3D echocardiography-derived LV volumes and LVEF have been published from a large cohort of subjects free of cardiovascular disease, hypertension and diabetes mellitus [9].

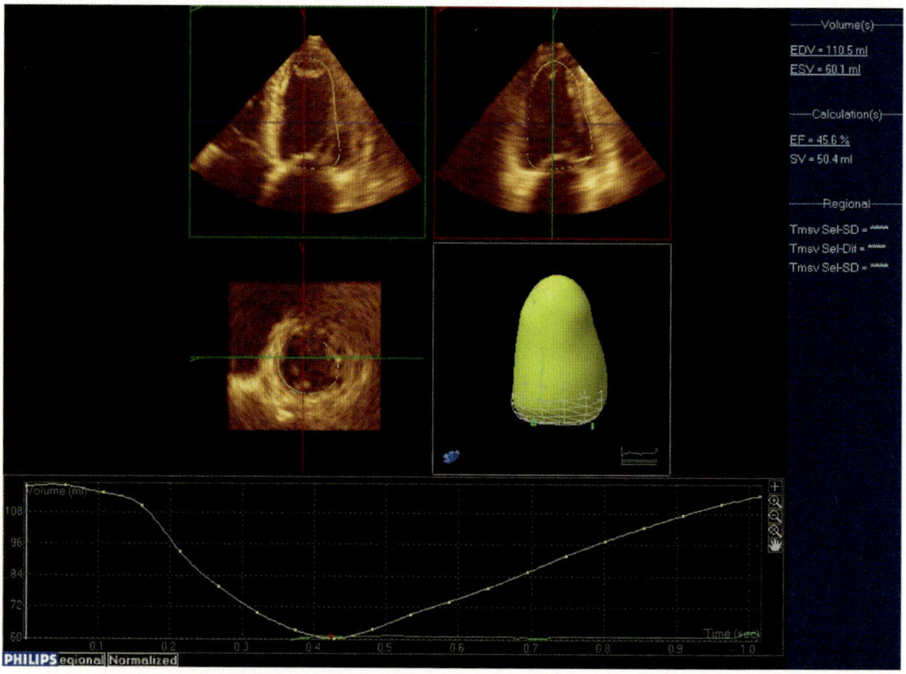

Fig. 3.1 Assessment of global LV volume

3.1.2 Assessment of Left Ventricular Mass

Echocardiography is more sensitive than electrocardiography in diagnosing LVH, and this is more important in patients with moderate total CV risk, as it may refine the risk evaluation by detecting LVH undetected by ECG [10].

It is well known that accurate assessment of LV mass in patients without major distortions of LV geometry is performed with an anatomically validated formula using primary measurement of left ventricular internal dimension [11], posterior wall thickness and septal wall thickness at end diastole, respectively. In patients with distorted LV geometry, LV mass can be assessed by the area-length formula and the truncated ellipsoid formula, from short-axis and apical four-chamber 2D echocardiographic views [11].

Measurement of LV mass relies on both endocardial and epicardial visualizations, with the latter being more difficult because of problems in identifying the epicardial border. As with measurements of LV volumes, there are also other limitations such as difficult assessment due to foreshortening. Several studies have reported significant improvement in the accuracy, inter- and intra-observer variability and reproducibility of estimation of LV mass with the use of 3D echocardiography compared to their traditional M-mode and 2D techniques [12, 13] (Fig. 3.2). It can also be applied in patients with ischaemic cardiomyopathy (IC) in whom the assessment of LV mass is challenging because it is based on geometric assumptions.

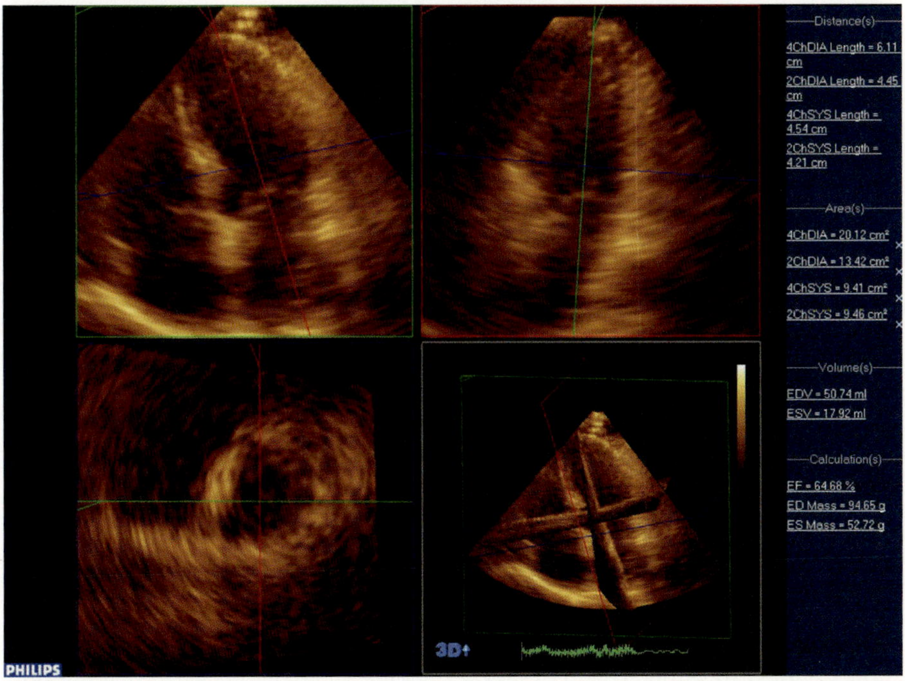

Fig. 3.2 Assessment of LV mass

In IC patients 3D echocardiography is more accurate and reliable considering the measurement of LV mass than 2D echocardiography [14].

Real-time 3DE has also been proved to be useful in detecting even a mild increase of the LV mass in new-onset arterial hypertension where the patients are too young to produce evidence of clear-cut LVH [15].

Accordingly, this has clinical implications for the serial assessments of the severity of LVH in patients with systemic hypertension.

3.1.3 Contrast-Enhanced Real-Time 3D Echocardiography

Recently, contrast-enhanced real-time 3D echocardiography (CE RT 3DE) has been shown to have improved the accuracy of left ventricular volumes and EF measurements in patients with poor acoustic windows without significantly affecting those in patients with optimal images. In addition, CE RT 3DE imaging improved the reproducibility of the measurements, as reflected by a decrease in intermeasurement variability [16]. This approach allows quantification of global as well as regional LV function, when used with selective dual triggering at end systole and end diastole to reduce the destructive effects of ultrasound on contrast-enhancing microbubble agents (Fig. 3.3). Thus, this methodology may become the new standard for LV size and function, which will be particularly important in patients with poor acoustic windows or contraindications to CMR.

3.1.4 3D Speckle Tracking

Technological advancement of real-time 3D echocardiography has developed software that tracks the motion of speckles irrespective of their direction and allows to obtain a homogeneous spatial distribution of all three components of the myocardial displacement vector [17]. The main advantage of 3D speckle tracking echocardiography is the possibility of analysing the whole left ventricle from a single volume of data obtained from the apical transducer position. In addition, its use considerably reduces the time duration of analysis to one-third in comparison with 2D speckle tracking echocardiography [18].

Global area 3D strain has recently been shown to be a comprehensive parameter of myocardial systolic deformation and is very sensitive to both changes of afterload and LV mass. In a recent study that included native, untreated hypertensive patients, global area 3D strain was precautiously reduced, and longitudinal and radial strain impaired, while circumferential strain was still preserved, supporting a normal LV chamber systolic function. Reduction of global area strain was independently associated with both pressure overload and magnitude of the LV mass [15]. Interestingly, global area 3D strain has been proven to be the only parameter which was at the same time an independent predictor of LV mass, 2D LV ejection fraction and LV global function. The 3D speckle tracking technique revealed that the subjects with high-normal blood pressure suffered subclinical impairment of LV

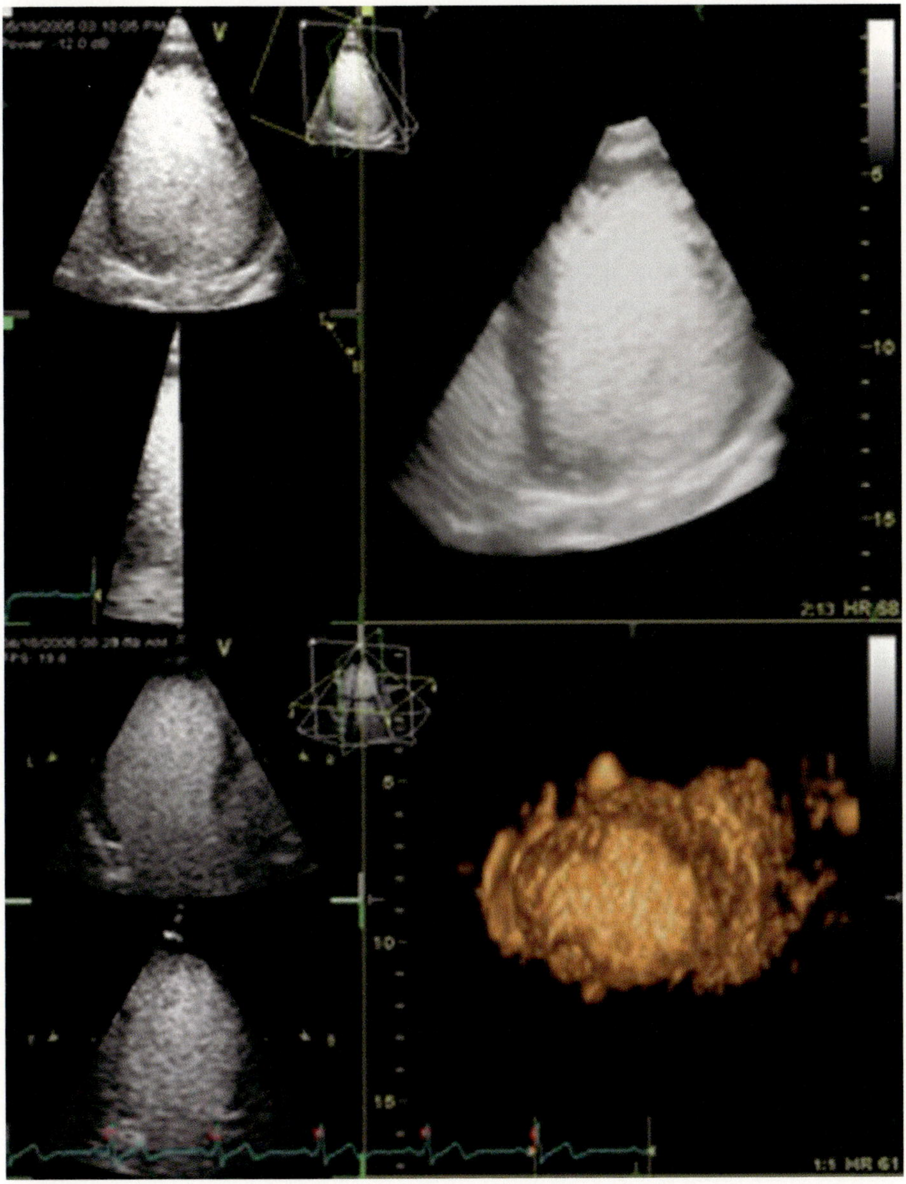

Fig. 3.3 Contrast-enhanced real-time 3D echocardiography

mechanics similar as the hypertensive patients [19]. 3D global longitudinal, circumferential, radial and area strains were also demonstrated to be significantly impaired in patients with uncontrolled and untreated hypertension in comparison with controls and well-controlled hypertensive patients, and functional capacity seems to be independently associated with 3D global longitudinal strain [20].

3.1.5 Diastolic Function

Hypertension predominantly affects diastolic LV function before altering systolic function. Echocardiography is the most widely used technique for the evaluation of LV filling, which mostly relies on Doppler evaluation of transmitral and pulmonic flow patterns as well as mitral annular velocities. Currently, no real-time 3D echocardiographic indices are recommended by the guidelines for the assessment of diastolic dysfunction.

Interestingly recently the following 3D indices have been used for the estimation of diastolic LV function [21]: volume at 25, 50 and 75 % of filling duration in per cent of end-diastolic volume (volume index) and rapid filling volume fraction. Temporal indices included filling duration in % of RR and rapid filling duration in % of filling duration. Additionally, longitudinal, radial and circumferential strains at 25, 50 and 75 % of filling duration were calculated. End-diastolic volume index and rapid filling volume fraction showed a biphasic pattern with the severity of diastolic dysfunction characterized by an initial decrease (grade 1), a pseudo-normalization (grade 2) and then an increase above normal (grade 3). Filling duration progressively decreased with the severity of diastolic dysfunction. Rapid filling duration was significantly increased in all 3 groups compared to normal. After normalization by peak systolic values, all three strain components showed a linear pattern with the severity of diastolic dysfunction, suggesting potential clinical usefulness.

3.1.6 Assessment of Left Atrial Structure and Function

Measurement of left atrial (LA) volume is an essential component of the comprehensive assessment of LV diastolic function [22]. Although LA volume by 2D echocardiography provides prognostic information, the misalignment of the 2D cutting plane of the left atrium could make the measurements inaccurate. LA volumes can be easily obtained by 3D echocardiography, and improved accuracy and reproducibility of the 3D approach have been demonstrated at the cost of more elaborate offline analysis in studies that compared 2D and 3D echocardiographic measurements of atrial volumes against an independent gold standard such as cardiovascular magnetic resonance imaging [23, 24] (Fig. 3.4). 3D echocardiography has been recently shown to classify LA dilatation more accurately than 2D echocardiography, resulting in fewer patients with undetected atrial enlargement and potentially undiagnosed diastolic dysfunction [25]. In another recent study minimum LA volume at end diastole measured by real-time 3D echocardiography has been shown to be more strongly correlated to LV diastolic function and LV filling pressure than maximum LA volume, and LV longitudinal systolic function has been demonstrated to be a strong determinant of the LA reservoir function [26].

Apart from estimation of LA structure, estimation of LA function remains a challenge. During the cardiac cycle, LA acts as a reservoir, receiving pulmonary

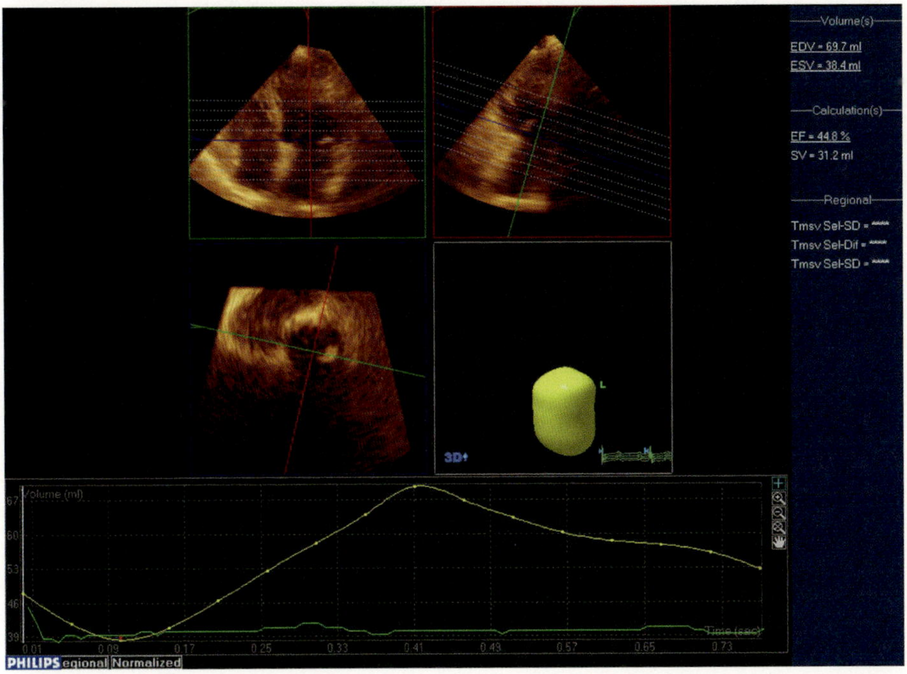

Fig. 3.4 Assessment of LA volume

venous return during LV systole; as a conduit, passively transferring blood to the LV during early diastole; and as a pump actively priming LV in late diastole. In normal subjects, the reservoir, passive conduit and pumping phases account for approximately 40, 35 and 25 % of the atrial contribution to stroke volume, respectively [27].

3D speckle tracking echocardiography has been used for quantitative evaluation of LA function in essential hypertension patients with different patterns of left ventricular geometric models. Left atrial booster pump function is demonstrated to decrease in patients with the eccentric hypertrophy pattern, while left atrial conduit function is reported to be unchanged in the normal pattern and the concentric remodelling pattern groups [28]. Additionally, 3D speckle tracking enables the measurement of both LA strain and synchrony with excellent reproducibility and appears to be more accurate compared with 2D LA strain for identifying hypertensive patients with paroxysmal atrial fibrillation [29].

Conclusively, 3D echocardiography is a novel technique that permits accurate and reproducible assessment of left ventricular mass and left ventricular volumes in comparison to the gold standard technique—CMR. Further studies are necessary for the implementation of 3D echocardiography in the evaluation of left atrial structure and function and left ventricular diastolic function.

3.2 Cardiac Computed Tomography in Hypertension

Cardiac computed tomography (CT) is not currently a first-line exam in the evaluation of hypertensive patients. Coronary CT angiography is considered to be its most popular and fascinating application since it permits the visualization of coronary anatomy in a non-invasive way.

According to the appropriateness criteria for cardiac computed tomography, CT angiography of the coronary arteries is generally acceptable for the evaluation of chest pain syndrome in patients with intermediate pretest probability of coronary artery disease who have either an inconclusive ECG or who cannot exercise [30]. Moreover, CT angiography is suggested for patients with acute chest pain with intermediate pretest probability of coronary artery disease with negative enzymes and without ECG changes [30]. The use of 64-slice multi-detector computed tomography (MDCT) has a sensitivity of 93 % and a specificity of 96 % in detecting coronary artery stenosis [31, 32]. In this regard, CT coronary angiography has an excellent negative predictive value, while positive predictive value is low, and therefore an exam with normal findings can practically rule out coronary artery disease [31].

Cardiac CT is additionally used for coronary plaque imaging. The straight relation between coronary arteries' amount of calcium and atherosclerotic plaque burden has already been established [31, 33]. Coronary artery calcium (CAC) can be observed with electron beam computed tomography (EBCT) as well as with MDCT, and for its quantification, among the different methods suggested, 'Agatston score' is the most common [31]. According to the 2010 ACCF/AHA guidelines for assessment of cardiovascular risk in asymptomatic adults, CAC evaluation can be performed in asymptomatic adults at intermediate risk (class II a), while adults at low risk have no benefit from this method [34].

Another application of cardiac CT is in the assessment of cardiac morphology and function; nevertheless, it is improbable to become the method of choice for this purpose. This is mostly due to the radiation exposure and the contrast material used [31]. As a matter of fact, myocardial mass, left and right end-systolic and end-diastolic volumes, ejection fraction and stroke volume can be calculated in this way with great accuracy [30, 31]. As far as calculation of left ventricular function is concerned, different studies have indicated the good correlation between CT and MRI as well as between CT and echocardiography in this field [31, 35–37].

In patients with atrial fibrillation, MDCT has been used in the evaluation of the pulmonary vein's anatomy preceding ablation procedures along with the assessment of pulmonary vein stenosis following the above procedure. Furthermore, the appropriateness criteria for cardiac CT suggest its use prior to ablation [30].

Moreover, the use of CT angiogram is appropriate for the estimation of a suspected thoracic aortic aneurysm or an aortic dissection, and CT can be also employed in the diagnosis of the secondary causes of hypertension [30].

3.3 Magnetic Resonance in Hypertension

The indications of cardiovascular magnetic resonance imaging (CMR) have been greatly broadened. However, CMR is not among the first diagnostic procedures followed in patients with systemic hypertension. In these patients, the assessment of target organ damage is without a doubt a very important objective. In this regard, the 2013 ESC/ESH guidelines for the management of arterial hypertension suggest that cardiac magnetic resonance imaging should be considered for the assessment of left ventricle size and mass when the image quality obtained by echocardiography is poor and when imaging of delayed enhancement would have therapeutic consequences [38]. In the same guideline's edition, stress cardiac magnetic resonance is recommended in hypertensive patients when the exercise electrocardiogram (ECG) results are inconclusive in order to achieve a valid identification of myocardial ischaemia [38]. The detection of identifiable causes of hypertension is also a major objective in hypertensive patients. The same guidelines suggest as an additional or confirmatory test for pheochromocytoma an MRI of the abdomen and pelvis as well as an MR angiography for the detection of renal artery stenosis [38].

CMR appears to contribute to a global assessment of hypertensive cardiovascular disease by the following means:

- It has been applied for the measurement of left and right ventricular dimensions, volumes, mass and systolic function. Furthermore, CMR has been proposed as the gold standard method for the assessment of ventricular volumes, mass and function due to its accuracy and reproducibility [39–41]. The standardized cardiovascular magnetic resonance protocols used for this purpose have been described in detail [42]. Additionally, reference ranges have been established [43]. Emphasis must be given to the fact that CMR can determine the pattern of LVH and provide an answer regarding its cause [39]. Moreover, focal myocardial fibrosis encountered in hypertensive heart disease can be visualized by late gadolinium enhancement (LGE) CMR, while other sequences are being tested in order to detect diffuse myocardial fibrosis [39].
- CMRI has also been proposed as the gold standard for the measurement of LA volume although 3D echocardiography seems to gain ground [44, 45]. In addition, references regarding left atrial dimensions and volumes have been published [46]. Different CMR techniques have been employed in order to assess diastolic function; nevertheless, in this field echocardiography remains the technique of choice [39].
- In addition CMRI offers an accurate evaluation of the hypertensive vascular disease. According to the clinical indications for CMR/Consensus Panel report, CMRI can be used for the diagnosis and the follow-up of thoracic aortic aneurysms (class I), diagnosis and stent treatment for abdominal aortic aneurysms (class II), diagnosis of acute aortic dissection (class I) and follow-up of the chronic form (class II) as well as for the diagnosis of aortic intramural haemorrhage (class I) [47]. Furthermore CMR/gadolinium MRA has been applied in the

evaluation of occlusive peripheral arterial disease. CMR is indicated for the assessment of renal, iliac, femoral and lower leg arteries as well as of the thoracic great vessel origins (class I) [47]. Extracranial carotid artery disease can also be evaluated by means of CMR angiography that can detect internal carotid stenosis similarly to X-ray angiography [47]. Arterial wall CMR offers the possibility to identify the composition as well as the anatomy of the plaque [47, 48]. Different studies have evaluated the regression of atherosclerotic plaques with lipid-lowering therapy by MRI [47, 48].

- CMRI can be used in order to identify the presence of coronary artery disease in hypertensive patients [47]. As mentioned previously, it is now the gold standard for the assessment of ventricular volumes and systolic function. Dobutamine stress CMR has shown superiority when compared to dobutamine stress echocardiography in detecting myocardial ischaemia [47]. LGE-CMR identifies myocardial scar with high accuracy and sensitivity [47].
- Moreover, with the use of CMR, some of the secondary causes of hypertension can be excluded. Thus, MRA is a very sensitive technique for renal artery stenosis, and CMR detects aortic coarctation in hypertensive adults as well as re-coarctation after surgery [39]. MRI is also considered for the detection of adenomas in hypertensive patients with primary hyperaldosteronism, taking into account the fact that it has comparable sensitivity to CT imaging [39]. When pheochromocytoma is suspected, MRI can determine the localization of the tumour [39]. Finally, in case of Cushing's syndrome when an ACTH-independent lesion is indicated, abdominal MRI can localize the site of the lesion [39].

References

1. Mancia G, et al. Reappraisal of European guidelines on hypertension management: a European Society of Hypertension Task Force document. J Hypertens. 2009;27:2121–58.
2. Hogg K, Swedberg K, McMurray J. Heart failure with preserved left ventricular systolic function; epidemiology, clinical characteristics, and prognosis. J Am Coll Cardiol. 2004;43:317–27.
3. Sehestedt T, Jeppesen J, Hansen TW, et al. Risk prediction is improved by adding markers of subclinical organ damage to SCORE. Eur Heart J. 2010;31:883–91.
4. Sehestedt T, Jeppesen J, Hansen TW, et al. Thresholds for pulse wave velocity, urine albumin creatinine ratio and left ventricular mass index using SCORE, Framingham and ESH/ESC risk charts. J Hypertens. 2012;30:1928–36.
5. Volpe M, Battistoni A, Tocci G, et al. Cardiovascular risk assessment beyond systemic coronary risk estimation: a role for organ damage markers. J Hypertens. 2012;30:1056–64.
6. Jenkins C, Bricknell K, Hanekom L, Marwick TH. Reproducibility and accuracy of echocardiographic measurements of left ventricular parameters using real-time three-dimensional echocardiography. J Am Coll Cardiol. 2004;44:878.
7. Jacobs LD, Salgo IS, Goonewardena S, et al. Rapid online quantification of left ventricular volume from real-time three-dimensional echocardiographic data. Eur Heart J. 2006;27:460.
8. Thavendiranathan P, Liu S, Verhaert D, et al. Feasibility, accuracy, and reproducibility of real-time full-volume 3D transthoracic echocardiography to measure LV volumes and systolic function: a fully automated endocardial contouring algorithm in sinus rhythm and atrial fibrillation. JACC Cardiovasc Imaging. 2012;5:239.

9. Chahal NS, Lim TK, Jain P, et al. Population-based reference values for 3D echocardiographic LV volumes and ejection fraction. JACC Cardiovasc Imaging. 2012;5:119.
10. ESH/ESC Guidelines for the management of arterial hypertension. The task force for the management of arterial hypertension of the European Society of Hypertension (ESH) and of the European Society of Cardiology (ESC). Eur Heart J. 2013. doi:10.1093.
11. Lang RM, Bierig M, Devereux R, et al. Recommendations for chamber quantification: a report from the American Society of Echocardiography's Guidelines and Standards Committee and the Chamber Quantification Writing Group, Developed in Conjunction with the European Association of Echocardiography, a Branch of the European Society of Cardiology. J Am Soc Echocardiogr. 2005;18:1440–63.
12. Chuang ML, Salton CJ, Hibberd MG, et al. Relation between number of component views and accuracy of left ventricular mass determined by three-dimensional echocardiography. Am J Cardiol. 2007;99:1321–32.
13. Pouleur AC, le Polain de Waroux JB, Pasquet A, et al. Assessment of left ventricular mass and volumes by three-dimensional echocardiography in patients with or without wall motion abnormalities: comparison against cine magnetic resonance imaging. Heart. 2008;94:1050–9.
14. Kusunose K, Kwon DH, Motoki H, et al. Comparison of three-dimensional echocardiographic findings to those of magnetic resonance imaging for determination of left ventricular mass in patients with ischemic and non-ischemic cardiomyopathy. Am J Cardiol. 2013;112:604–11.
15. Galderisi M, Esposito R, Lomoriello V, et al. Correlates of global area strain in native hypertensive patients: a three-dimensional speckle-tracking echocardiography study. Eur Heart J Cardiovasc Imaging. 2012;13:730–8.
16. Coon PD, Pollard H, Furlong K, et al. Quantification of left ventricular size and function using contrast-enhanced real-time 3D imaging with power modulation: comparison with cardiac MRI. Ultrasound Med Biol. 2012;38(11):1853–8.
17. Mor-Avi V, Lang RM, Badano LP, et al. Current and evolving echocardiographic techniques for the quantitative evaluation of cardiac mechanics: ASE/EAE consensus statement on methodology and indications endorsed by the Japanese Society of Echocardiography. Eur J Echocardiogr. 2011;12:167–205.
18. De Isla LP, Balcones DV, Fernandez-Golfin C, et al. Three-dimensional wall motion tracking: a new and faster tool for myocardial strain assessment: comparison with two-dimensional wall motion tracking. J Am Soc Echocardiogr. 2009;22:325–30.
19. Tadic M, Majstorovic A, Pencic B, et al. The impact of high-normal blood pressure on left ventricular mechanics: a three-dimensional and speckle tracking echocardiography study. Int J Cardiovasc Imaging. 2014;30:699–711.
20. Celic V, Tadic M, Suzic-Lazic J, et al. Two- and three-dimensional speckle tracking analysis of the relation between myocardial deformation and functional capacity in patients with systemic hypertension. Am J Cardiol. 2014;113:832–9.
21. Yodwut C, Lang R, Weinert L, et al. Three-dimensional echocardiographic quantitative evaluation of left ventricular diastolic function using analysis of chamber volume and myocardial deformation. Int J Cardiovasc Imaging. 2013;29:285–93.
22. Nagueh S, Appleton C, Gillebert T, et al. Recommendations for the evaluation of left ventricular diastolic function by echocardiography. J Am Soc Echocardiogr. 2009;22:107–33.
23. Cameli M, Lisi M, Righini FM, et al. Novel echocardiographic techniques to assess left atrial size, anatomy and function. Cardiovasc Ultrasound. 2012;10:4. doi:10.1186/1476-7120-10-4.
24. Buechel RR, Stephan FP, Sommer G, et al. Head-to-head comparison of two-dimensional and three-dimensional echocardiographic methods for left atrial chamber quantification with magnetic resonance imaging. J Am Soc Echocardiogr. 2013;26:428–35.
25. Mor-Avi V, Yodwut C, Jenkins C, et al. Real-time 3D echocardiographic quantification of left atrial volume: multicenter study for validation with CMR. JACC Cardiovasc Imaging. 2012;5:769.
26. Russo C, Zhezhen J, Shunichi H, et al. Left atrial minimum volume and reservoir function as correlates of left ventricular diastolic function: impact of left ventricular systolic function. Heart. 2012;98:813–20.

27. Todaro CM, Choudouri I, Belohlavec M. New echocardiographic techniques for evaluation of left atrial mechanics. Eur Heart J Cardiovasc Imaging. 2012;13:973–84.
28. Wang Y, et al. Assessment of left atrial function by full volume real-time three-dimensional echocardiography and left atrial tracking in essential hypertension patients with different patterns of left ventricular geometric models. Chin Med Sci J. 2013;28(3):152–8. doi:10.1016/j.echo.2012.10.003. Epub 2012 Nov 8.
29. Mochizuki A, Yuda S, Oi Y, et al. Assessment of left atrial deformation and synchrony by three-dimensional speckle-tracking echocardiography: comparative studies in healthy subjects and patients with atrial fibrillation. J Am Soc Echocardiogr. 2013;26:165–74.
30. Hendel RC, Patel MR, Kramer CM, Poon M, Hendel RC, Carr JC, Gerstad NA, Gillam LD, Hodgson JM, Kim RJ, Kramer CM, Lesser JR, Martin ET, Messer JV, Redberg RF, Rubin GD, Rumsfeld JS, Taylor AJ, Weigold WG, Woodard PK, Brindis RG, Hendel RC, Douglas PS, Peterson ED, Wolk MJ, Allen JM, Patel MR, American College of Cardiology Foundation Quality Strategic Directions Committee Appropriateness Criteria Working Group; American College of Radiology; Society of Cardiovascular Computed Tomography; Society for Cardiovascular Magnetic Resonance; American Society of Nuclear Cardiology; North American Society for Cardiac Imaging; Society for Cardiovascular Angiography and Interventions; Society of Interventional Radiology. ACCF/ACR/SCCT/SCMR/ASNC/NASCI/SCAI/SIR2006 appropriateness criteria for cardiac computed tomography and cardiac magnetic resonance imaging. A report of the American College of Cardiology Foundation Quality Strategic Directions Committee Appropriateness Criteria Working Group, American College of Radiology, Society of Cardiovascular Computed Tomography, Society for Cardiovascular Magnetic Resonance, American Society of Nuclear Cardiology, North American Society for Cardiac Imaging, Society for Cardiovascular Angiography and Interventions, and Society of Interventional Radiology. J Am Coll Cardiol. 2006;48(7):1475–97.
31. Schroeder S, Achenbach S, Bengel F, et al. Cardiac computed tomography: indications, applications, limitations, and training requirements. Eur Heart J. 2008;29:531–56.
32. Vanhoenacker PK, et al. Diagnostic performance of multidetector CT angiography for assessment of coronary artery disease: meta-analysis. Radiology. 2007;224(2):419–28.
33. Perrone-Filardi P, Achenbach S, Möhlenkamp S, Reiner Z, Sambuceti G, Schuijf JD, Van der Wall E, Kaufmann PA, Knuuti J, Schroeder S, Zellweger MJ. Cardiac computed tomography and myocardial perfusion scintigraphy for risk stratification in asymptomatic individuals without known cardiovascular disease. A position statement of the Working Group on Nuclear Cardiology and Cardiac CT of the European Society of Cardiology. Eur Heart J. 2011;32:1986–93.
34. ACCF/AHA guideline for assessment of cardiovascular risk in asymptomatic adults. The ACCF/AHA task force members developed in collaboration with the American Society of Echocardiography, American Society of Nuclear Cardiology, Society of Atherosclerosis Imaging and Prevention, Society for Cardiovascular Angiography and Interventions, Society of Cardiovascular Computed Tomography, and Society for Cardiovascular Magnetic Resonance. J Am Coll Cardiol. 2010;56(25):e50–103. doi:10.1016/j.jacc2010.09.001.
35. Heuschmid M, et al. Assessment of left ventricular myocardial function using 16-slice multidetector- row computed tomography: comparison with magnetic resonance imaging and echocardiography. Eur Radiol. 2006;16(3):551–9.
36. Juergens KU, et al. Multi-detector row CT of left ventricular function with dedicated analysis software versus MR imaging: initial experience. Radiology. 2004;230(2):403–10.
37. Dewey M, et al. Evaluation of global and regional left ventricular function with 16-slice computed tomography, biplane cineventriculography, and two-dimensional transthoracic echocardiography: comparison with magnetic resonance imaging. J Am Coll Cardiol. 2006;48(10):2034–44.
38. Mancia G, Fagard R, Narkiewicz K, Redón J, Zanchetti A, Böhm M, Christiaens T, Cifkova R, De Backer G, Dominiczak A, Galderisi M, Grobbee DE, Jaarsma T, Kirchhof P, Kjeldsen SE, Laurent S, Manolis AJ, Nilsson PM, Ruilope LM, Schmieder RE, Sirnes PA, Sleight P, Viigimaa M, Waeber B, Zannad F, Task Force Members. 2013 ESC/ESH Guidelines for the

management of arterial hypertension. The Task Force for the management of arterial hypertension of the European Society of Hypertension (ESH) and of the European Society of Cardiology (ESC). J Hypertens. 2013;31:1281–357.
39. Maceira AM, Mohiaddin R. Cardiovascular magnetic resonance in systemic hypertension. J Cardiovasc Magn Reson. 2012;14:28.
40. Myerson SG, Bellenger NG, Pennell DJ. Assessment of left ventricular mass by cardiovascular magnetic resonance. Hypertension. 2002;39:750–5.
41. Grothues F, et al. Comparison of interstudy reproducibility of cardiovascular magnetic resonance with two-dimensional echocardiography in normal subjects and in patients with heart failure or left ventricular hypertrophy. Am J Cardiol. 2002;90(1):29–34.
42. Kramer CM, et al. Standardized cardiovascular magnetic resonance (CMR) protocols 2013 update. J Cardiovasc Magn Reson. 2013;15:91.
43. Maceira AM, et al. Normalized left ventricular systolic and diastolic function by steady state free precession. J Cardiovasc Magn Reson. 2006;8:417–26.
44. Tops LF, Schalij MJ, Bax JJ. Imaging and atrial fibrillation: the role of multimodality imaging in patient evaluation and management of atrial fibrillation. Eur Heart J. 2010;31:542–51.
45. de Groot NM, Schalij MJ. Imaging modalities for measurements of left atrial volume in patients with atrial fibrillation: what do we choose? Europace. 2010;12:766–7. doi:10.1093/europace/euq140.
46. Maceira AM, et al. Reference left atrial dimensions and volumes by steady state free precession cardiovascular magnetic resonance. J Cardiovasc Magn Reson. 2010;12:65–72.
47. Pennell DJ, et al. Clinical indications for cardiovascular magnetic resonance (CMR): Consensus Panel report. Eur Heart J. 2004;25:1940–65.
48. Choudhury RP, et al. MRI and characterization of atherosclerotic plaque: emerging applications and molecular imaging. Arterioscler Thromb Vasc Biol. 2002;22(7):1065–74.

Part II

Large Arteries

Ultrasound: Carotid Intima-Media Thickness and Plaque (2D–3D)

4

Enrico Agabiti Rosei, Massimo Salvetti, and Maria Lorenza Muiesan

4.1 How to Assess

High-resolution ultrasound of the carotid arteries allows the measurement of the intima-media complex in the arterial wall, according to a validated method, and carotid IMT (C-IMT) is the most widely accepted noninvasive marker of subclinical atherosclerosis [1, 2]. Ultrasound methodology has manifest benefits, being real time, noninvasive, low cost, reliable, and safe.

C-IMT represents the combined thickness of the intima and media layers of the carotid artery wall, which are technically indistinguishable. IMT is defined as a double-line pattern visualized by ultrasound on both walls of the carotid arteries in a long-axis view. It consists of two parallel anatomical boundaries referred to as the lumen-intima and media-adventitia interfaces. Ultrasound waves are reflected differently by blood (vessel lumen) and wall layers because of their differences in density and elasticity; the lack of reflection of ultrasound waves by blood (vessel lumen) and by the tunica media allows the detection of the lumen-intima (LI) interface and of the media-adventitia (MA) interface. Intima-media thickness corresponds to the distance between the lumen-intima and the media-adventitia interface.

The carotid ultrasound examination is performed in the patient supine, with the neck in partial extension and turned to the side opposite to the measurement. The carotid artery may be usually divided into three segments: the common carotid (CCA), the carotid bifurcation, and the internal carotid artery (ICA). Each of these segments has approximately a 1 cm length. The most proximal segment is the CCA and may be identified as the 1 cm segment proximal to the divergence of the near and far walls. The focal widening of carotid bifurcation (or bulb) extends over approximately 1 cm, and then it bifurcates into its internal and external carotid

E. Agabiti Rosei, MD (✉) • M. Salvetti • M.L. Muiesan
Department of Clinical and Experimental Sciences, Clinica Medica,
University of Brescia, Piazzale Spedali Civili 1, 25121 Brescia, Italy
e-mail: enrico.agabiti@unibs.it; massimo.salvetti@unibs.it; marialorenza.muiesan@unibs.it

E. Agabiti Rosei, G. Mancia (eds.), *Assessment of Preclinical Organ Damage in Hypertension*, DOI 10.1007/978-3-319-15603-3_4

arteries; the distal margin of the bifurcation is identified by the tip of the flow divider separating the diverging internal and external carotid artery. The third final segment is the proximal 1 cm of the ICA.

The CCA far wall is the easiest segment to be examined and can be measured in almost all subjects. It is the most commonly used measurement in clinical studies because of its greater feasibility and reproducibility, especially at the site of the far wall [2]. However, measurements of C-IMT at multiple angles of both the near and far walls may provide the best balance between reproducibility, evaluation of extent of subclinical atherosclerosis, and assessment of rate of C-IMT progression and of treatment effect. The other most frequently used measurements in clinical trials are as follows: (1) mean of the maximum IMT of the 4 far walls of the carotid bifurcations and distal common carotid arteries (CBM max), (2) mean maximum thickness (M max) of up to 12 different sites (right and left, near and far walls, distal common, bifurcation, and proximal internal carotid), and (3) overall single maximum IMT (T max).

The essential drawbacks of ultrasound are the B-mode image low signal-to-noise ratio and the use of a manual cursor for measurements of IMT from the ultrasound scan images, with a significant operator dependent methodology. Clinical and epidemiological studies have given useful informations on the reproducibility of IMT repeated measurements. Salonen and Salonen have indicated that between observers and intraobservers variation coefficients resulted 10.5 and 8.3 %, respectively [3]. In the ACAPS study [4], the mean replicate difference was 0.11 mm, and in the Multicenter Isradipine Diuretic Atherosclerosis Study (MIDAS) [5] 0.12 mm. In the MIDAS, arithmetic difference in replicate scans mean max IMT was calculated as 0.003 ± 0.156 mm. More recently, the ELSA (European Lacidipine Study of Atherosclerosis) included more than 2,000 patients, in whom the cross-sectional reproducibility of ultrasound measurements at baseline was calculated: the overall coefficient of reliability (R) was 0.859 for CBM max, 0.872 for M max, and 0.794 for T max; intra- and inter-reader reliability were 0.915 and 0.872, respectively [6].

Analysis of C-IMT may be performed now by automated computerized edge detection, in order to optimize reproducibility; with this method, IMT measurement is restricted to the far wall of the distal segment of the common carotid artery, thus providing about 3 % of relative difference between two successive measurements.

A new echo-tracking technology based on up to 128 radio-frequency lines may allow a more rapid and precise measurement of IMT [7]. By means of this technique, it is also possible to investigate the carotid wall mechanical properties; the circumferential and longitudinal stress may exert a direct action on carotid plaque stability and composition [8] (Fig. 4.1).

The normal IMT values are influenced by age and sex. IMT normal values may be defined in terms of statistical distribution within a healthy population [9].

More recently, C-IMT reference values by echo-tracking were obtained in a cohort of 24,871 individuals from 24 research centers worldwide [8] and allowed estimation of C-IMT age- and sex-specific percentiles in a healthy population of the 4,234 individuals without CV disease, CV risk factors, and blood pressure-, lipid-, and/or glucose-lowering medication. These reference values will favor the use of C-IMT assessment in clinical practice, possibly for a better risk classification particularly concerning C-IMT modifications over time.

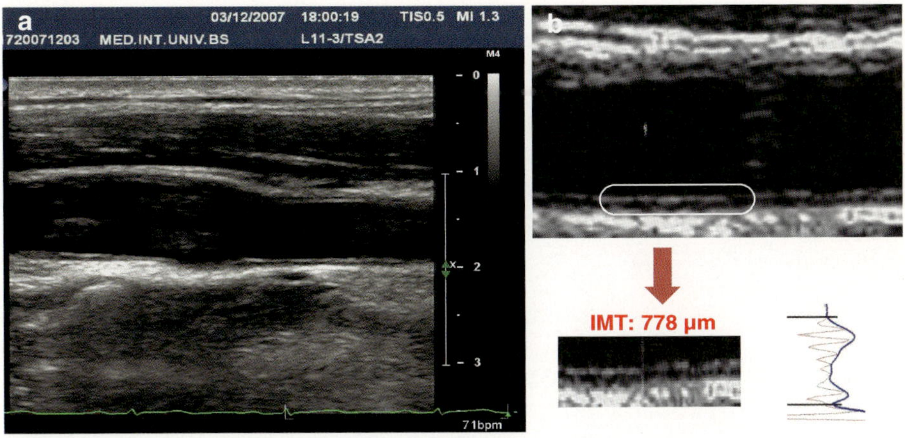

Fig. 4.1 Examples of ultrasound image (**a**) and of echo-tracking radio-frequency image (**b**) of the carotid vessels

The increase in IMT may be better defined in terms of increased risk, and available data indicate that IMT > 0.9 mm, by the use of caliper measurements of B-mode images, represents a risk of myocardial infarction and/or cerebrovascular disease [10–16]. No data are presently available on IMT values obtained by the echo-tracking technique as related to the risk of CV events.

Ultrasound may also identify the presence of plaques, defined by the Manheim consensus [2] as a focal structure encroaching into the arterial lumen of at least 0.5 mm or 50 % of the surrounding IMT value, or demonstrate a thickness >1.5 mm as measured from the media-adventitia interface to the intima-lumen interface.

Ultrasonic plaque morphology may add useful information on plaque stability and may correlate with symptoms. In addition to the visual judgment of plaque echolucency and homogeneity, the use of noninvasive methods that may quantify tissue composition of vascular wall (such as videodensitometry or the analysis of integrated backscatter signal) has been proposed for the assessment of cellular composition of atherosclerotic plaque, particularly of earlier lesions [17, 18].

In addition, plaque volume assessment by three-dimensional reconstruction of ultrasound or nuclear magnetic resonance images has been proposed to better evaluate atherosclerotic lesions changes and stratify patients' risk [19, 20] (Fig. 4.2).

4.2 Prevalence

Population studies, such as the Rotterdam [10] and the Cardiovascular Health Study [16] or the Vobarno study [21], have clearly demonstrated that systolic blood pressure is a major determinant of the increase of intima-media thickness in the carotid arteries, particularly in hypertensive patients.

Data collected in the VHAS (Verapamil in Hypertension and Atherosclerosis Study) [22] and the ELSA studies [23] have shown a high prevalence of carotid wall

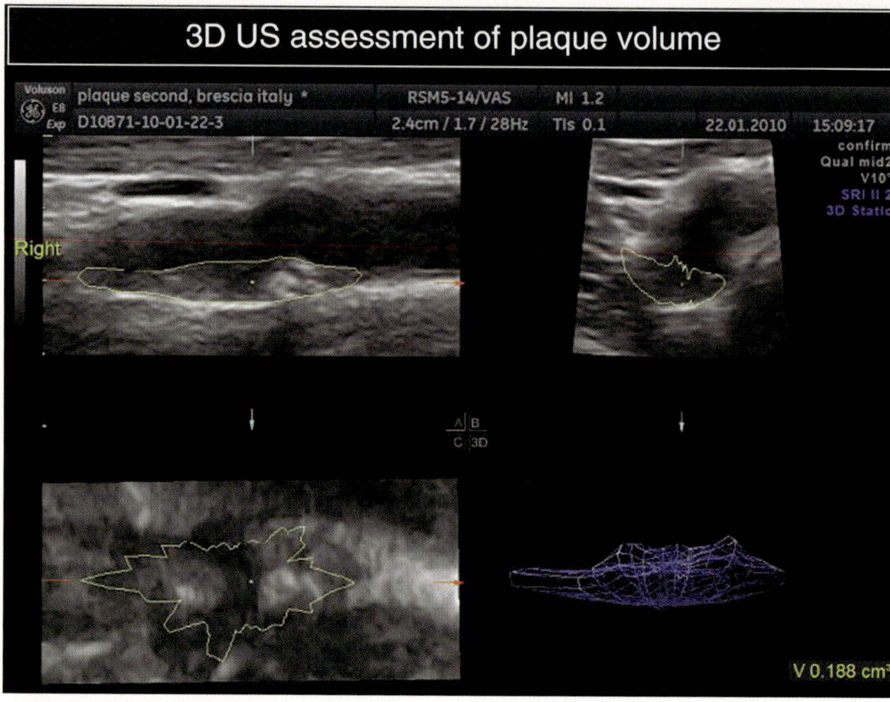

Fig. 4.2 3D reconstruction of a carotid plaque

structural changes in hypertensive patients; in the VHAS study, 40 % of the patients had a plaque (i.e., an intima-media thickness >1.5 mm) in at least 1 site along the carotid arteries, and only 33 % of patients had normal carotid arteries walls. In the ELSA study, 82 % of 2,259 essential hypertensives had a plaque (i.e., an intima-media ≥ 1.3 mm). Moreover, in the RIS study (Risk Intervention Study), patients with severe essential hypertension and high cardiovascular risk had a significantly higher prevalence of atherosclerotic lesions in respect to control subjects [24]. In patients with resistant hypertension, the presence of a carotid plaque has been identified in up to 97 % of subjects [25].

4.3 Change with Treatment (Criteria for Significant Change, Incidence During Treatment)

Therapeutic double-blind trials have shown that antihypertensive drugs may have a more or less marked effect on carotid IMT progression. A large meta-regression analysis [26], including 22 randomized controlled trials, has evaluated the effects of an antihypertensive drug versus placebo or another antihypertensive agent of a different class on carotid intima-media thickness. The results have shown that, compared with no treatment, diuretics/±beta-blockers, or ACE inhibitors, CCBs attenuate the rate of progression of carotid intima-media thickening. In the prevention of carotid intima-media thickening, calcium antagonists are more effective than ACE inhibitors, which in turn are more effective than placebo or no treatment, but not more active than diuretics/±beta-blockers. The odds ratio for all fatal and non-fatal cardiovascular events in trials comparing active treatment with placebo reached statistical significance ($P=0.007$).

Few studies, including a relatively small number of patients, have shown a lower thickness of intima-media during treatment with angiotensin II antagonists in respect with patients treated with beta-blockers [27].

Several randomized, comparative studies performed in the late 1990s have shown an effect of statin treatment on IMT progression. A first meta-analysis published in 2004 [28], evaluating 10 trials with 3,443 individuals (age range from 30 to 70 years) and follow-up for 1–4 years, has shown that conventional statin treatment reduces IMT progression as compared to placebo (8 studies) and that aggressive cholesterol reduction with high-dose statin may be more effective than conventional dosages.

A more recent meta-analysis [29] has examined 21 randomized controlled trials involving 6,317 individuals. The pooled weighted mean difference between statin therapy and placebo or usual care on CCA-IMT was −0.029 mm (95 % CI: −0.045, −0.013), and subgroup analyses showed a greater decrease in mean CCA-IMT in the setting of secondary prevention versus primary prevention, in younger patients versus older patients, and in studies with a greater proportion of male patients .

In other recent studies (ENHANCE, RADIANCE1, and RADIANCE2), no significant differences in IMT between treatment groups were observed in patients with familial hypercholesterolemia, even while significant decreases in LDL levels and increased HDL were observed, perhaps because patients had been previously long-term and optimally treated with statins and no difference in IMT occurred.

The results of the PHYLLIS study have reported that in hypertensive and hypercholesterolemic patients, the administration of pravastatin prevents the progression of carotid intima-media thickness seen in patients treated with hydrochlorothiazide, but the combination of pravastatin and the ACE-inhibitor fosinopril had no additive effect [30].

The greater reduction of plaque volume with the angiotensin II blocker in respect to the beta-blocker was demonstrated by a study (Multicenter Olmesartan Atherosclerosis Regression Evaluation (MORE)) assessing the effect of long-term treatment with an AT1 receptor antagonist (olmesartan) and with a beta-blocker (atenolol) on carotid atherosclerosis, with the use of the noninvasive 3D plaque measurement [31]. A significant change in 3D plaque volume was also observed during short-term treatment with a high-dose statin in a small group of 20 patients [32].

No significant changes in plaque composition were observed after 4 years of treatment with either lacidipine or atenolol in patients participating into the ELSA study, suggesting that treatment with a calcium antagonist may slow IMT progression, without influencing the characteristics of plaque tissue [33].

4.4 Prognostic Value of Baseline and of Changes of IMT and Plaque

Traditional risk factors, including male sex, ageing, being overweight, elevated blood pressure, diabetes, smoking, are all positively associated with carotid IMT in observational and epidemiological studies. Hypertension, and particularly, high systolic BP values, seems to have the greatest effect on IMT [34].

Some new risk factors, including various lipoproteins, plasma viscosity, and hyperhomocysteinemia, have demonstrated an association with increased IMT. Patients with metabolic syndrome have higher IMT than patients with individual metabolic risk factors. Carotid IMT has also been found to be associated with preclinical cardiovascular alterations in the heart, in the brain, in the kidney, and in the lower limb arteries.

Several studies have demonstrated and confirmed the important prognostic significance of intima-media thickness, as measured by ultrasound. In their prospective study, Salonen et al. [11] have observed, in 1,288 Finnish male subjects, that the risk for coronary events was exponentially related to the increase of intima-media thickness in the common carotid and in the carotid bifurcation. In a larger sample of middle-age subjects (13,780) enrolled into the ARIC (Atherosclerotic Risk in Communities) study [12], intima-media thickness, measured by ultrasound, was associated to an increased prevalence of cardiovascular and cerebrovascular diseases. In the Rotterdam study [13], the intima-media thickness was shown to predict the risk of myocardial infarction and cerebrovascular events during a mean follow-up period of 2.7 years. The results of the CHS [16] have prospectively evaluated 4,400 subjects aged more than 65 years for a follow-up period of 6 years; the annual incidence of myocardial infarction or stroke increased in the highest quintiles of intima-media thickness measured in the common and the internal carotid arteries even in this large group of elderly subjects.

A recent meta-analysis of data collected in eight studies in general populations, including 37,197 subjects who were followed up for a mean of 5.5 years, has demonstrated that for an absolute carotid IMT difference of 0.1 mm, the future risk of myocardial infarction increases by 10–15 % and the stroke risk increases by 13–18 % [14].

A second meta-analysis that evaluated CCA-IMT alone and excluded CCA or bulb IMT or plaques in 45,828 patients from 14 population-based studies showed that the addition of C-IMT does not add clinically meaningful information to the standard prediction modalities [15]. The net reclassification index with the addition of CCA-IMT was only 0.8 % for the overall cohort and 3.6 % for those at intermediate risk.

A high heterogeneity in the assessment of C-IMT in the different studies (number of carotid segments, type of measurements, number of imaging angles, inclusion of plaques in IM thickness, the use of adjusted or unadjusted models, and the different arbitrary cutoff points for C-IMT and for plaque) may explain the different results related to risk prediction. CCA-IMT measurement at sites not containing plaque and IMT measurement in the carotid bulb and ICA, inclusive of plaque

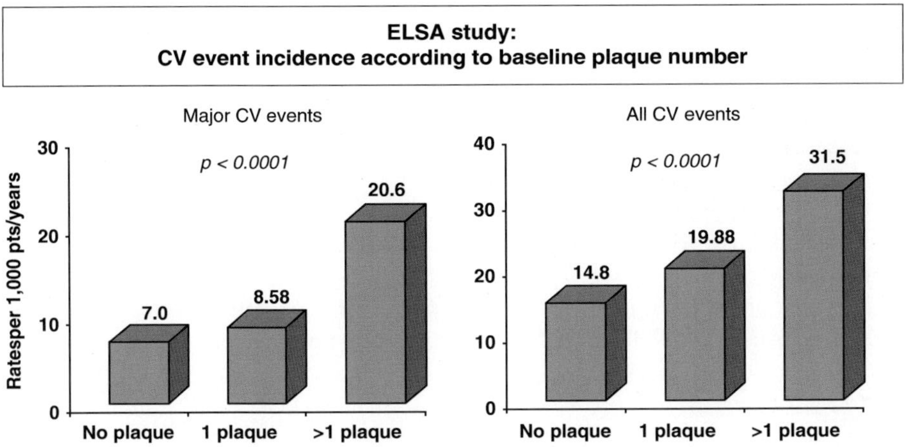

Fig. 4.3 Association of plaque number with cardiovascular events in the European Lacidipine Study on Atherosclerosis (ELSA) (Data from [39])

(if present), represent two separate phenotypes, with different association to the risk of cardiac and cerebrovascular events.

In fact, the assessment of carotid plaque appears to be a more powerful predictor of CV events than C-IMT alone, as suggested by a meta-analysis of 11 population-based studies including 54,336 patients [35]. The plaque number or the quantitative measurement of plaque thickness, area, or 3D volume may parallel the sensitivity in CV risk-predictive value [36] (Fig. 4.3).

The additional effect of C-IMT on CV risk stratification has been confirmed in some, but not all studies. About 30 % of hypertensive subjects may be mistakenly classified as at low or moderate added risk without ultrasound for carotid arteries thickening or plaque, whereas vascular damage places them in the high added risk group [21, 34, 37].

It has been therefore proposed that IMT may be proposed as a surrogate endpoint for cardiovascular events [38]. However, available studies have not been conducted to demonstrate whether a decrease of IMT progression may be associated with a reduction of cardiovascular events and an improvement in prognosis; the retrospective analysis of some studies has given conflicting results [15, 39, 40]. It has to be acknowledged that the estimation of C-IMT in the vast majority of the studies was obtained manually by calipers, without the use of an automatic approach for the measurement, suggesting that the accuracy of C-IMT and, particularly, of its changes over time might have important consequences in the clinical setting. The use of RF C-IMT measurements has been recently shown to have an additional stratification power for coronary artery disease, in addition to the Framingham risk score [41].

Furthermore, changes in plaque composition characteristics seem to have additional prognostic significance [20].

Conclusions

An ultrasound examination of the common bifurcation and internal carotid arteries should be performed in hypertensive patients with concomitant risk factors, such as smoking, dyslipidemia, diabetes, and family history for cardiovascular diseases. However, methodological standardization for IMT measurement needs to be further implemented for the routine measurement of IMT in clinical practice for stratifying cardiovascular risk.

Quantitative B-mode ultrasound of carotid arteries requires appropriate training.

In the presence of increased IMT or plaque in the carotid arteries, an aggressive approach to risk factor modifications should be considered.

References

1. Bots M, Evans G, Riley W, Grobbee DE. Carotid intima-media thickness measurements in intervention studies design options, progression rates, and sample size considerations: a point of view. Stroke. 2003;34:2985–94.
2. Touboul PJ, Hennerici MG, Meairs S, Adams H, Amarenco P, Bornstein N, Csiba L, Desvarieux M, Ebrahim S, Fatar M, Hernandez Hernandez R, Jaff M, Kownator S, Prati P, Rundek T, Sitzer M, Schminke U, Tardif JC, Taylor A, Vicaut E, Woo KS, Zannad F, Zureik M. Mannheim Carotid Intima-Media Thickness Consensus (2004–2006). An update on behalf of the advisory board of the 3rd and 4th watching the risk symposium 13th and 15th European Stroke Conferences, Mannheim, Germany, 2004, and Brussels, Belgium, 2006. Cerebrovasc Dis. 2006;23:75–80.
3. Salonen R, Haapanen A, Salonen JT. Measurement of intima-media thickness of common carotid arteries with high resolution B-mode ultrasonography: inter and intra-observer variability. Ultrasound Med Biol. 1991;17:225–30.
4. Furberg CD, Adams Jr HP, Applegate WB, Byington RB, Espeland MA, Hartwell T, et al. Effect of Lovastatin on early carotid atherosclerosis and cardiovascular events. Asymptomatic Carotid Artery Progression Study (ACAPS) research group. Circulation. 1994;90:1679–87.
5. Borhani NO, Mercuri M, Borhani PA, Buckalow VM, et al. Final outcome results of the Multicenter Isradipine Diuretic Atherosclerosis Study (MIDAS). JAMA. 1996;276:785–91.
6. Tang R, Henning M, Thomasson B, Scherz R, Ravinetto R, Cattalini R, et al. Baseline reproducibility of B mode ultrasonic measurement of carotid artery intima-media thickness: the European Lacidipine Study on Atherosclerosis (ELSA). J Hypertens. 2000;18:197–201.
7. Paini A, Boutouyrie P, Calvet D, Zidi M, Agabiti-Rosei E, Laurent S. Multiaxial mechanical characteristics of carotid plaque: analysis by multiarray echotracking system. Stroke. 2007;38:117–23.
8. Engelen L, Ferreira I, Stehouwer CD, Boutouyrie P, Laurent S, Reference Values for Arterial Measurements Collaboration. Reference intervals for common carotid intima-media thickness measured with echotracking: relation with risk factors. Eur Heart J. 2013;34(30):2368–80.
9. Howard G, Sharrett AR, Heiss G, Evans GW, Chambless LE, Riley WA, et al. Carotid artery intimal-medial thickness distribution in general populations as evaluated by B-mode ultrasound: ARIC investigators. Stroke. 1993;24:1297–304.
10. Bots ML, Hoes AW, Koudstaal PJ, Hofman A, Grobbee DE. Common carotid intima-media thickness and risk of stroke and myocardial infarction the Rotterdam Study. Circulation. 1997;6(5):1432–7.
11. Salonen JT, Salonen R. Ultrasonographically assessed carotid morphology and the risk of coronary heart disease. Arterioscler Thromb. 1991;11:1245.

12. Chambeless LE, Heiss G, Folsom AR, Rosamond W, Szklo M, Sharret AR, Clegg LX. Association of coronary heart disease incidence with carotid arterial wall thickness and major risk factors: the Atherosclerosis Risk in Communities (ARIC) Study. 1987–1993. Am J Epidemiol. 1997;146:483–94.
13. Hodis HN, Mack WJ, LaBree L, Selzer RH, Liu CR, Liu CH, Azen SP. The role of arterial intima-media thickness in predicting clinical coronary events. Ann Intern Med. 1998;128(4):262–9.
14. Lorenz M, Markus H, Bots M, Rosvall M, Sitzer M. Prediction of clinical cardiovascular events with carotid intima-media thickness: a systematic review and meta-analysis. Circulation. 2007;115:459–67.
15. Den Ruijter HM, Peters SA, Anderson TJ, et al. Common carotid intima-media thickness measurements in cardiovascular risk prediction: a meta-analysis. JAMA. 2012;308:796–803.
16. O'Leary DH, Polak JF, Kronmal RA, Manolio TA, Burke GL, Wolfson SK, for the Cardiovascular Health Study Collaborative research Group. Carotid intima and media thickness as a risk factor for myocardial infarction and stroke in older adults. N Engl J Med. 1999;340:14–22.
17. Puato M, Faggin E, Rattazzi M, et al.; on behalf of the Study Group on Arterial Wall Structure. In vivo non invasive identification of cell composition of intimal lesions: a combined approach with ultrasonography and immunocytochemistry. J Vasc Surg. 2003;38:1390–5.
18. Ciulla M, Paliotti R, Ferrero S, et al. Assessment of carotid plaque composition in hypertensive patients by ultrasonic tissue characterization: a validation study. J Hypertens. 2002;20: 1589–96.
19. Wannarong T, Parraga G, Buchanan D, Fenster A, House AA, Hackam DG, Spence JD. Progression of carotid plaque volume predicts cardiovascular events. Stroke. 2013;44(7):1859–65.
20. van Engelen A, Wannarong T, Parraga G, Niessen WJ, Fenster A, Spence JD, de Bruijne M. Three-dimensional carotid ultrasound plaque texture predicts vascular events. Stroke. 2014;45(9):2695–701.
21. Muiesan ML, Pasini GF, Salvetti M, Calebich S, Zulli R, Castellano M, Rizzoni D, et al. Cardiac and vascular structural changes: prevalence and relation to ambulatory blood pressure in a middle aged general population in northern Italy: the Vobarno Study. Hypertension. 1996;27:1046–53.
22. Zanchetti A, Agabiti-Rosei E, Dal Palu' C, Leonetti G, Magnani B, Pessina A, for the Verapamil in Hypertension and Atherosclerosis Study (VHAS) Investigators. The Verapamil in Hypertension and Atherosclerosis Study (VHAS): results of long-term randomized treatment with either verapamil or chlortalidone on carotid intima-media thickness. J Hypertens. 1998;16:1667–76.
23. Zanchetti A, Bond MG, Hennig M, Neiss A, Mancia G, Dal Palu' C, et al. Calcium antagonist lacidipine slows down progression of asymptomatic carotid atherosclerosis: Principal results of the European Lacidipine Study on Atherosclerosis (ELSA), a randomized, double-blind, long-term trial. Circulation. 2002;106:2422–7.
24. Suurkula M, Agewall M, Fagerberg B, Wendelhalg I, Widgren B, Wikstrand J. Ultrasound evaluation of atherosclerotic manifestations in the carotid artery in high risk hypertensive patients. Risk intervention Study (RIS) Group. Arterioscler Thromb. 1994;14(8):1297–304.
25. Muiesan ML, Salvetti M, Rizzoni D, Paini A, Agabiti-Rosei C, Aggiusti C, Agabiti Rosei E. Resistant hypertension and target organ damage. Hypertens Res. 2013;36(6):485–91.
26. Wang JG, Staessen JA, Li Y, Van Bortel LM, Nawrot T, Fagard R, Messerli FH, Safar M. Carotid intima-media thickness and antihypertensive treatment a meta-analysis of randomized controlled trials. Stroke. 2006;37:1933–40.
27. Agabiti-Rosei E, Muiesan ML, Rizzoni D. Angiotensin II antagonists and protection against subclinical cardiac and vascular damage. In: Mancia G, editor. Angiotensin II receptors antagonists. 2nd ed. Boca Raton: Taylor & Francis; 2006. p. 111–26.
28. Kang S, Wu Y, Li X. Effects of statin therapy on the progression of carotid atherosclerosis: a systematic review and meta-analysis. Atherosclerosis. 2004;177:433–42.

29. Huang Y, Li W, Dong L, Li R, Wu Y. Effect of statin therapy on the progression of common carotid artery intima-media thickness: an updated systematic review and meta-analysis of randomized controlled trials. J Atheroscler Thromb. 2013;20(1):108–21.
30. Zanchetti A, Crepaldi G, Bond G, Gallus G, Veglia F, Mancia G, Ventura S, Baggio G, Sampietri L, Rubba P, Sperti G, Magni A, on behalf of PHYLLIS Investigators. Different effects of antihypertensive regimens based on Fosinopril or hydrochlorothiazide with or without lipid lowering by pravastatin on progression of asymptomatic carotid atherosclerosis principal results of PHYLLIS—a randomized double-blind trial. Stroke. 2004;35:2807–12.
31. Stumpe KO, Agabiti-Rosei E, Zielinski T, et al.; MORE Study Investigators. Carotid intima-media thickness and plaque volume changes following 2-year angiotensin II-receptor blockade. The Multicentre Olmesartan atherosclerosis Regression Evaluation (MORE) study. Ther Adv Cardiovasc Dis. 2007;1(2):97–106.
32. Krasinski A, Chiu B, Spence JD, Fenster A, Parraga G. Three-dimensional ultrasound quantification of intensive statin treatment of carotid atherosclerosis. Ultrasound Med Biol. 2009;35(11):1763–72.
33. Paliotti R, Ciulla M, Hennig M, Tang R, Bond G, Mancia G, Magrini F, Zanchetti A. Carotid wall composition in hypertensive patients after 4-year treatment with lacidipine or atenolol: an echoreflectivity study. J Hypertens. 2005;23:1203–9.
34. Cuspidi C, Ambrosioni E, Mancia G, Pessina AC, Trimarco B, Zanchetti A. Role of echocardiography and carotid ultrasonography in stratifying risk in patients with essential hypertension: the assessment of prognostic risk observational survey. J Hypertens. 2002;20:1307–14.
35. Inaba Y, Chen JA, Bergmann SR. Carotid plaque, compared with carotid intima-media thickness, more accurately predicts coronary artery disease events: a meta-analysis. Atherosclerosis. 2012;220:128–33.
36. Spence JD. Carotid plaque measurement is superior to IMT: invited editorial comment on: carotid plaque, compared with carotid intima-media thickness, more accurately predicts coronary artery disease events: a meta-analysis—Yoichi Inaba, M.D., Jennifer A. Chen M.D., Steven R. Bergmann M.D., Ph.D. Atherosclerosis. 2012;220:34–5.
37. Sehestedt T, Jeppesen J, Hansen TW, Wachtell K, Ibsen H, Torp-Pedersen C, Hildebrandt P, Olsen MH. Risk prediction is improved by adding markers of subclinical organ damage to SCORE. Eur Heart J. 2010;31(7):883–91.
38. Espeland MA, O'Leary DH, Terry JG, Morgan T, Evans G, Mudra H. Carotid intimal-media thickness as a surrogate for cardiovascular disease events in trials of HMG-CoA reductase inhibitors. Curr Control Trials Cardiovasc Med. 2005;6(1):3.
39. Zanchetti A, Hennig M, Hollweck R, Bond G, Tang R, Cuspidi C, Parati G, Facchetti R, Mancia G. Baseline values but not treatment-induced changes in carotid intima-media thickness predict incident cardiovascular events in treated hypertensive patients: findings in the European Lacidipine Study on Atherosclerosis (ELSA). Circulation. 2009;120(12):1084–90.
40. Costanzo P, Perrone-Filardi P, Vassallo E, Paolillo S, Cesarano P, Brevetti G, Chiariello M. Does carotid intima-media thickness regression predict reduction of cardiovascular events? A meta-analysis of 41 randomized trials. J Am Coll Cardiol. 2010;56(24):2006–20.
41. Moreo A, Gaibazzi N, Faggiano P, Mohammed M, Carerj S, Mureddu G, Pigazzani F, Muiesan ML, Salvetti M, Cesana F, Faden G, Facchetti R, Giannattasio C, Rigo F. Multiparametric carotid and cardiac ultrasound compared with clinical risk scores for the prediction of angiographic coronary artery disease: a multicenter prospective study. J Hypertens. 2015 [Epub ahead of print].

Echocardiographic Assessment of the Aorta and Coronary Arteries in Hypertensive Patients

5

Costas P. Tsioufis

5.1 Aorta

5.1.1 How to Assess

Ultrasound techniques for imaging of the aorta (aortic root, tubular ascending aorta, aortic arch, descending thoracic aorta) in hypertensive patients include transthoracic echocardiography (TTE), transesophageal echocardiography (TOE), and rarely intravascular ultrasound (IVUS).

5.1.1.1 Transthoracic Echocardiographic

Evaluation of the aorta is a routine part of the standard echocardiographic examination. Using different acoustic windows, the proximal ascending aorta is visualized in the left and right parasternal long-axis views and, to a lesser extent, in basal short-axis views. The long-axis view affords the best opportunity for measuring aortic root diameters in the following levels: outflow track, Valsalva sinuses, sinotubular junction, and tubular ascending aorta, by taking advantage of the superior axial image resolution. The ascending aorta is also visualized in the apical long-axis and modified apical five-chamber views. However, in these views the aortic walls are seen with suboptimal lateral resolution [1].

The suprasternal view is of paramount importance for evaluation of the thoracic aorta. This view primarily depicts the aortic arch and the three major supra-aortic vessels (innominate, left carotid and left subclavian arteries), as well as variable lengths of the descending and, to a lesser degree, the ascending aorta. Although this view may be obstructed, particularly in patients with emphysema or short wide necks, it should be systematically sought when aortic disease is evaluated. The

C.P. Tsioufis
First Cardiology Clinic, Hippokration Hospital, University of Athens,
114 Vas. Sofias Ave, 11527 Athens, Greece
e-mail: ktsioufis@hippocratio.gr

E. Agabiti Rosei, G. Mancia (eds.), *Assessment of Preclinical Organ Damage in Hypertension*, DOI 10.1007/978-3-319-15603-3_5

entire thoracic descending aorta is not well visualized by TTE. From the apical window a short-axis cross section of the descending aorta is seen lateral to the left atrium in the four-chamber view and a long-axis stretch in the two-chamber view. By 90° transducer rotation, a long-axis view is obtained visualizing a mid part of the descending aorta [2].

5.1.1.2 Transesophageal Echocardiography

The proximity of the esophagus and the thoracic aorta permits high-resolution images from higher-frequency TOE. The indications for performing TOE are the evaluation of native valve disease, prosthetic heart valve function, cardiac masses, patients with hemodynamic instability, congenital heart disease, and the thromboembolic risk in patients with atrial fibrillation and inadequate anticoagulation. Other indications are the detection of aortic dissection, endocarditis complications, and potential etiologies of stroke, while it is also useful as an adjunct to percutaneous cardiac procedures and cardiac surgical procedures. The most important transesophageal views of the ascending aorta, aortic root, and aortic valve are the high transesophageal long-axis (at 120–150°) and short-axis (at 30–60°) views. The descending aorta is easily visualized in short-axis (0°) and long-axis (90°) views from the celiac trunk to the left subclavian artery. Further withdrawal of the probe shows the aortic arch, where the inner curvature and anterior arch wall are usually well seen all the way to the ascending aorta. In the distal part of the arch, the origin of the subclavian artery is easily visualized [3].

5.1.1.3 Measurement of Aorta Dimensions

Measurements of the aortic diameter by echocardiography are accurate and reproducible when a true perpendicular dimension is obtained and gain settings are appropriate. Two-dimensional (2D) aortic measurements are preferable to M-mode, as the cyclic motion of the heart and the resultant changes in M-mode cursor location result in systematic underestimation by 1–2 mm of aortic diameter by M-mode in comparison with the 2D aortic diameter. Standard diameter measurements are at the level of the aortic annulus, of Valsalva sinuses, and of the sinotubular junction. Aortic annular diameter is measured between the hinge points of the aortic valve leaflets in the left parasternal long-axis view, during systole, which reveals the largest aortic annular diameter. In a normal ascending aorta, the diameter at sinus level is the largest, followed by the sinotubular junction and the aortic annulus level [4].

The aorta size is related most strongly to body surface area (BSA) and age. Therefore, BSA may be used to predict aortic root diameter in several age intervals. Some groups have suggested indexing by height to avoid the influence of overweight on BSA [5]. Aortic root dilatation at the sinuses of Valsalva is defined as an aortic root diameter above the upper limit of the 95 % confidence interval of the distribution in a large reference population. In adults a diameter of 2.1 cm/m^2 has been considered to be the upper normal range in ascending aorta. TTE is satisfactory for the quantification of maximum aortic root and proximal ascending aorta diameters, when the acoustic window is adequate. Nevertheless, the technique is more limited for measuring the remaining aortic segments. TOE overcomes part of

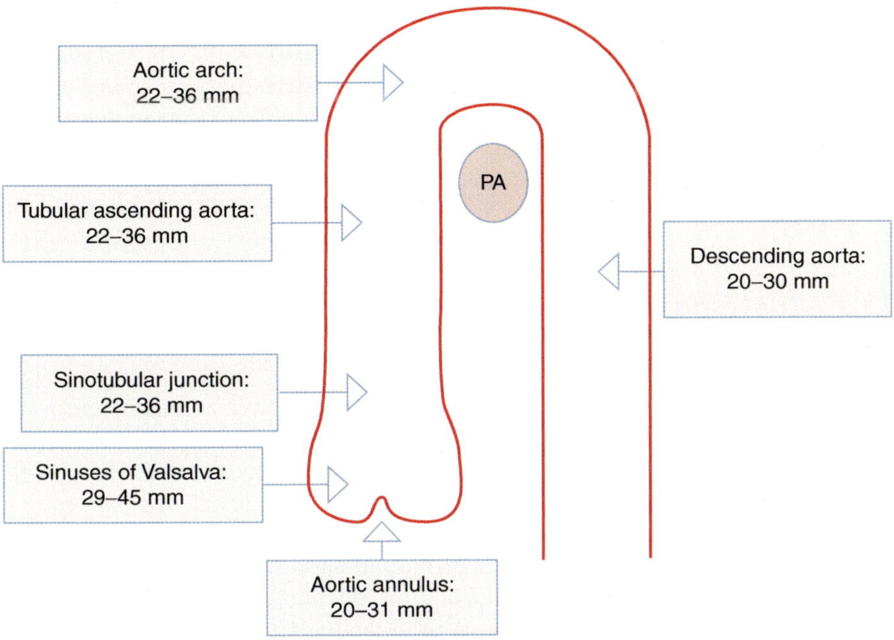

Fig. 5.1 Normal size of thoracic aortic segments. The thoracic aorta can be divided into three segments: the ascending aorta that extends from the aortic annulus to the innominate artery and is typically measured at the level of the aortic annulus, the sinuses of Valsalva, the sinotubular junction, and the proximal ascending aorta; the aortic arch that extends from the innominate artery to the ligamentum arteriosum; and the descending aorta that extends from the ligamentum arteriosum to the level of the diaphragm. *PA* right pulmonary artery

these TTE limitations by affording better measurement of aortic arch and descending thoracic aorta size. The absolute and indexed normal values of the various aortic segments are shown in Fig. 5.1 [6].

5.1.1.4 Aortic Pressure-Dimension Relationship

An increase in distending pressure during systole induces an increase in aortic dimension which is directly related to the elastic properties of the aorta [7]. Diameter or area changes can be determined using TTE or TOE, but the estimation of the pressure changes at the same site may be unreliable because of the amplification of the pulse pressure and the inaccuracy of all cuff sphygmomanometer systems, particularly in young subjects. However, studies have shown a good correlation between aortic distensibility calculated using echocardiography and noninvasive brachial artery blood pressure (BP) measurements and aortic distensibility calculated invasively using contrast aortography and direct aortic pressure recordings. Changes in arterial diameter can be measured at the level of the ascending aorta ~3 cm above the aortic valve in 2D-guided M-mode of parasternal long-axis view, with the diastolic aortic diameter measured at the peak of the QRS complex and systolic aorta diameter measured at the maximal anterior motion of the aorta [8, 9].

There are several indices derived from aortic or arterial dimensions and pressures, used for the estimation of the elastic properties of the aorta. The indices most frequently used are the aortic/arterial distensibility (the relative change in a diameter or area for pressure change), the compliance (the absolute change in diameter or area for pressure change), and the non-dimensional index of local arterial stiffness named the β-index which is less affected by arterial pressure changes and is easily measured using echo-tracking devices [10].

5.1.2 The Aorta and Blood Pressure

Although early case reports and pathological series suggest that hypertension might directly contribute to the enlargement of the aorta, more recent pathological and M-mode echocardiographic studies have not found an association between BP and aortic size when the confounding influence of aging is considered. Thus, aortic diameter is strongly related to age, and senescence may result in cystic medial necrosis [11]. In contrast, other M-mode echocardiographic studies have noted significant relations of aortic diameter to systolic and diastolic BP.

As mentioned before, studies evaluating the relation of aortic root size to BP have yielded conflicting results [12]. In the Framingham Heart Study, scientists using two-dimensionally guided M-mode measurement of the sinuses of Valsalva found that diastolic pressure was directly related to aortic diameter, whereas both systolic and pulse pressures were inversely related to aortic diameter after adjustment for age, height, and weight [13]. In the Cardiovascular Health Study, a relation was found between diastolic, but not systolic, BP and M-mode echocardiographic aortic dimensions when the entire elderly cohort was analyzed. However, when the healthier subgroup was examined (subjects not receiving antihypertensive therapy or without coronary heart disease), aortic diameter was not associated with BP. Other researchers have shown either no relation of BP to M-mode aortic measurements or a relationship only to systolic BP [14].

There are few studies showing a correlation between aortic root diameter and hemodynamic load. A progressive enlargement in aortic dimension was found only at the supra-aortic ridge and ascending aorta according to the quartiles of casual systolic blood pressure, while all aortic diameters were found to significantly increase according to the quartiles of casual diastolic pressure, with the most significant increases occurring in the more distal segments [15].

Four previous studies have reported inverse associations between aortic diameter and pulse pressure (PP). In the Framingham cohort an independent inverse association was found between aortic diameter and PP, and it was speculated that intimal-medial hypertrophy or reflex smooth muscle activation induced by an increased PP may underlie this association [13]. Similarly, a substudy of the Losartan Intervention for Endpoint Reduction Trial observed an inverse association between aortic diameter and PP and hypothesized that the higher compliance of the aortic root may reduce the rise in systolic pressure and thus result in lower PP [16]. In a subgroup of the stroke prevention, an inverse association between aortic diameter and PP was also found. Furthermore in a smaller study, it was shown that aortic dimensions were inversely associated with carotid PP (but not brachial) in the healthy control group but were positively associated with PP in subjects with Marfan syndrome who have known alterations in their aortic wall properties. The authors speculated that this inverse association between aortic diameter and carotid PP in the healthy cohort was due to the reduced wave reflection, accruing from the higher aortic compliance of subjects with larger aortic diameters [17, 18].

5.1.3 Relationship Between 24-h Ambulatory Blood Pressure and Aortic Dimensions

The impact of ambulatory BP and its circadian components on aortic diameter in hypertensive patients has never been prospectively investigated in large studies. In a small series of 48 hypertensive patients, it was shown that awake diastolic BP was independently correlated with aortic diameter measured at four different locations [19]. In a study of a larger sample, it was observed that nocturnal BP may have an independent role in determining aortic dimension. This observation is further supported by the progressive reduction in the prevalence of a normal nocturnal BP pattern with advancing aortic root size. This finding is also in line with the evidence that nocturnal BP has superior prognostic value than awake BP in predicting cardiovascular morbidity and mortality in both normotensive and hypertensive individuals. The reasons of the prognostic superiority of nighttime over daytime BP are not clear. However, there is a hypothesis suggesting that the excessive variability of diurnal BP may reduce its prognostic value compared to that of nocturnal BP [20].

Individuals with obstructive sleep apnea (OSA) are usually non-dippers and have aortic dilatation in echocardiography. During each apneic episode there is a marked increase in transmural pressure of the aortic wall, resulting in aortic dilatation. An animal study showed that the thoracic aorta can be distended during the diastolic phase in the setting of negative intrathoracic pressure, probably due to diminished antegrade flow out of the thorax. Furthermore, cyclical fluctuations in sympathetic activity and BP, which have been shown to progressively increase during apneic episodes in patients with OSA, may result in aortic dilatation [21, 22].

5.1.4 Modifications of the Aorta and Cardiovascular Events

Although anatomical changes of the aortic root are likely to reflect the effects of hypertension and atherosclerosis, few data are available on the predictive value of aortic root dimension for cardiovascular events. In the Cardiovascular Health Study, it was shown that a large aortic root dimension is associated with an increased risk for incident congestive heart failure, stroke, and cardiovascular mortality but not for myocardial infarction. The lack of association between aortic root dimension and incident myocardial infarction may suggest that an increased aortic root is not a consequence of acute myocardial infarction, but of the interaction of age, hypertension, and atherosclerosis over time [23]. The Rotterdam Study observed that the presence of atheromatous plaques in the aorta was strongly correlated with decreased aortic distensibility. In contrast, other studies have found no relation between arterial stiffness and aortic atherosclerosis. However, the elevation of systolic blood pressure, causing a rise in left ventricular afterload and myocardial work, and the decrease in diastolic blood pressure, which reduces coronary perfusion, result in subendocardial ischemia [24, 25].

5.2 Coronary Arteries

5.2.1 Coronary Artery Remodeling in Hypertension

In essential hypertension remodeling of the small arteries (100–300 mm of diameter) is the most prevalent and earliest form of target organ damage. At the level of the coronary artery tree, it causes increased vascular reactivity and a reduction in coronary flow reserve (CFR) at maximal vasodilation [26–28]. Coronary remodeling in the form of media thickening is mainly caused by complex hemodynamic and neurohumoral interactions [26, 28]. The dimensions of the epicardial coronary arteries remain constant resulting in an elevated coronary flow velocity [29]. This may increase longitudinal shear stress, causing premature atherosclerosis. It should be noted that changes in microcirculation maintain the increase in vascular resistance that is common in hypertension [30]. However, it is still under investigation whether these microcirculatory abnormalities are the cause or effect in the hypertensive setting [31].

Blood vessels react to physiologic or pathologic conditions with changes in their size and structure [32]. Exposure of the large coronary arteries to high pulsatile pressure and blood flow velocity can lead to an increase in endothelial shear stress, resulting in endothelial dysfunction responsible for the increase in the endothelial permeability and deposition of lipoproteins in the arterial wall and eventually the formation of atherosclerotic plaques [33].

Coronary remodeling in hypertensive patients can be distinguished as positive and negative. Compensatory or positive remodeling (described by Glagov) delays the onset of luminal narrowing because the vessel expands with plaque enlargement [34], while in the case of negative remodeling, the vessel's cross-sectional area is much less compared to the adjacent normal reference segment contributing to the development of focal coronary artery stenosis [35]. Based on the presence or not of stenosis, coronary remodeling may be also defined as adequate or inadequate, respectively.

Arterial remodeling is considered to be initiated by the detection of signals related to changes in hemodynamic conditions such as blood flow, wall stretch, and shear stress as well as signals related to humoral factors that include cytokines and vasoactive substances [32]. These signals which are relayed to the endothelium and transmitted to adjacent cells can lead to the synthesis or the activation of substances that influence cell growth and apoptosis. The extracellular matrix also appears to have an important role in the remodeling response on account of a group of enzymes (matrix metalloproteinases) that regulate the composition of the matrix by selective degradation of its components. Inflammation plays a key role in coronary remodeling and the atherosclerotic process, contributing to the formation of the vulnerable plaque prone to rupture leading to acute coronary syndromes [32, 34]. In contrast, fibrotic changes could lead to a reduced risk of plaque rupture and to plaque stabilization.

5.2.2 Methods for Assessment

Although contrast coronary angiography offers excellent visualization of the configuration of the long axes of the blood vessel lumen, it lags in information on the structure, morphology, and consistence of the coronary arterial wall [35, 36]. Intravascular ultrasound (IVUS) can provide information on the arterial wall under the endothelial surface and can help detect structural and functional changes of the coronary vessels in hypertensive patients [37]. By using IVUS in the coronary arteries, we can evaluate the lumen area and geometry, the wall tissue characteristics and thickness, the branch points, the degree of calcification, and the location and the extent of atherosclerotic lesions [38, 39]. Occult plaques can be concealed in segments of an apparent and angiographically normal coronary artery, and only intravascular imaging modalities like IVUS can identify them [34].

Intravascular US consists of an ultrasound catheter that incorporates a polyethylene shaft and a phased array transducer tip. The multielement array yields an image perpendicular to the axis of the catheter. The field of view is adjustable from 8 to 16 mm in diameter, and images may be acquired up to 10 frames/second [38].

Intravascular US studies have demonstrated that arterial remodeling could be bidirectional and it is a plaque-specific rather than a patient-specific process. That means that in the same coronary artery, the degree of the remodeling varies from plaque to plaque [34]. The use of IVUS is valuable to understand the nature and the characteristics of the coronary wall during the process of remodeling. Indeed IVUS imaging has demonstrated an expansion or a shrinkage of the external elastic membrane area in the case of positive or negative remodeling, respectively [32].

5.2.3 Coronary Circulation: Functional Changes

In hypertensive patients, the structural alterations of the intramyocardial arteries of the coronary tree contribute to the reduced coronary vasodilator capacity and to an increased minimal coronary resistance independently of the presence of left ventricular hypertrophy [37]. Studies have documented a reduced coronary reserve in most of the hypertensive patients even in the absence of coronary artery disease. Responsible of this impaired coronary vasodilator reserve are considered mainly the intramyocardial arterioles that largely contribute in the coronary vascular resistance and the autoregulation of myocardial perfusion. Arterial hypertension increases the wall-to-lumen ratio of the intramyocardial arteries by inducing arterial medial hypertrophy that in turn leads to wall thickening and lumen reduction. Moreover, the coronary vasodilator capacity can be influenced by vascular tone, endothelial dysfunction, increase of vascular collagen biosynthesis, interstitial and periarteriolar fibrosis, or/and noxious interactions between structural and functional components of a thickened arterial wall. In addition, studies have revealed that the lumen size of the major coronary arteries of hypertensive patients do not match with the increased coronary flow [40]. This mismatch can be influenced by the vascular tone, but it is more related to the absence of structural enlargement.

5.2.4 How to Perform Coronary Flow Reserve Measurements

It is established that microvascular function can be accurately assessed by CFR measured either invasively [41] or noninvasively [42].

5.2.4.1 Invasive

A 0.014 in. Doppler guidewire (FloWire, Cardiometrics) is advanced into the proximal part of the left anterior descending artery. ECG, coronary ostial pressure, instantaneous spectral peak velocity, and time-averaged spectral peak flow velocity are continuously and simultaneously recorded. Then an intracoronary bolus of 60 μg adenosine is administered into the left coronary artery, and further measurements are obtained under peak hyperemic conditions. CFR is calculated as the ratio of hyperemic to baseline time-averaged spectral peak flow velocity. All measurements should be performed twice, and mean values should be calculated.

5.2.4.2 Noninvasive

Parts of coronary arteries can be visualized using TTE. The anatomy and pathophysiology of the coronary arteries can be rivaled based on two-dimensional evaluation, but the introduction of Doppler velocity measurements has allowed the assessment of the function of the coronary arteries, and TTE has been introduced in the detection of coronary flow velocity and coronary flow velocity reserve (CFVR) [42]. CFR can be quantified using flow velocity-derived methods. Three types of Doppler techniques can be applied to coronary flow measurement: pulse wave Doppler in which intermittent bursts of ultrasound are transmitted, continuous wave Doppler where ultrasounds are transmitted and received continuously, and color flow mapping which uses simple sampling volumes to record shifts [42].

CFR can be quantificated by inducing maximal hyperemia with the use of pharmacological agents such as adenosine, ATP, and dipyridamole. CFR can be affected by epicardial stenosis and microcirculation. In the absence of stenosis in the epicardial arteries, CFVR depicts the reactivity of the microcirculation. To level out the effect of microcirculation on CFR measurements in stenosed vessels, the relative flow reserve has been developed. It is calculated by comparing the flow velocity reserve distal to the stenosis in the target vessel with the velocity reserve to a non-stenosed reference vessel [42].

5.2.4.3 Changes of CFR in Hypertension

Notably, abnormal CFR often accompanies hypertension even in the absence of left ventricular hypertrophy [43]. The observed reduction in CFR in hypertension is attributed to remodeling of the coronary small arteries and arterioles as well as to interstitial fibrosis [37]. This pathological alteration has been suggested to cause angina-like chest pain in noncoronary artery disease patients with [43] or without hypertension [44, 45] and is regarded as a microvascular disturbance. End-organ damage in the form of left ventricular hypertrophy has a strong contribution to the attenuation of CFR [46]. Carotid intima-media thickness (IMT) has been shown to correlate with traditional risk factors for atherosclerosis and the presence and severity of coronary artery disease, as well as with left ventricular mass in patients with hypertension [47, 48]. Interestingly, carotid atherosclerosis, measured by IMT, not only reflects coronary morphological changes (coronary IMT measured by intravascular ultrasound) [49] but also coronary functional changes (reduced CFR) [50].

Using the more sensitive method of optical coherence tomography (OCT) in never-treated hypertensive patients, it was again confirmed that reduced CFR was not related to increased coronary IMT in the absence of echocardiographically evident left ventricular hypertrophy [46]. Moreover, no significant difference was found between patients with low and normal CFR with respect to OCT-measured IMT and IT with the values of the latter being in agreement with past works [51, 52]. Therefore, adverse functional microcirculatory changes occur independently from and possibly precede vascular remodeling in hypertension.

5.2.4.4 Clinical Perspectives

Considering that the adverse functional microcirculatory changes could cause insufficient coronary perfusion and impaired wall function during stress, the presence of attenuated CFR even in hypertensive patients without left ventricular hypertrophy identifies a subgroup at greater risk. Moreover, repeated stress and regional ischemia lead to fibrosis, which also impairs cardiac function leading to heart failure in the absence of obstructive coronary disease. Interestingly, CFR attenuation might constitute the earlier phase of the hypertensive insult to the arterial coronary tree.

Finally, from a therapeutical point of view, in selected patients with blunted CFR, the use of specific drugs, such as candesartan and nebivolol, that exert favorable effects on the microcirculation can induce not only BP reduction per se, but it might also attenuate target organ progression and ameliorate overall prognosis [53, 54].

References

1. Evangelista A, Flachskampf FA, Erbel R, Antonini-Canterin F, Nihoyannopoulos P, et al. Echocardiography in aortic diseases: EAE recommendations for clinical practice. Eur J Echocardiogr. 2010;11:645–58.
2. Oh JK, Seward JB, Talik AJ. The echo manual. 3rd ed. Philadelphia: Lippincott Williams & Wilkins; 2006.

3. Pearson AC, Guo R, Orsinelli DA, Binkley PF, Pasierski TJ. Transesophageal echocardiographic assessment of the effects of age, gender, and hypertension on thoracic aortic wall size, thickness, and stiffness. Am Heart J. 1994;128(2):344–5.
4. Feigenbaum H, Echocardiography. 4th Ed., 1986. Lea & Febiger. Philadelphia.
5. Mirea O, Maffessanti F, Gripari P, Tamborini G, Muratori M, Fusini L, Claudia C, Fiorentini C, Plesea IE, Pepi M. Effects of aging and body size on proximal and ascending aorta and aortic arch: inner edge-to-inner edge reference values in a large adult population by two-dimensional transthoracic echocardiography. J Am Soc Echocardiogr. 2013;26(4):419–27.
6. Inga V, Michael J-H, Jürgen H, Eileen P, Christopher H, Dominik Daniel G, Jan Hinnerk H, Colin P, Hans-Heiner K, Carsten R. Normal values of aortic dimensions, distensibility, and pulse wave velocity in children and young adults: a cross-sectional study. J Cardiovasc Magn Reson. 2012;14:77.
7. Stefanadis C, Dernellis J, Toutouzas P. Mechanical properties of the aorta determined by the pressure-diameter relation. Pathol Biol (Paris). 1999;47(7):696–704.
8. Khanafer K, Schlicht MS, Berguer R. How should we measure and report elasticity in aortic tissue? Eur J Vasc Endovasc Surg. 2013;45(4):332–9.
9. Schultz MG, Davies JE, Hardikar A, Pitt S, Moraldo M, Dhutia N, Hughes AD, Sharman JE. Aortic reservoir pressure corresponds to cyclic changes in aortic volume: physiological validation in humans. Arterioscler Thromb Vasc Biol. 2014;34(7):1597–603.
10. Heerman JR, Segers P, Roosens CD, Gasthuys F, Verdonck PR, Poelaert JI. Echocardiographic assessment of aortic elastic properties with automated border detection in an ICU: in vivo application of the arctangent Langewouters model. Am J Physiol Heart Circ Physiol. 2005;288(5):H2504–11.
11. Dahan M, Paillole C, Ferreira B, Gourgon R. Doppler echocardiographic study of the consequences of aging and hypertension on the left ventricle and aorta. Eur Heart J. 1990;11(Suppl G):39–45.
12. Kim M, Roman MJ, Cavallini MC, Schwartz JE, et al. Effect of hypertension on aortic root size and prevalence of aortic regurgitation. Hypertension. 1996;28:47–52.
13. Vasan RS, Larson MG, Levy D. Determinants of echocardiographic aortic root size The Framingham Heart Study. Circulation. 1995;91:734–40.
14. Tell GS, Rutan GH, Kronmal RA, Bild DE, Polak JF. Correlates of blood pressure in community-dwelling older adults. The Cardiovascular Health Study. Cardiovascular Health Study (CHS) Collaborative Research. Hypertension. 1994;23:59–67.
15. Aars H. Relationship between blood pressure and diameter of ascending aorta in normal and hypertensive rabbits. Acta Physiol Scand. 1969;75(3):397–405.
16. Bella JN, Wachtell K, Boman K, Palmieri V, Papademetriou V, Gerdts E, Aalto T, Olsen MH, Olofsson M, Dahlof B, Roman MJ, Devereux RB. Relation of left ventricular geometry and function to aortic root dilatation in patients with systemic hypertension and left ventricular hypertrophy (the LIFE study). Am J Cardiol. 2002;89:337–41.
17. Agmon Y, Khandheria BK, Meissner I, Schwartz GL, Sicks JD, Fought AJ, O'Fallon WM, Wiebers DO, Tajik AJ. Is aortic dilatation an atherosclerosis-related process? Clinical, laboratory, and transesophageal echocardiographic correlates of thoracic aortic dimensions in the population with implications for thoracic aortic aneurysm formation. J Am Coll Cardiol. 2003;42:1076–83.
18. Jondeau G, Boutouyrie P, Lacolley P, Laloux B, Dubourg O, Bourdarias JP, Laurent S. Central pulse pressure is a major determinant of ascending aorta dilation in Marfan syndrome. Circulation. 1999;99:2677–81.
19. Cuspidi C, Meani S, Valerio C, Esposito A, Sala C, Maisaidi M, Zanchetti A, Mancia G. Ambulatory blood pressure, target organ damage and aortic root size in never-treated essential hypertensive patients. J Hum Hypertens. 2007;21(7):531–8.
20. Ohkubo T, Iami Y, Tsuji I, Nagai K, Watanabe N, Minami N, et al. Relation between nocturnal decline in blood pressure and mortality: the Ohasama Study. Am J Hypertens. 1997;10:1201–7.
21. Baguet JP, Minville C, Tamisier R, Roche F. Increased aortic root size is associated with nocturnal hypoxia and diastolic blood pressure in obstructive sleep apnea. Sleep. 2011;34(11): 1605–7.

22. Lee LC, Torres MC, Khoo SM, Chong EY, Lau C. The relative impact of obstructive sleep apnea and hypertension on the structural and functional changes of the thoracic aorta. Sleep. 2010;33(9):1173–6.
23. Gardin JM, Arnold AM, Polak J, Jackson S, Smith V, Gottdiener J. Usefulness of aortic root dimension in persons ≥ 65 years of age in predicting heart failure, stroke, cardiovascular mortality, all-cause mortality and acute myocardial infarction. Am J Cardiol. 2006;2:270–5.
24. Guize L, Ducimetiere P, Benetos A, Laurent S, Boutouyrie P, Asmar R, Gautier I, Laloux B. Aortic stiffness is an independent predictor of all-cause and cardiovascular mortality in hypertensive patients. Hypertension. 2001;37:1236–41.
25. Kongola K, Coppack SW, Gosling RG, Lehmann ED, Hopkins KD, Rawesh A, Joseph RC. Relation between number of cardiovascular risk factors/events and noninvasive doppler ultrasound assessments of aortic compliance. Hypertension. 1998;32:565–9.
26. Park JB, Schiffrin EL. Small artery remodeling is the most prevalent (earliest?) form of target organ damage in mild essential hypertension. J Hypertens. 2001;19(5):921–30.
27. Rizzoni D, Palombo C, Porteri E, Muiesan ML, Kozakova M, La Canna G, Nardi M, Guelfi D, Salvetti M, Morizzo C, Vittone F, Rosei EA. Relationships between coronary flow vasodilator capacity and small artery remodelling in hypertensive patients. J Hypertens. 2003;21(3):625–31.
28. Erdogan D, Yildirim I, Ciftci O, Ozer I, Caliskan M, Gullu H, Muderrisoglu H. Effects of normal blood pressure, prehypertension, and hypertension on coronary microvascular function. Circulation. 2007;115(5):593–4. Nitenberg A, Antony I. Epicardial coronary arteries are not adequately sized in hypertensive patients. J Am Coll Cardiol. 1996;27(1):115–23.
29. Kozakova M, Paterni M, Bartolomucci F, Morizzo C, Rossi G, Galetta F, Palombo C. Epicardial coronary artery size in hypertensive and physiologic left ventricular hypertrophy. Am J Hypertens. 2007;20(3):279–84.
30. Struijker Boudier HA, le Noble JL, Messing MW, Huijberts MS, le Noble FA, van Essen H. The microcirculation and hypertension. J Hypertens Suppl. 1992;10(7):S147–56.
31. Levy BI, Ambrosio G, Pries AR, Struijker-Boudier HA. Microcirculation in hypertension: a new target for treatment? Circulation. 2001;104(6):735–40.
32. Schoenhagen P, Ziada KM, Vince DG, Nissen SE, Tuzcu EM. Arterial remodeling and coronary artery disease: the concept of "dilated" versus "obstructive" coronary atherosclerosis. J Am Coll Cardiol. 2001;38(2):297–306. © 2001 by the American College of Cardiology.
33. Davies MJ. Glagovian remodelling, plaque composition, and stenosis generation. Heart. 2000;84:461–2.
34. Achenbach S, Ropers D, Hoffmann U, MacNeill B, Baum U, Pohle K, Brady TJ, Pomerantsev E, Ludwig J, Flachskampf FA, Wicky S, Jang I-k, Daniel WG. Assessment of coronary remodeling in stenotic and nonstenotic coronary atherosclerotic lesions by multidetector spiral computed tomography. J Am Coll Cardiol. 2004;43(5):842–7. © 2004 by the American College of Cardiology Foundation.
35. Little WC, Constantinescu M, Applegate RJ, Kutcher MA, Burrows MT, Kahl FR, Santamore WP. Can coronary angiography predict the site of a subsequent myocardial infarction in patients with mild-to-moderate coronary artery disease? Circulation. 1988;78:1157–66.
36. Mintz GS, Popma JJ, Pichard AD, Kent KM, Satler LF, Chuang YC, DeFalco RA, Leon MB. Limitations of angiography in the assessment of plaque distribution in coronary artery disease. A systematic study of target lesion eccentricity in 1446 lesions. Circulation. 1996;93:924–31.
37. Schwartzkopff B, Motz W, Frenzel H, Vogt M, Knauer S, Strauer BE. Structural and functional alterations of the intramyocardial coronary arterioles in patients with arterial hypertension. Circulation. 1993;88:993–1003.
38. Hodgson JMB, Graham SP, Savakus AD, Dame SG, Stephens DN, Dhillon PS, Brands D, Sheehan H, Eberle MJ. Clinical percutaneous imaging of coronary anatomy using an over-the-wire ultrasound catheter system. Int J Card Imaging. 1989;4(2–4):187–93. Kluwer Academic Publishers. Printed in the Netherlands.
39. Roelandt JRTC, Serruys PW, Bom N, Gussenhoven WG, Lancee CT, ten Hoff H. Intravascular real-time, two-dimensional echocardiography. Int J Card Imaging. 1989;4:63–7. Kluwer Academic Publishers. Primed in the Netherlands.

40. Nitenberg A, Antony I. Epicardial coronary arteries are not adequately sized in hypertensive patients. J Am Coll Cardiol. 1996;27(1):115–23.
41. Kern MJ, Lerman A, Bech JW, De Bruyne B, Eeckhout E, Fearon WF, Higano ST, Lim MJ, Meuwissen M, Piek JJ, Pijls NH, Siebes M, Spaan JA, American Heart Association Committee on Diagnostic and Interventional Cardiac Catheterization, Council on Clinical Cardiology. Physiological assessment of coronary artery disease in the cardiac catheterization laboratory: a scientific statement from the American Heart Association Committee on Diagnostic and Interventional Cardiac Catheterization, Council on Clinical Cardiology. Circulation. 2006;114(12):1321–4.
42. Kiviniemi T. Assessment of coronary blood flow and the reactivity of the microcirculation non-invasively with transthoracic echocardiography. Clin Physiol Funct Imaging. 2008;28:145–55.
43. Brush Jr JE, Cannon 3rd RO, Schenke WH, Bonow RO, Leon MB, Maron BJ, Epstein SE. Angina due to coronary microvascular disease in hypertensive patients without left ventricular hypertrophy. N Engl J Med. 1988;319(20):1302–7.
44. Reis SE, Holubkov R, Lee JS, Sharaf B, Reichek N, Rogers WJ, Walsh EG, Fuisz AR, Kerensky R, Detre KM, Sopko G, Pepine CJ. Coronary flow velocity response to adenosine characterizes coronary microvascular function in women with chest pain and no obstructive coronary disease. Results from the pilot phase of the Women's Ischemia Syndrome Evaluation (WISE) study. J Am Coll Cardiol. 1999;33(6):1469–75.
45. Camici PG. Is the chest pain in cardiac syndrome X due to subendocardial ischaemia? Eur Heart J. 2007;28(13):1539–40.
46. Hamasaki S, Al Suwaidi J, Higano ST, Miyauchi K, Holmes Jr DR, Lerman A. Attenuated coronary flow reserve and vascular remodeling in patients with hypertension and left ventricular hypertrophy. J Am Coll Cardiol. 2000;35(6):1654–60.
47. Kallikazaros I, Tsioufis C, Sideris S, Stefanadis C, Toutouzas P. Carotid artery disease as a marker for the presence of severe coronary artery disease in patients evaluated for chest pain. Stroke. 1999;30(5):1002–7.
48. Chambless LE, Heiss G, Folsom AR, Rosamond W, Szklo M, Sharrett AR, Clegg LX. Association of coronary heart disease incidence with carotid arterial wall thickness and major risk factors: the Atherosclerosis Risk in Communities (ARIC) Study, 1987–1993. Am J Epidemiol. 1997;146(6):483–94.
49. Amato M, Montorsi P, Ravani A, Oldani E, Galli S, Ravagnani PM, Tremoli E, Baldassarre D. Carotid intima-media thickness by B-mode ultrasound as surrogate of coronary atherosclerosis: correlation with quantitative coronary angiography and coronary intravascular ultrasound findings. Eur Heart J. 2007;28(17):2094–101. Epub 2007 Jun 27.
50. Campuzano R, Moya JL, Garcia-Lledo A, Tomas JP, Ruiz S, Megias A, Balaguer J, Asín E. Endothelial dysfunction, intima-media thickness and coronary reserve in relation to risk factors and Framingham score in patients without clinical atherosclerosis. J Hypertens. 2006;24(8):1581–8.
51. Prati F, Regar E, Mintz GS, Arbustini E, Di Mario C, Jang IK, Akasaka T, Costa M, Guagliumi G, Grube E, Ozaki Y, Pinto F, Serruys PW, Expert's OCT Review Document. Expert review document on methodology, terminology, and clinical applications of optical coherence tomography: physical principles, methodology of image acquisition, and clinical application for assessment of coronary arteries and atherosclerosis. Eur Heart J. 2010;31(4):401–15.
52. Kume T, Akasaka T, Kawamoto T, Watanabe N, Toyota E, Neishi Y, Sukmawan R, Sadahira Y, Yoshida K. Assessment of coronary intima–media thickness by optical coherence tomography: comparison with intravascular ultrasound. Circ J. 2005;69(8):903–7.
53. Galderisi M, D'Errico A, Sidiropulos M, Innelli P, de Divitiis O, de Simone G. Nebivolol induces parallel improvement of left ventricular filling pressure and coronary flow reserve in uncomplicated arterial hypertension. J Hypertens. 2009;27(10):2108–15.
54. Tomás JP, Moya JL, Barrios V, Campuzano R, Guzman G, Megías A, Ruiz-Leria S, Catalán P, Marfil T, Tarancón B, Muriel A, García-Lledó A. Effect of candesartan on coronary flow reserve in patients with systemic hypertension. J Hypertens. 2006;24(10):2109–14.

Pulse Wave Velocity and Central Blood Pressure

6

Stéphane Laurent and Pierre Boutouyrie

6.1 Introduction

In hypertension, large arteries stiffen and central blood pressure increases, due to wave reflections. A major reason for measuring pulse wave velocity (PWV) and central blood pressure (cBP) 'routinely' in clinical practice in hypertensive patients comes from the recent demonstration that they have predictive value for cardiovascular events [1, 2]. A large body of evidence has been published during the last decade, concerning the epidemiology, pathophysiology and pharmacology of large arteries in hypertension. In addition, although the gold standard for measuring blood pressure (BP) and diagnosing hypertension is the brachial cuff that favours a distal site accessible to non-invasive measurement, two concepts have gained an important audience these last years: pressure amplification between central and peripheral arteries and higher damaging effect of central BP than brachial BP on target organs in hypertensive patients.

The aims of this chapter are (1) to describe the various non-invasive methods currently available to measure PWV and cBP in clinical practice (2), to detail the normal values in a healthy population and the reference values in a population of hypertensive patients with cardiovascular risk factors (3), to report the amplitude of changes under antihypertensive treatment in clinical trials (4) and to detail the prognostic values of changes. Since PWV and cBP are two parameters strongly linked by their interdependency for the haemodynamic status of hypertensive patients, they will be addressed in parallel.

S. Laurent (✉) • P. Boutouyrie
Department of Pharmacology and INSERM U 970, Hôpital Européen Georges Pompidou, Assistance Publique – Hôpitaux de Paris, Université Paris-Descartes, 20, rue Leblanc, 75015 Paris, France
e-mail: stephane.laurent@egp.aphp.fr; pierre.boutouyrie@egp.aphp.fr

E. Agabiti Rosei, G. Mancia (eds.), *Assessment of Preclinical Organ Damage in Hypertension*, DOI 10.1007/978-3-319-15603-3_6

6.2 How to Assess Arterial Stiffness and Central Blood Pressure

6.2.1 How to Assess Arterial Stiffness

Arterial stiffness can be evaluated at the systemic, regional and local levels. In contrast to systemic arterial stiffness, which can only be estimated from models of the circulation, regional and local arterial stiffness can be measured directly, and non-invasively, at various sites along the arterial tree. A major advantage of the regional and local evaluations of arterial stiffness is that they are based on direct measurements of parameters strongly linked to wall stiffness. Reviews have been published on methodological aspects [3, 4]. Table 6.1 gives the main features of the various methods currently available.

Table 6.1 Device and methods used for determining regional, local and systemic arterial stiffness and wave reflections

Year of first publication	Device	Methods	Measurement site
Regional stiffness			
1984[a]	Complior®	Mechanotransducer	Aorta, cf PWV[b]
1990[a]	Sphygmocor®	Tonometer	Aorta, cf PWV[b]
1991	WallTrack®	Echo-tracking	Aorta, cf PWV[b]
1994	QKD	ECG+	Aorta, cf PWV[b]
1997[a]	Cardiovascular Eng. Inc®	Tonometer	Aorta, cf PWV[b]
2002	Artlab®	Echo-tracking	Aorta, cf PWV[b]
2002	Ultrasound systems	Doppler probes	Aorta, cf PWV[b]
2002	Omron VP-1000®	Pressure cuffs	Aorta, ba PWV[b]
2007	CAVI-Vasera®	ECG + pressure cuffs	Aorta, ca PWV[b]
2008	Arteriograph®	Arm pressure cuff	Aorta, aa PWV[b]
2009	MRI, ArtFun®	MRI	Aorta, aa PWV[b]
2009	Vicorder®	Cuffs	Aorta, cf PWV[b]
2010	Mobil-O-Graph®	Arm pressure cuff	Aorta, cf PWV[b]
Local stiffness			
1991	WallTrack®	Echo-tracking	CCA[c], CFA, BA
1992	NIUS®	Echo-tracking	RA
2002	Artlab®	Echo-tracking	CCA[c], CFA, BA
	Various ultrasound system	Echography	CCA[c], CFA, BA
2009	MRI, ArtFun®	Cine-MRI	AA, DA
Systemic stiffness			
1989	Area method	Diastolic decay	
1995	HDI PW CR-2000®	Modif. Windkessel	
1997[a]	Cardiovascular Eng. Inc®	Tonometer/Doppler/echo	

Adapted from [3], with permission

[a]Apparatus used in pioneering epidemiological studies showing the predictive value of aortic stiffness for CV events; *PWV* pulse wave velocity

[b]*cf* carotid-femoral, *ba* brachial-ankle, *ca* cardiac-ankle, *aa* aortic arch, *ft* finger-toe

[c]All superficial arteries, including particularly those mentioned; *Ao* aorta, *CCA* common carotid artery, *CFA* common femoral artery, *BA* brachial artery, *RA* radial artery, *AA* ascending aorta, *DA* descending aorta

6.2.1.1 Regional Measurements of Arterial Stiffness

The measurement of pulse wave velocity (PWV) is generally accepted as the most simple, non-invasive, robust and reproducible method with which to determine arterial stiffness [3]. It is recommended by the 2013 ESH-ESC Guidelines for the Management of Hypertension [4]. Carotid-femoral PWV is a direct measurement, and it corresponds to the widely accepted propagative model of the arterial system. Measured along the aortic and aortoiliac pathway, it is the most clinically relevant, since the aorta and its first branches are what the left ventricle 'sees' and are thus responsible for most of the pathophysiological effects of arterial stiffness. Carotid-femoral PWV has been used in epidemiological studies demonstrating the predictive value of aortic stiffness for CV events [1, 2].

PWV is usually measured using the foot-to-foot velocity method from various waveforms. These are usually obtained transcutaneously at the right common carotid artery and the right femoral artery (i.e. 'carotid-femoral' PWV), and the time delay (Δt, or transit time) is measured between the feet of the two waveforms. The 'foot' of the wave is defined at the end of diastole, when the steep rise of the wavefront begins. The transit time is the time of travel of the 'foot' of the wave over a known distance. A variety of different waveforms can be used including pressure, distension and Doppler [3, 5]. The distance (D) covered by the waves is usually assimilated to the surface distance between the two recording sites, i.e. the common carotid artery (CCA) and the common femoral artery (CFA). The direct distance DD is (CFA to CCA). PWV is calculated as PWV = D (metres)/Δt (seconds). However, since the descending thoracic aorta is reached by the pressure wave at the time another pressure wave, originating from the same cardiac contraction, arrives at the carotid site, it has been recommended to calculate the distance between the suprasternal notch (SSN) and the common femoral artery (CFA) and to subtract from this distance the small length between carotid transducer and SSN. The so-called subtracted distance is (SSN to CFA) – (SSN to CCA). A recent consensus paper [6] stated that investigator should either use the subtracted distance or, best, measure the direct distance and apply a 0.8 coefficient, to take into account the different pathways of the pressure wave described above.

6.2.1.2 Local Determination of Arterial Stiffness

Local arterial stiffness of superficial arteries can be determined using ultrasound devices. Carotid stiffness may be of particular interest, since in that artery, atherosclerosis is frequent. All types of classical, bi-dimensional vascular ultrasound systems can be used in determining diameter at diastole and stroke changes in diameter, but most of them are limited in the precision of measurements because they generally use a video-image analysis. Echo-tracking devices were developed to measure diameter in end-diastole and stroke change in diameter with a very high precision. The two first devices were the Wall Track System® and the NIUS 02® (Table 6.1). These apparatus use the radio-frequency (RF) signal to obtain a precision six to ten times higher than with video-image systems, which are limited by the spatial resolution of pixel analysis.

At present, some researchers also measure local arterial stiffness of deep arteries like the aorta using cine magnetic resonance imaging (MRI). However, most of pathophysiological and pharmacological studies have used echo-tracking techniques. Most of these parameters required measurement of blood pressure. This should be local pressure, which is usually obtained by applanation tonometry of the vessel in question and calibration of the waveform to brachial mean and diastolic pressures obtained by integration of the brachial or radial waveform or automatic calculation using transfer function processing. All the superficial arteries are suitable for the geometrical investigation and particularly the common carotid, common femoral and brachial arteries.

6.2.1.3 Systemic Arterial Stiffness

Methods used for the non-invasive determination of systemic arterial stiffness are based on analogies with electrical models combining capacitance and resistance in series (Table 6.1). As such they rely on numerous theoretical approximations following direct measurement of one peripheral, and often distal, parameter. Their theoretical, technical and practical limitations that impact on their widespread application in the clinical setting have been discussed and compared with methods used for the non-invasive determination of regional stiffness [3]. Until now, they did not provide evidence, in a longitudinal study, that systemic arterial stiffness or systemic arterial compliance has independent predictive value for CV events.

6.2.2 How to Assess Central Blood Pressure

A large number of reviews have made recommendations for adequate measurements of central BP [3, 7–9]. Arterial pressure waveform should be analysed at the central level, i.e. the ascending aorta, since it represents the true load imposed to the heart, the brain and the kidney and more generally to central large artery walls. Table 6.2 details the various methods currently used for determining central BP [8]. The pressure waveform can be recorded non-invasively with a pencil-type probe incorporating a high-fidelity Millar strain gauge transducer (SPT-301, Millar Instruments). The most widely used approach is to perform radial artery tonometry and then apply a transfer function (Sphygmocor, AtCor, Sydney Australia) to calculate the aortic pressure waveform from the radial waveform (Table 6.2). Indeed, the radial artery is well supported by bony tissue, making optimal applanation easier to achieve. The algorithm used to apply the transfer function revealed to be robust for accurately determining central BP even during haemodynamic perturbations, including exercise, Valsalva manoeuvre, nitroglycerin, beta-adrenergic stimulation, angiotensin II and noradrenaline [9]. However, this procedure may underestimate central systolic BP at higher heart rates (e.g. above 100 bpm), and major error can be created by using inaccurate upper arm cuff BP values to calibrate the pressure waveforms. Careful attention to correctly measuring brachial cuff BP can help alleviate, but not entirely deal with this problem, particularly as there may be additional systolic BP amplification from the brachial to radial arterial beds [8, 9]. Despite these limitations, radial tonometry is popular since it is simple to perform and well tolerated.

Table 6.2 Device and methods used for determining central blood pressure and wave reflections

Year of first publication	Device	Method	Parameter	Measurement site
Central pressure waveform				
1984	Millar strain gauge®[a]	Tonometer, direct	cSBP, cPP, cAIx	Radial, carotid
1990	Sphygmocor®[a]	Tonometer, transfer function	cSBP, cPP, cAIx	Radial, carotid
1997	Cardiovascular Eng. Inc®[a]	Tonometer, cardiac echo, impedance	cSBP, cPP, cAIx, Zc, fW, bW	Radial, carotid
2004	Pulse Pen®	Tonometer, direct	cSBP, cPP, cAIx	Carotid
Central SBP				
2008	Arteriograph®	Oscillometric	cSBP, cPP, cAIx	Brachial
2009	Omron HEM-9001A I®	Tonometer	cSBP, rAIx	Radial
2010	Mobil-O-Graph®	Oscillometric	cSBP, cPP, cAIx	Brachial

Adapted from [8], with permission
[a]Apparatus used in pioneering epidemiological studies showing the predictive value of central BP for CV events; *cSBP* central systolic blood pressure, *cPP* central pulse pressure, *cAIx* central augmentation index, *rAIx* radial artery augmentation index, *Zc* characteristic impedance, *fW* forward pressure wave, *bW* backward pressure wave

A part from methods determining the pressure waveform at the central site, novel methods have been developed, which aim at determining the discrete value of central SBP instead of the whole pressure waveform at central site [3, 8] (Table 6.2). Estimation of central BP without a transfer function is possible from the second systolic peak (SBP2) on the radial or brachial pressure waveform. The radial method relies on accurate calibration using brachial cuff BP.

6.3 Prevalence

A prerequisite to a wide implementation of pulse wave velocity and central blood pressure measurements into clinical practice is the availability of normal and reference values based on a large population, established through standardisation of methodology for measurement.

6.3.1 Normal and Reference Values of Pulse Wave Velocity

These values have been established by *The Reference Values for Arterial Measurements Collaboration* in 16,867 subjects and patients originating from 13 different centres across eight European countries [10]. Of these, 11,092 individuals

Table 6.3 Distribution of pulse wave velocity (m/s) according to the age category in the normal values population (1,455 subjects)

Age category (years)	Mean (±2 SD)	Median (10–90 pc)
<30	6.2 (4.7–7.6)	6.1 (5.3–7.1)
30–39	6.5 (3.8–9.2)	6.4 (5.2–8.0)
40–49	7.2 (4.6–9.8)	6.9 (5.9–8.6)
50–59	8.3 (4.5–12.1)	8.1 (6.3–10.0)
60–69	10.3 (5.5–15.0)	9.7 (7.9–13.1)
≥70	10.9 (5.5–16.3)	10.6 (8.0–14.6)

Adapted from [10], with permission
SD standard deviation, *10 pc* the upper limit of the 10th percentile, *90 pc* the lower limit of the 90th percentile

Table 6.4 Distribution of pulse wave velocity (PWV) values (m/s) in the reference value population (11,092 subjects) according to age and blood pressure category

Age category	Blood pressure category				
PWC as median (10–90 pc)	Optimal	Normal	High normal	Grade I HT	Grade II/III HT
<30	6.0 (5.2–7.0)	6.4 (5.7–7.5)	6.7 (5.8–7.9)	7.2 (5.7–9.3)	7.6 (5.9–9.9)
30–39	6.5 (5.4–7.9)	6.7 (5.3–8.2)	7.0 (5.5–8.8)	7.2 (5.5–9.3)	7.6 (5.8–11.2)
40–49	6.8 (5.8–8.5)	7.4 (6.2–9.0)	7.7 (6.5–9.5)	8.1 (6.8–10.8)	9.2 (7.1–13.2)
50–59	7.5 (6.2–9.2)	8.1 (6.7–10.4)	8.4 (7.0–11.3)	9.2 (7.2–12.5)	9.7 (7.4–14.9)
60–69	8.7 (7.0–11.4)	9.3 (7.6–12.2)	9.8 (7.9–13.2)	10.7 (8.4–14.1)	12.0 (8.5–16.5)
≥70	10.1 (7.6–13.8)	11.1 (8.6–15.5)	11.2 (8.6–15.8)	12.7 (9.3–16.7)	13.5 (10.3–18.2)

Adapted from reference [10] with permission
SD standard deviation, *10 pc* the upper limit of the 10th percentile, *90 pc* the lower limit of the 90th percentile, *HT* hypertension

were free from overt CV disease, nondiabetic, and untreated by either antihypertensive or lipid-lowering drugs and constituted the reference value population, of which the subset with optimal/normal blood pressures ($n = 1,455$) is the normal value population. Subjects were categorised by age decade and further subdivided according to BP categories. Pulse wave velocity increases with age and BP category, the increase with age being more pronounced for higher BP categories and the increase with BP being more important for older subjects (Tables 6.3 and 6.4).

6.3.2 Normal and Reference Values of Central Blood Pressure

These data have been established by *The Reference Values for Arterial Measurements Collaboration* in 45,436 subjects out of 82,930 that were gathered from 77 studies of 53 centres [11]. Of these, 27,253 individuals were free from overt CV disease, nondiabetic, and untreated by either antihypertensive or lipid-lowering drugs and constituted the reference value population, and another subset with optimal/normal

Table 6.5 Central systolic blood pressure values according to age categories, for males and females, in the normal and reference populations

	Normal population		Reference population	
Age category	Female	Male	Female	Male
<20 (n=1,104)	97 (86, 91, 102, 109)	105 (95, 99, 109, 113)	99 (88, 93, 105, 120)	109 (96, 102, 117, 127)
	n=350	n=290	n=182	n=282
20–29 (n=4,157)	95 (80, 88, 102, 110)	103 (92, 97, 109, 115)	101 (88. 94, 110, 124)	110 (95, 102, 120, 130)
	n=1,411	n=880	n=888	n=974
30–39 (n=6,386)	98 (84, 90, 108, 119)	103 (88, 95, 112, 120)	111 (92, 100, 127, 141)	114 (95, 103, 129, 144)
	n=1,860	n=1,259	n=1,373	n=1,889
40–49 (n=9,595)	102 (87, 93, 113, 123)	106 (90, 97, 114, 123)	116 (95, 104, 133, 146)	118 (97, 106, 132, 144)
	n=2,318	n=2,068	n=2,196	n=2,995
50–59 (n=11,950)	110 (93, 100, 119, 127)	110 (96, 102, 118, 126)	120 (100, 109, 134, 148)	123 (102, 111, 137, 150)
	n=2,002	n=1,997	n=4,251	n=3,646
60–69 (n=7,779)	114 (97, 105, 122, 129)	114 (97, 105, 122, 128)	128 (105, 115, 141, 154)	128 (105, 115, 142, 155)
	n=1,057	n=1,410	n=2,656	n=2,629
70+ (n=4,445)	118 (100, 109, 126, 131)	116 (99, 107, 124, 130)	138 (113, 126, 152, 164)	135 (113, 124, 147, 160)
	n=530	n=747	n=1,567	n=1,592

Adapted from [11], with permission
Values given here are referred, respectively, to the 50th (10th, 25th, 75th and 90th) percentiles

blood pressures (n=18,133) was the normal value population. Values of cSBP were stratified by brachial blood pressure categories and age decade in turn, both being stratified by sex. Central SBP increases with ageing in healthy subjects. The age-induced increase in PWV cSBP is exaggerated in patients with cardiovascular risk factors (Table 6.5).

6.4 Changes with Treatment

6.4.1 Changes in Pulse Wave Velocity with Antihypertensive Drugs

Numerous studies have been published on the effect of antihypertensive drugs on arterial stiffness and are summarised in Table 6.6. Recent reviews [3, 12] underlined important differences between the effects of various classes of antihypertensive drugs. The general view is that drugs antagonising the renin-angiotensin system (RAS) [i.e. angiotensin-converting enzyme inhibitors (ACEIs) and angiotensin

Table 6.6 Comparison of the effect on pulse wave velocity (PWV) and wave reflection by various antihypertensive drug classes

ACE inhibitors	PWV	Wave reflection	Angiotensin receptor blockers	PWV	Wave reflection
Captopril	↓	↓	Losartan	↓	↓
Ramipril	↓	↓	Telmisartan	↓	↓
Trandolapril	↓	↓/↔	Valsartan	↓	↓
Quinapril	↓	↓	Candesartan	↓	↓
Lisinopril	↔	↔	Olmesartan	↓	
Perindopril	↓	↓			
Enalapril	↓	↓	*Calcium channel blockers*		
Aldosterone antagonists			Amlodipine	↔	↓
Canrenoate	↔		Nitrendipine	↓	↓
Spironolactone	↔/↓	↓	Nifedipine		↓
Eplerenone	↓		Felodipine	↓	↓
			Lacidipine	↔/↓	↓
α-Blockers			Verapamil	↓	
Doxazosin	↔/↓	↓			
			β-Blockers		
Diuretics			Atenolol	↓	↔↓/↑
Hydrochlorothiazide	↔	↔	Metoprolol	↔	
Indapamide	↔	↔	Propranolol	↓	↑
Bendroflumethiazide	↔	↔	Bisoprolol	↓	↑
Nitrates			Dilevalol	↓	↓
Nitroglycerin	↔	↓	Nebivolol	↓	↔/↓
Isosorbide mononitrate	↔	↓			

Reproduced from [12], with permission

receptor blockers (ARBs)] are superior in reducing arterial stiffness than other classes including calcium channel blockers (CCBs), diuretics and beta-blockers. This may be because the RAS system is a potent pro-fibrotic system. While most CCBs lower PWV and reduce wave reflection, their effect is far less than that of drugs blocking the RAS. Diuretics have been shown in most studies to have no beneficial effect on arterial stiffness or wave reflection. The special case of β-blockers is examined below.

6.4.2 Drugs and BP-Independent Destiffening of Large Artery

An increasing body of evidence suggests that only part of aortic stiffness could be reduced through the normalisation of BP by pharmacological treatment, and further reduction of aortic stiffness would require long-term arterial remodelling, including reduction in collagen density and rearrangement of the wall materials.

The demonstration has been given by a recent meta-analysis of double-blind randomised controlled trials [13], a long-term observational studies in humans [14] and two pharmacological mechanistic studies [15, 16] which are detailed here. These studies demonstrate that BP-independent large artery destiffening could be obtained with most antihypertensive drugs, particularly with RAS blockers, and that these BP-independent changes are amplified with a higher dose and long-term treatment.

6.4.3 Change in Central Blood Pressure with Antihypertensive Drugs

Whether pharmacological classes, and specific molecules within a given pharmacological class, differ in their ability to lower central BP has been addressed in several studies [7–9, 12]. Protogerou et al. [17] analysed the ability of drug treatment to lower central BP beyond the reduction in peripheral (brachial) BP, by computing the effects of drugs on BP amplification, according to either its absolute (peripheral PP *minus* central PP, in mmHg) or relative (peripheral PP/central PP) expression. There are several mechanisms by which drugs may differently alter central and peripheral BP, thus BP amplification. They include large artery stiffness, vascular resistance, stroke volume and heart rate.

The pharmacological classes which reduce wave reflection, thus central BP, and increase amplification are ACEIs, ARBs and CCBs, whereas diuretics are less efficacious (Table 6.6). Non-vasodilating beta-blockers (such as propranolol and atenolol) are the least effective agents for reducing wave reflection and central BP. Nitrates, which are not indicated for hypertension, reduce wave reflection, thus central BP and increase SBP amplification (Table 6.6).

6.5 Prognostic Value of Change

6.5.1 Prognostic Value of the Changes in Pulse Wave Velocity

An important issue is whether the reduction in arterial stiffness translates into a reduction in CV events. There is only very little indirect evidence. To our knowledge, only one study reported CV outcomes in patients having repeated measurements of PWV along several years [18]: 150 patients (aged 52 ± 16 years) with end-stage renal disease (ESRD) were monitored for 51 ± 38 months for blood pressure and PWV. Fifty-nine deaths occurred, including 40 cardiovascular and 19 non-cardiovascular events. Cox analyses demonstrated that the lack of PWV decrease in response to BP reduction was a strong independent predictor of all-cause (RR 2.59 [1.51–4.43]) and cardiovascular mortality (RR 2.35[1.23–4.41]). However, this study suffers several limitations: this was not a randomised clinical trial but rather a post hoc retrospective analysis; baseline PWV was different in the two groups, and there is no mention that statistical analysis was adjusted to it; finally this study included patients at very high risk, and results cannot be extrapolated to other (milder) clinical situations, as discussed thereafter.

Thus, it remains to be shown in a population of hypertensive patients at lower CV risk that a therapeutic strategy aiming at normalising arterial stiffness proves to be more effective in preventing CV events than usual care. Such a study requires a large number of patients, benefiting from a long-term follow-up. It has been started in France [19].

6.5.2 Prognostic Value of the Changes in Central Blood Pressure

Such randomised studies with the aim of targeting central BP reduction are needed because a consistent limitation of all the above-mentioned central BP prognostic studies is that they are observational and causality between elevated central BP and CV risk cannot be inferred. The only randomised intervention trial with recording of central BP and CV events was the Conduit Artery Function Evaluation (CAFE) study, an ancillary study of the ASCOT study in 2,199 patients with hypertension and multiple CV risk factors [3, 8]. The CAFE study showed that a therapeutic regimen based on amlodipine was more effective than an atenolol-based regimen to lower central BP, despite similar brachial SBP between treatment groups. Because the ASCOT study showed that the amlodipine-based regimen prevented more major CV events than the atenolol-based regimen, it was tempting to attribute, at least in part, this superiority to a higher efficacy on the reduction in central BP. However, such a conclusion cannot be drawn since central BP was not measured at baseline in the CAFE study; thus, no change in central BP could be calculated [3, 8].

In a prospective, open-label, blinded-endpoint study in hypertensive patients randomised to treatment decisions guided by best-practice usual care or, in addition, by central BP intervention, Sharman et al. [20] showed that central BP intervention leads to less use of medication to achieve BP control. Such a clinical trial should also take into account the cardiovascular complications.

Conclusion

In conclusion, the measurement of pulse wave velocity and central systolic pressure, which is recommended by the current guidelines for the management of hypertension, benefits from well-established methodologies, using validated apparatus. Measured values can be compared with normal and reference values obtained in very large cohorts. Further studies should determine whether pulse wave velocity and central systolic pressure are true surrogate endpoints.

References

1. Ben-Shlomo Y, Spears M, Boustred C, et al. Aortic pulse wave velocity improves cardiovascular event prediction: an individual participant meta-analysis of prospective observational data from 17,635 subjects. J Am Coll Cardiol. 2014;63:636–46.
2. Vlachopoulos C, Aznaouridis K, O'Rourke MF, Safar ME, Baou K, Stefanadis C. Prediction of cardiovascular events and all-cause mortality with central haemodynamics: a systematic review and meta-analysis. Eur Heart J. 2010;31:1865–71.

3. Laurent S, Cockcroft J, Van Bortel L, Boutouyrie P, Giannattasio C, Hayoz D, Pannier B, Vlachopoulos C, Wilkinson I, Struijker-Boudier H. Expert consensus document on arterial stiffness: methodological aspects and clinical applications. Eur Heart J. 2006;27:2588–605.
4. Mancia G, Fagard R, Narkiewicz K, Redón J, Zanchetti A, Böhm M, Christiaens T, Cifkova R, DeBacker G, Dominiczak A, Galderisi M, Grobbee DE, Jaarsma T, Kirchhof P, Kjeldsen SE, Laurent S, Manolis AJ, Nilsson PM, Ruilope LM, Schmieder RE, Sirnes PA, Sleight P, Viigimaa M, Waeber B, Zannad F. 2013 ESH/ESC guidelines for the management of arterial hypertension: the task force for the management of arterial hypertension of the European Society of Hypertension (ESH) and of the European Society of Cardiology (ESC). Eur Heart J. 2013;34:2159–219.
5. Laurent S, Mousseaux E, Boutouyrie P. Arterial stiffness as an imaging biomarker: are all pathways equal? Hypertension. 2013;62:10–2.
6. Van Bortel LM, Laurent S, Boutouyrie P, et al.; on behalf of the Artery Society, the European Society of Hypertension Working Group on Vascular Structure and Function and the European Network for Noninvasive Investigation of Large Arteries. Expert consensus document on the measurement of aortic stiffness in daily practice using carotid-femoral pulse wave velocity. J Hypertens. 2012;30:445–8.
7. McEniery C, Cockroft J, Roman M, Franklin S, Wilkinson I. Central blood pressure: current evidence and clinical importance. Eur Heart J. 2014;35:1719–925.
8. Giannatasio C, Laurent S. Central blood pressure. In: Mancia G, Grassi G, Redon J, editors. Textbook of hypertension. Informa Healthcare; 2014 London, UK.
9. Sharman JE, Laurent S. Value of central blood pressure in the management of hypertension. J Hum Hypertens. 2013;27:405–11.
10. Reference Values for Arterial Stiffness' Collaboration. Determinants of pulse wave velocity in healthy people and in the presence of cardiovascular risk factors: 'establishing normal and reference values'. Eur Heart J. 2010;31:2338–50.
11. Herbert A, Cruickshank K, Laurent S, Boutouyrie P, on behalf of The Reference Values for Arterial Measurements Collaboration. Establishing reference values for central blood pressure and its amplification in a general healthy population and according to cardiovascular risk-factors. Eur Heart J. 2014;35(44):3122–33.
12. Boutouyrie P, Lacolley P, Briet M, Reignault V, Stanton A, Laurent S, Mahmud A. Pharmacological modulation of arterial stiffness. Drugs. 2011;71:1689–701.
13. Ong KT, Delerme S, Pannier B, Safar M, Benetos A, Laurent S, Boutouyrie P. Aortic stiffness is reduced beyond blood pressure lowering by short- and long-term antihypertensive treatment: a meta-analysis of individual data in 294 patients. J Hypertens. 2011;29:1034–42.
14. Ait-Oufella H, Collin C, Bozec E, Ong KT, Laloux B, Boutouyrie P, Laurent S. Long-term reduction in aortic stiffness: a 5.3-year follow-up in routine clinical practice. J Hypertens. 2010;28:2336–41.
15. Tropeano AI, Boutouyrie P, Pannier B, Joannides R, Balkestein E, Katsahian S, Laloux B, Thuillez C, Struijker-Boudier H, Laurent S. Brachial pressure-independent reduction in carotid stiffness after long-term angiotensin-converting enzyme inhibition in diabetic hypertensives. Hypertension. 2006;48:80–6.
16. Laurent S, Boutouyrie P. Dose-dependent arterial destiffening and inward remodeling after olmesartan in hypertensives with metabolic syndrome. Hypertension. 2014;64(4):709–16. pii: HYPERTENSIONAHA.114.03282.
17. Protogerou AD, Stergiou GS, Vlachopoulos C, et al. The effect of antihypertensive drugs on central blood pressure beyond peripheral blood pressure. Part II: evidence for specific class-effects of antihypertensive drugs on pressure amplification. Curr Pharm Des. 2009;15:272–89.
18. Guerin AP, Blacher J, Pannier B, Marchais SJ, Safar ME, London GM. Impact of aortic stiffness attenuation on survival of patients in end-stage renal failure. Circulation. 2001;20(103):987–92.
19. Laurent S, Briet M, Boutouyrie P. Arterial stiffness and central pulse pressure as surrogate markers: needed clinical trials. Hypertension. 2012;60:518–22.
20. Sharman JE, Marwick TH, Gilroy D, Otahal P, Abhayaratna WP, Stowasser M, Value of Central Blood Pressure for GUIDing ManagEment of Hypertension Study Investigators. Randomized trial of guiding hypertension management using central aortic blood pressure compared with best-practice care: principal findings of the BP GUIDE study. Hypertension. 2013;62:1138–45.

7 Ankle-Brachial Index (ABI)

Denis L. Clement

7.1 Introduction

Peripheral artery disease (PAD) has remained for a long time the most neglected part in the domain of cardiovascular diseases. The fact that the disease can remain completely asymptomatic for many years in a large number of patients plays an important role in this respect. However, even when intermittent claudication of the lower limbs which is the most common clinical manifestation of peripheral artery disease is present, it is often considered by physicians as a minor problem. This is surprising as in many patients, intermittent claudication profoundly affects the quality of their life. As a result of all of this, no efforts are made to clarify the diagnosis, to look for confounding clinical states, and to elucidate the causes of the problem. Therefore, quite often, PAD is only detected when complications arise or when, sometimes by chance, a good clinical examination is performed implemented by noninvasive tests such as measurement of the ankle-brachial pressure index (ABI).

7.2 How to Assess Ankle Blood Pressure and Calculating the Ankle-Brachial Index?

Diagnosis of PAD can be made quite easily at the consultation by palpation and auscultation of the arteries in the limbs. However, this needs time and expertise. Measuring the ankle-brachial index (ABI) is an easy and cheap alternative, totally noninvasive, that can elegantly be performed during the consultation. It is expressed as the systolic blood pressure measured at the ankle divided by systolic pressure at the arm. Although recently automated systems have been developed to get

D.L. Clement, MD, PhD
Department of the Dean, Ghent University Hospital,
185 De Pintelaan, B-9000 Ghent, Belgium
e-mail: denis.clement@UGent.be

E. Agabiti Rosei, G. Mancia (eds.), *Assessment of Preclinical Organ Damage in Hypertension*, DOI 10.1007/978-3-319-15603-3_7

Table 7.1 ABI and severity of arterial stenosis

Mild stenosis: 0.9–0.7
Moderate stenosis: 0.6–0.5
Severe stenosis: lower than 0.5

information from upper and lower extremities simultaneously, in general, a portable Doppler device is sufficient to perform these measurements.

The technique has excellent records [1–3]: the actual sensitivity and specificity have been estimated, respectively, at 79 and 96 %. For diagnosis in primary care, an ABI <0.8 or the mean of three ABIs <0.90 had a positive predictive value of ≥95 %; an ABI = 1.10 or the mean of three ABIs >1.00 had a negative predictive value of ≥99 %. Sensitivity can further be improved by making measurements after a short exercise such as a brief walk on treadmill. The most confounding condition is that of severe hardening of the arterial wall such as seen in diabetic patients or in the elderly. If that occurs, ABI should be replaced by more complex techniques such as pressure measurement or oscillation recordings at the toe.

Information obtained by ABI recordings is not like an all or none; increasing severity of the vascular obstruction is accompanied by progressive decrease of the index (Table 7.1). In case of the presence of an arterial ulcer, the chances for healing, spontaneous or by medical means, can be estimated by measuring the systolic pressure at the ankle; below 50 mmHg, there rarely is spontaneous healing, also with careful medical therapy; in diabetic patients, even higher figures (like 80 mmHg) are needed to allow for a successful healing of the ulcers.

Measuring an ABI has also been used in large-scale studies to detect PAD in the population or at the consultation of the general practitioner. In the PARTNERS study [4], the diagnosis of PAD was missed in 86 % of the cases, as long as only clinical history and symptoms were used; ABI was an excellent tool to improve on the detection of PAD in this very large group of patients; however, in many cases, physicians were totally unaware of the presence of PAD.

7.3 Epidemiology

According to the Rose questionnaire, the prevalence of PAD in males is approximately 1.5 % in men under the age of 50 and reaches 4–5 % in the age group of 50 and older. In females under the age of 50, the prevalence is lower than in men, but contrary to common belief, it is as high and even higher as in males over the age of 60 [5]. Moreover, in women, the clinical picture of PAD is more peculiar and in particular, the symptoms are more severe, more often leading to more profound ischemia and ulceration.

Hypertension is a risk factor for vascular disorders such as PAD; follow-up data from the Framingham study [6] demonstrated an almost doubling of intermittent claudication in hypertensive men and women; in elderly patients, similar data have been shown. Of hypertensives at presentation, about 2–5 % have intermittent claudication, with increasing prevalence with age [7–9]. Conversely, 35–55 % of patients with PAD at presentation also show hypertension, and this is particularly thru in elderly patients. Thus, in patients with PAD there is a higher prevalence of hypertension [10]; among several possible mechanisms, the presence of associated renal artery disease in many patients plays an important role.

When making up these figures, it is important to remember that the prevalence of asymptomatic PAD is clearly higher than that of symptomatic PAD [7–9]. Remarkably, as said above, at least half to two-thirds of individuals with PAD are asymptomatic or have atypical limb exertional symptoms, especially in female patients; this will in any way further increase the figures on prevalence published so far.

7.4 Changes of Ankle Pressure and of ABI with Treatment

Ankle-brachial pressure *expressed as an index* will not significantly change with the treatment of arterial hypertension [7].

However, ankle pressure by itself is depending on the central blood pressure and its changes besides the local hemodynamic conditions; as said above, it can change in function of time with age, diabetes, etc. [9]. In all of these, the increase in stiffness of the arteries will increase the measured value of ankle pressure, while in reality, local perfusion is not significantly altered; the higher value of ankle pressure in such case is due to the lower compressibility of the arteries resulting in a false higher number; this phenomenon, also seen at the brachial arteries but to a lesser degree, can lead to very high figures of ankle pressure and consequently of ABI what is most often encountered in diabetic patients. Real values can be obtained in such cases by measurements at the toe by oscillography or pulse/volume recordings. Because ABI in these conditions can become surprisingly high, the problem, in most cases, is easily detected.

Much more misleading is when there is hardening of the arteries in patients with a minor degree of obstruction in the arteries; this can increase the calculated index, for example, from 0.8 to 1.1, and lead to a false "normal" value and in fact causing under diagnosis or underestimation of an existing arterial stenosis. It is not well known how frequently such a phenomenon misleads the physician in regular practice. Most likely, it only plays a role in borderline cases. Other information, for example, coming from palpation of the arteries, should help to correct such a "false normal" reading.

Another problem to be mentioned here is the situation of a severe stenosis in the arterial tree of the lower limbs, in a patient with systemic hypertension; treatment of the high blood pressure can in such condition bring the ankle perfusion pressure to lower than 50 mmHg, what can lead to critical ischemia. This phenomenon needs to be known by the physician and is by itself a good reason to measure ankle blood pressure in every hypertensive patient, especially in elderly people and diabetic patients.

Finally, a significant improvement and even normalization of a low ABI due to arterial stenosis is only realized by interventional treatment of the existing stenosis by balloon dilatation (PTA) or by surgery. Therefore, measurement of ABI immediately after such interventions is an excellent tool to estimate the success of it and also is most helpful in the further follow-up.

7.5 Prognostic Value of ABI

Although, as said above, the prognostic value of the change in ABI is largely linked to the local changes in the arterial circulation, several well-documented studies have illustrated the long-term prognostic value of ABI as a single reading. There is a surprising, well-fitting, and graded inverse correlation between the decrease in ABI and the risk to develop a cardiovascular event (Fig. 7.1) [7–11]. Such correlation holds true even after adjustment for the regular cardiovascular risk factors [11]. Statisticians have sometimes criticized the robustness of this correlation; still, recently, its value was again clearly confirmed in a recent study on a large, well-controlled group of patients, followed over a long period of time [3].

Moreover, it was also shown that not only a low but also an elevated ABI (more than 1.3) could predict a worsened prognosis [12]. The relationship between ABI and cardiovascular events therefore is not rectilinear but rather U-shaped (see Fig. 7.1).

Such information is extremely useful in general but more especially during the outpatient consultation at the cardiologist's office [11]. It is fitting very well with the present views as the actual approach and management of cardiovascular patients largely is guided by the patient's total cardiovascular risk [2]. PAD is carrying a surprisingly elevated risk; at middle age, yearly mortality is around 5 % [10]. Such impressive figure is further increased by the presence of other risk factors such as hypertension and lipid disorders and by associated clinical conditions such as

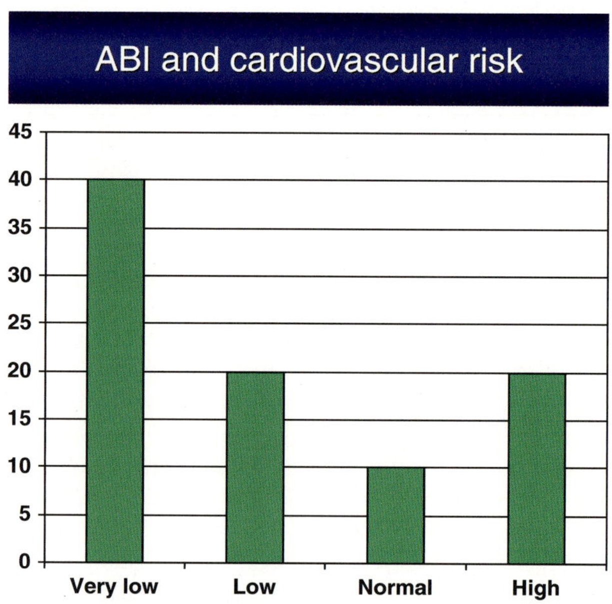

Fig. 7.1 Inverse relationship of ABI and 5-year risk of developing cardiovascular events and death. Schematic representation of information and data given in references [5–7, 10]. Cardiovascular risk increases when ABI moves from normal values to low and very low values. Notice that risk also increases when ABI value is above normal (above 1.3)

coronary artery disease; this holds true whatever the presentation as stable angina pectoris or previous myocardial infarction. Finally, physicians should bear in mind that PAD patients with no or atypical symptoms also carry this elevated risk; this also explains why the risk of PAD often is strongly underestimated.

Conclusions

The prevalence of peripheral artery disease (PAD) is increased by hypertension. Measurement of ankle pressure and calculating ankle-brachial blood pressure index (ABI) is an excellent tool to diagnose the presence of peripheral arterial disease and its severity. It also is very useful in the follow-up after vascular intervention like angioplasty with or without stent placement or vascular surgery. However, it also provides the physician with an easy estimation of the existing cardiovascular risk in a PAD patient. This totally noninvasive and cheap technique has shown not only the large prevalence of PAD in the western population but also, at the same time, the low detection rate of PAD and low awareness of the medical community. Experts in hypertension and in vascular medicine should join efforts to increase awareness toward this important clinical problem. Measurement of ankle-brachial index is an excellent tool to help reaching this goal.

References

1. McDermott MM, Greenland P, Liu K, Guralnik JM, Criqui MH, Dolan NC, Chan C, Celic L, Pearce WH, Schneider JR, Sharma L, Clark E, Gibson D, Martin GJ. Leg symptoms in peripheral arterial disease: associated clinical characteristics and functional impairment. JAMA. 2001;286:1599–606.
2. Tendera M, Aboyans V. 2011 ESC Guidelines on the diagnosis and treatment of patients with peripheral artery diseases. Eur Heart J. 2011;32:2851–906.
3. Diehm C, Allenberg JR, Pittrow D, et al. German epidemiological trial on ankle brachial index Study Group. Circulation. 2009;24:2053–61.
4. Hirsch AT, Criqui MH, Treat-Jacobson D, Regensteiner JG, Creager MA, Olin JW, Krook SH, Hunninghake DB, Comerota AJ, Walsh ME, McDermott MM, Hiatt WR. Peripheral arterial disease detection, awareness, and treatment in primary care. JAMA. 2001;286(11):1317–24.
5. Duprez D. Natural history and evolution of peripheral obstructive arterial disease. Int Angiol. 1992;11:165–8.
6. Murabito JM, Evans JC, D'Agustino Sr RB, Wilson PW, Kannel WB. Temporal trends in the incidence of intermittent claudication from 1950 to 1999. Am J Epidemiol. 2005;162:430–7.
7. De Buyzere M, Clement DL. Management of hypertension in peripheral arterial disease. Prog Cardiovasc Dis. 2008;50:238–63.
8. Clement DL. Control of hypertension in patients with peripheral artery disease. European Society of Hypertension Newsletter. Update Hypertens Manag. 2011;12:26.
9. Norgren L, Hiatt WR, et al. Intersociety consensus for the management of peripheral artery disease (TASCII). J Vasc Surg. 2007;45(suppl A):S1–68.
10. Steg PG, Bhatt DL, Wilson PWF, et al. One-year cardiovascular event rates in outpatients with atherothrombosis. JAMA. 2007;297:1197–206.
11. Fowkes FG, Murray GD, Butcher J, et al. Ankle brachial index combined with Framingham Risk Score to predict cardiovascular events and mortality: a meta-analysis. JAMA. 2008;300:197–208.
12. Wohlfahrt P, Palous D, Ingrischová M, Krajcoviechová A, Seidlerová J, Galovcová M, Bruthans J, Jozífová M, Adámková V, Filipovsky J, Cífková R. A high ankle-brachial index is associated with increased pulse wave velocity: the Czech post-Monica study. Eur J Cardiovasc Prev Rehabil. 2011;32:2851–906.

8 Atherosclerosis and General Principles of Arterial Imaging

Isabel Gonçalves, Nuno V. Dias, and Peter M. Nilsson

8.1 Early Stages of Atherosclerosis

The large arteries are frequent targets for disease development in patients with hypertension. Atherosclerotic plaques develop along the years as focal thickenings of the intima of the arterial wall. These thickenings are mainly present in the carotid, iliac, femoral and coronary arteries as well as in the aorta. These thickenings consist initially of lipid-rich macrophages and are often called fatty streaks. Fatty streaks have mostly been assessed with ultrasound. In the early stage of the atherosclerotic process, the intima and the media get thicker and can be seen with ultrasound as the intima-media thickness.

The intima-media thickness (IMT) has been thoroughly studied and used in numerous trials and related to a myriad of risk factors and interventions. IMT has been considered one of the most common surrogate markers that predicts cardiovascular events [1]. However, the importance of the evaluation of change of IMT over time and its biological meaning has been more controversial. Nevertheless, this structure of the vessel wall has been easily measured, mostly non-invasively in carotid or femoral arteries with ultrasound. The vessel wall thickness can actually be measured by other techniques, as long as one can delineate the vessel wall layers,

I. Gonçalves, MD, PhD
Department of Cardiology, Clinical Sciences Malmö, Lund University, Skåne University Hospital, Malmö, Sweden

N.V. Dias, MD, PhD
Vascular Center, Skåne University Hospital Malmö, Ruth Lundsskogsgatan 10, 205 02 Malmö, Sweden

P.M. Nilsson, MD, PhD (✉)
Clinical Research Unit, Department of Internal Medicine and Clinical Sciences, Skåne University Hospital, IM Nilssons gata 42, S-205 02 Malmö, Sweden
e-mail: Peter.Nilsson@med.lu.se

E. Agabiti Rosei, G. Mancia (eds.), *Assessment of Preclinical Organ Damage in Hypertension*, DOI 10.1007/978-3-319-15603-3_8

such as with magnetic resonance (MR) [2] or computed tomography (CT) [3]. It may also be measured invasively with intravascular ultrasound (IVUS), but in that case, the cheap cost, low risk and high comfort for the individual are lost.

8.2 Later Stages of Atherosclerosis

The early phase of the disease is, however, silent. What leads to clinical events such as myocardial infarction or stroke is a much later phenomenon: thrombosis.

Thrombosis occurs when an atherosclerotic plaque ruptures or suffers surface erosion, leading to platelet activation. The pathophysiology of the atherosclerosis is complex and slow over many decades. Recently, we have shown in living humans for the first time that turnover time of human plaque tissue is very long and may explain why regression of atherosclerotic plaque size is difficult to attain [4].

So why do some plaques rupture and the others do not? The answer is unfortunately not known, but some of the characteristics of the plaques that are more prone to rupture have been unveiled. These plaques that have higher risk for rupture - causing events are often called vulnerable or high-risk plaques (VP) (Fig. 8.1). In 2003, Naghavi et al. [5] summarized several of their characteristics:

1. Large inflammatory activity with agglomerates of macrophages. High macrophage content has been suggested with more than 25 cells per 0.3 mm diameter of the plaque field [6].
2. Large lipid core, occupying more than 40 % of the total plaque volume, covered by a thin fibrous cap [7]. In 95 % of the coronary plaque ruptures, the cap has been thinner than 65 μm [8].

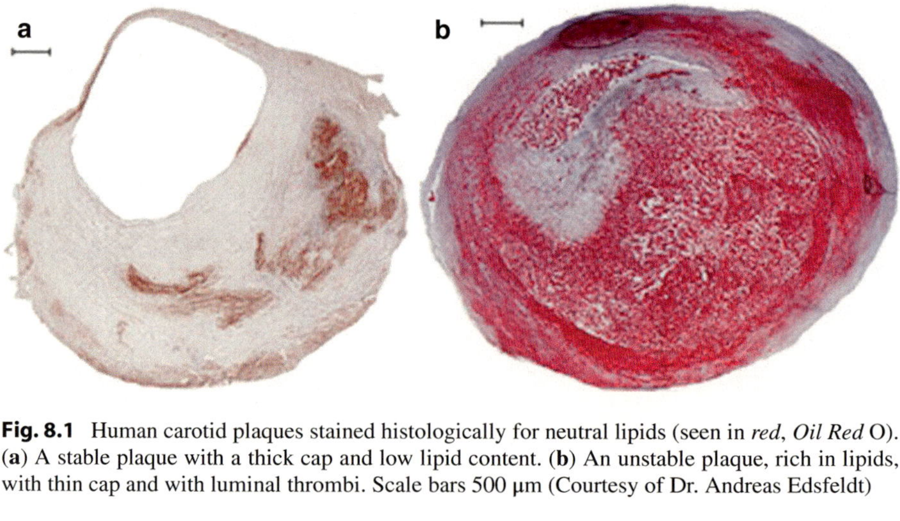

Fig. 8.1 Human carotid plaques stained histologically for neutral lipids (seen in *red*, *Oil Red* O). (**a**) A stable plaque with a thick cap and low lipid content. (**b**) An unstable plaque, rich in lipids, with thin cap and with luminal thrombi. Scale bars 500 μm (Courtesy of Dr. Andreas Edsfeldt)

3. Superficial erosion with possible endothelial damage or dysfunction, leading to increased attachment of inflammatory cells, deficient vasodilation and enhanced platelet aggregation.
4. Fissured caps as lateral tears that lift a part of the intimal layer, exposing the thrombogenic core. These may stand for 15 % of the acute coronary deaths [9].
5. High grade of stenosis. Even though most of the culprit lesions causing the symptoms do not show a significant grade of stenosis, a high-grade stenosis is a marker for advanced disease and for the presence of more plaques [10].
6. Calcified nodule located close to the lumen, as it is highly thrombogenic.
7. Intraplaque haemorrhage, often arising from friable neovessels that are quickly formed as a response to the hypoxic and necrotic environment of the core. These neovessels and haemorrhages are common in advanced plaques and are associated with the expansion of the core. Additionally, the erythrocyte debris increases the oxidative burden and cholesterol crystal amount, further perpetuating inflammation [11]. Intraplaque haemorrhage has been considered an independent predictor for cardiovascular events [12].
8. Outward or positive remodelling, as the increase of size is towards the adventitia of the vessel. It is an early sign of the disease, considering that only when more than 40 % of the diameter is reduced does the lumen start to be affected by the following negative remodelling [13]. Plaques with more inwards or negative remodelling have more lipids and macrophages than those with positive remodelling.

Besides these characteristics, there are certainly many more that have been tested and are to be found. Nevertheless, it would be a major clinical gain if we could detect at least some of these properties in plaques before they cause events. Several approaches can be taken, using, for instance, circulating biomarkers, certainly a cheaper approach, but demanding large amounts of individuals to be cost-effective, or using imaging techniques, more expensive but potentially more specific, ideal for subgroups of risk stratification.

8.3 How Can the Characteristics of the Vulnerable Plaques Be Assessed?

We will focus initially on intravascular invasive methods and finally move on to the three most common non-invasive methods used for plaque characterization:

8.3.1 Intravascular Ultrasound (IVUS), Optical Coherence Tomography (OCT) and Near-Infrared Spectroscopy (NIRS)

IVUS uses a transducer on the end of a flexible, steerable catheter inside the arteries allowing ultrasound of the vessels from the inside out. It is routinely used clinically to delineate plaque morphology, lesion length and obstruction severity when coronary angiography and/or pressure data are ambiguous. Additionally, it may help to guide percutaneous coronary interventions and detect in-stent restenosis. IVUS allows the actual visualization of the plaques – which the angiography actually does not allow, as it is simply a lumenography.

The main pitfalls of IVUS are its invasiveness with its inherent risks, high costs and being time-consuming and the fact that it demands particularly trained human resources. Additionally, only a segment of the coronary tree is assessed at a time, and there is no consensual direct evidence linking changes in the coronaries' plaque and clinical events. Studies to assess this would have to include large numbers of subjects to be then followed up with a non-risk-free technique. Nevertheless, IVUS has been widely used in smaller cohorts to test statin effects [14–16], as well as other therapies [17], with particular focus on the volume and size of the atheroma [18, 19].

Deriving from IVUS, several applications have been developed from the different manufacturers, such as virtual histology IVUS (Volcano Therapeutics), iMAP (Boston Scientific), integrated backscatter IVUS and automated differential echogenicity. Focusing again in plaque composition, tissue maps have been created that correspond to four major components: fibrous (green), fibrofatty (light green), dense calcium (white) and necrotic core (red) [20, 21]. Calcium appears as bright echoes with acoustic shadowing, as dense calcium obstructs the penetration of ultrasound. Therefore, IVUS detects only the leading edge and not the thickness of the calcification. However, it is a good technique to assess remodelling, both positive and negative. Thrombus, either fresh or organized, is the ultimate pathological feature leading to acute events. Unfortunately, none of the IVUS-based imaging modalities available can reliably identify thrombus as it varies largely in its aspect. Recently, there have been attempts to create scores that would distinguish culprit lesions and plaques causing stable angina, such as the Liverpool Active Plaque Score, which was based in a combination of plaque characteristics, namely, core and calcium ratio, minimum lumen area, remodelling index and thin-cap fibroatheroma [22].

More recently, the validation of some of these approaches has been questioned [23], which together with the pitfalls mentioned above contributed to the partially decreased interest in these approaches in many centres.

OCT is a fast-acquisition technique that has submicron resolution, at the expense of reaching very small depths, such as 1–2 mm. It is based on an optical beam that is directed at the tissue. A small part of this light reflects from features under the surface and is collected back. The light is in the near-infrared range, not visible to the human eye. No radiation is involved. Its major advantage is the very high resolution, ca ten times better than IVUS. OCT does not allow visualization through blood so it has to be flushed from the field of view, which in itself can cause complications. Just like IVUS, it is an invasive, catheter-based technique, with the subsequent risks and cost.

In atherosclerosis, it became particularly popular to study the coronaries, providing images of the fibrous cap [24, 25], particularly if ruptured and for very detailed assessment of stents [26]. OCT is quite good for assessing thrombus and even to distinguish red (red blood cell-rich) thrombus from white (platelet-rich) thrombus [26]. A thin cap and thrombosis are two important characteristics of VP. On the other hand, other characteristics are more challenging to detect. Macrophages may only be seen sometimes if in larger agglomerates. The lipid or necrotic core is a signal-poor region within the plaque, with poorly delineated borders [25, 26].

Potentially better to assess plaques with lipid-rich cores is *NIRS*. NIRS, as its name reveals, is also an optical technique that uses the near-infrared region of the electromagnetic spectrum. NIRS is actually widely used to determine the chemical content of substances. First tested in autopsies [27], NIRS could detect lipid pool, thin fibrous cap and inflammatory cells in human aortic atherosclerotic plaques. Soon after, the catheter-based spectroscopy system was implemented further, using wavelengths that can penetrate blood, fast enough to cope with cardiac motion. This system became particularly popular to identify lipid core coronary plaques in patients [28]. Results are usually depicted as chemograms – coloured maps showing the probability of the presence of lipid core plaques. Further studies are needed to establish the possible clinical role of NIRS. Nevertheless, it is an invasive technique with its implicit risks and costs.

8.3.2 Ultrasound

Ultrasonography is based on the emission of ultrasound waves that have higher frequency than 20 kHz (maximal frequency that can be heard by humans). Ultrasounds generated by the transducer propagate through the tissues and, depending on the tissue composition, can be partly reflected in different structures. They are then received back as vibratory mechanical energy, which is finally converted into electric signals and presented as images on the screen. The different acoustic impedance of tissues allows the detection of acoustic interfaces, allowing the definition of their echogenicity. The bigger the impedance differences between two tissues, the better the ultrasonographic discrimination between them. High emitted frequency allows a better definition of the structures that are more superficial. With ultrasound, distances can be quantified by measuring the time between transmission and reception of the signal, as the velocity of propagation of ultrasound in soft tissue can be considered constant (1,540 m/s) [29].

Ultrasonography, which is not intravascular, is a non-invasive method, without known toxicity or radiation. It can be done quickly at the "bedside", and it is cheap when compared with other techniques. Moreover, it allows both functional and morphological evaluations of the whole vessel wall, in contrast to angiography where only the lumen is outlined. It has become widely used as a standard diagnostic modality for carotid stenosis evaluation. No technique is totally perfect, and carotid ultrasonography may have limitations in discriminating subtotal from total occlusion in assessing plaques that have an acoustic shadow and in patients with short neck, high carotid bifurcation or severe arterial kinking. Operator dependency has been the most important limitation of ultrasonography.

Several subjective classifications for the ultrasonographic aspect of plaques have been proposed along the years. Gray-Weale et al. [30] divided plaques in echolucent, predominantly echolucent, predominantly echogenic and echogenic ones, inspiring other adaptations of this classification.

However, the need for objective criteria was more and more urged. Thus, standardization methods to process plaque images were created to overcome differences in the evaluation of plaque echogenicity between the different equipments and observers. One of the most used standardization methods was based on the greyscale values of pixels in a scale of grey intensities (0 darkest and 255 brightest). They

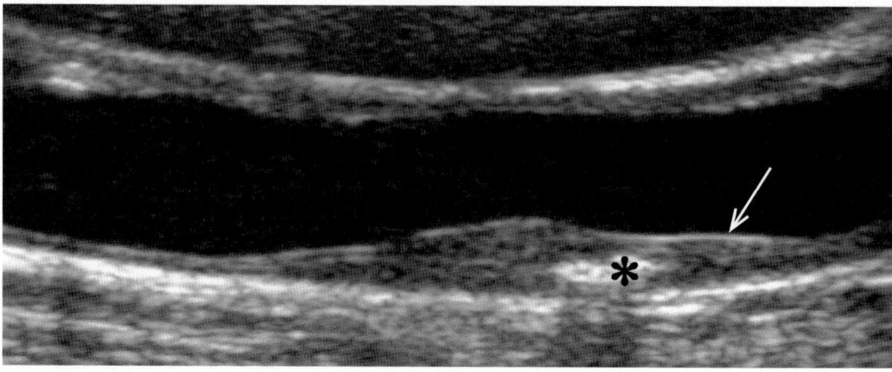

Fig. 8.2 Human carotid plaque, longitudinal image, with B-mode ultrasound. The fibrous cap is shown by the *arrow*. The white region marked with an * is calcified, causing a shadow cone

used the greyscale median (GSM) as a score of global echogenicity. The reference values were the blood as 0 (the darkest structure in the image) and the adventitia as 190 (the brightest structure in the image). The whole plaque image outlined would be processed by linear scaling, compressing the scale. Making the blood and adventitia of all the images have the same values allowed the comparison of different plaques, assessed with different equipments, set-ups and observers. Intra- and interobserver variabilities improved considerably [31].

Plaques with low GSM have been associated with higher incidence of cerebral infarction [32, 33]. Gronholdt et al. [34] showed that echolucent plaques causing stenosis >50 % are associated with increased risk of stroke in symptomatic but not asymptomatic individuals. The association between echolucency and high risk for ipsilateral symptoms has also been verified in other studies, though the influence of the degree of stenosis was not always accepted [35, 36]. Whereas some suggested hypertension and progressive lesions to be important additional determinants of risk [37], others proposed that echolucent plaques were associated with increased risk of neurological events, even independently of degree of stenosis and cardiovascular risk factors [38].

Some other studies evaluated heterogeneity of the plaque image and found that heterogenous and/or echolucent plaques are associated with higher risk of stroke [39–44]. The ability of ultrasonography to study other characteristics that could be associated with the presence of symptoms has been intensively studied. The identification of ulceration by ultrasonography in different studies showed large variation. Rubin et al. [45], using ultrasonography, detected 93 % of the ulcerated lesion, whereas Comerota et al. [46] argued that the possibility of detecting ulceration varied with different degrees of stenosis, being particularly difficult in high-grade stenoses. Bassiouny et al. [47] found that the proximity of plaque necrotic core to the lumen is associated with clinical ischaemic events. Our group [48] showed that in heterogenous plaques, juxtaluminal location of the echolucent region was associated with increased risk (Fig. 8.2). On the contrary, in homogenous plaques, the absence of an echogenic cap and disruption of the plaque surface correlated with symptoms. In an attempt to determine the relative importance of the ultrasonographic structural characteristic of the plaques, besides GSM, an activity index was calculated. This activity index was associated with symptoms [49]. The parameters associated with the presence of ipsilateral symptoms were surface disruption, severe stenosis and low GSM and, in heterogenous plaques, the presence of a juxtaluminal echolucent area. Though all these results are interesting, large-scale studies on different ultrasonographic aspects that can reflect risk and on the natural history of the plaques are needed.

Although the association of echolucent plaques with higher neurological risk has become accepted, no ultrasonographic characteristics have been associated with a single type of symptom. The majority of the studies did not separate those end points. TIA patients showed more hypoechoic carotid plaques with longitudinal motion. The association between plaque radial and longitudinal motion and neurological events was demonstrated in other studies [50].

We [51, 52] and other groups [53–56] have characterized the composition of the echolucent plaques by being richer in lipids, necrosis, haemorrhage and inflammatory cells and poorer in calcification and fibrosis than the echogenic plaques. The presence of neovessels in the plaque branches from the vasa vasorum, which may lead to intraplaque haemorrhage, may be seen with ultrasound, particularly if using contrast [57].

8.3.2.1 Effects of Drug Interventions

Besides the very common use in clinical trials of the intima-media thickness, plaque ultrasound has also started to be used as a tool to monitor the effect of therapeutic interventions, such as statins [58–60] and beta-blockers [61], or even risk for carotid stenting [62]. Further studies on new algorithms for plaque characterization are warranted and will be of great use in risk stratification and to follow up interventions in a cheap, non-invasive, contrast- and radiation-free approach in the future.

8.3.3 Computed Tomography (CT)

CT is a widely spread technique, available in most institutions, with a higher spatial resolution than MR, freedom from flow-related artefacts and simple and fast acquisition, demanding less patient-dependent modifications. The newer machines with multiple detectors and ECG triggering require very small timings of acquisition and need only short injections of contrast.

CT major pitfalls besides radiation and contrast are metal artefacts and, which concerns plaques in particular, calcifications. Calcifications, particularly if very large, may provide blooming artefacts. Other issues that might hamper the quality of the CT images are arrhythmias and fast heart rates, which motivate frequent use of beta-blockers before the scan.

Coronary calcification increases with age and is considered a marker of atherosclerotic burden [63], even though it does not reflect the rupture risk of individual plaques. There have been several approaches to quantify the calcium burden, but the one that became more popular and used in the clinical routine is the Agatston calcium score [64] – calculated by multiplying the lesion area by a weighted attenuation coefficient corresponding with the measured peak CT attenuation or by the volume and mass scores.

Nevertheless, it is now consensual in several position articles from the American Heart Association that coronary artery calcium correlates with greater overall

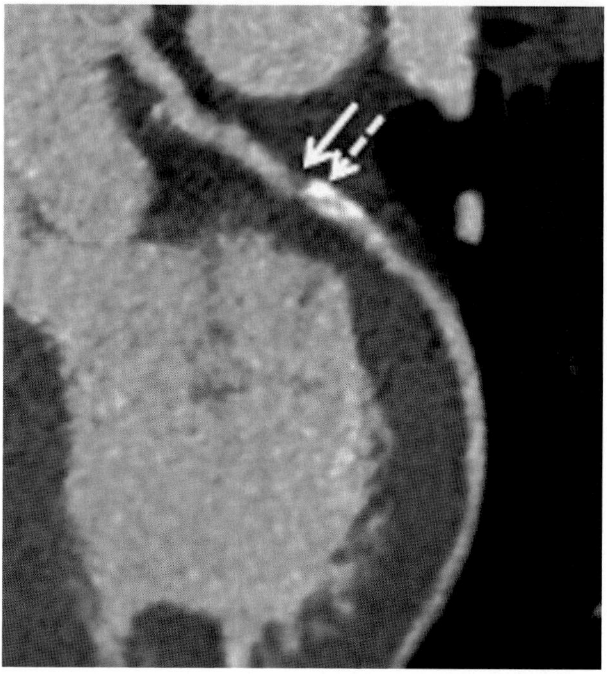

Fig. 8.3 Human coronary plaque in the left anterior descending artery, with a non-calcified part (*filled arrow*) and with a calcified part (*dashed arrow*), assessed with CT 64 detectors

severity of the atherosclerotic process and with the probability of coronary stenosis somewhere within the coronary circulation. Simultaneously, higher calcium scores are related to a higher overall risk for a future cardiac event. However, most interesting is the high negative predictive value for nonsignificant coronary disease of the absence of coronary calcium [65]. This makes CT an excellent method to rule out disease, particularly in patients with low to intermediate risk.

To evaluate the lumen as an angiography, CT is quite feasible, allowing good visualization of native vessels, coronary anomalies, chronic total occlusions, bypass grafts and even stents particularly if larger (>3 mm) [66]. However, as mentioned above, metallic clips and stent nets may cause artefacts creating interpretation difficulties.

CT may also be used for functional purposes, such as assessing the left ventricular function or even perfusion [67], but these aims can generally be obtained, at least as well, with MRI or ultrasound with the beneficial aspect of no use of radiation. More recently, it has become possible to assess the coronary flow reserve noninvasively with CT [68], which despite needing further validation is an extremely promising approach for the future.

Using contrast, it is possible to see both calcified and non-calcified plaques in the arterial tree (Fig. 8.3). More and more studies have tried to assess plaque composition with CT. Plaques in heart specimens with low densities consist mostly of lipids, while those with high densities have more fibrous tissue [69]. Thrombus may look like non-calcified lesions which may be a problem in the interpretation of plaque composition [70]. Carotid plaque CT signal attenuation correlates with the amount of calcification histologically and not with the lipids or haemorrhage [71]. Calcium scores in the carotids may represent an independent marker for luminal stenoses and symptoms [72], with lower calcium content associated with a greater prevalence of symptoms [73]. Hoffman et al. [74] showed that CT can detect non-invasively differences in lesion morphology and plaque composition between culprit lesions in acute coronary syndrome and stable lesions. The culprit lesions giving rise to acute coronary syndromes have larger areas, more remodelling and less calcified plaques than the stable lesions. Another particularly interesting study conducted by Motoyama et al. [75] demonstrated prospectively (follow-up of 27 months) that patients with positively remodelled coronary segments with low-attenuation plaques on CT angiography were at a higher risk for acute coronary syndrome.

A ringlike attenuation pattern of coronary plaques termed as napkin-ring sign was described in the CT of patients who had acute coronary syndromes. This sign was independently related to the size of the core and of the plaque and to the vessel area, measured histologically in seven autopsy specimens [76]. This concept was further reinforced by a recent longitudinal study [77] where the napkin-ring sign could predict future acute coronary syndromes, independent of the presence of positive remodelling and obstructive or low-attenuation plaques.

Taken together, one can recognize several of the characteristics of the VP by being now detected with CT.

8.3.4 Magnetic Resonance (MR)

MR has recently almost become the new gold standard for plaque composition, even though it might overestimate the degree of stenosis. Several protocols in varied field strengths and manufacturers have been implemented. For plaque characterization, dedicated coils have been developed.

The major pitfalls of MR are flow and motion artefacts as well as metal susceptibility artefacts. It is an expensive technique, both time-consuming and demanding a good degree of technical expertise for plaque characterization using multiple sequences. Many patients tend to feel claustrophobic and discomfort with the noise. For MR, nephrotoxic contrast may be used, which makes it less attractive for renal insufficiency or prior contrast reaction cases. Nevertheless, it may be slightly better for renal insufficiency patients than CT.

MR differentiates plaque components on the basis of biophysical and biochemical parameters, such as chemical composition and concentration, water content, physical state, molecular motion and diffusion. As it needs no ionizing radiation, it can be repeated over time, which has made it very attractive for clinical intervention trials where the imaging follow-up is of interest. Most of the in vivo studies have used a multi-contrast approach, using different sequences, allowing the detection of several components simultaneously.

In what concerns how MR can assess plaque composition, studies have been blooming in the last decade, particularly in the carotid territory (Fig. 8.4), as it is more accessible than the coronaries, but it has been tested at least for research

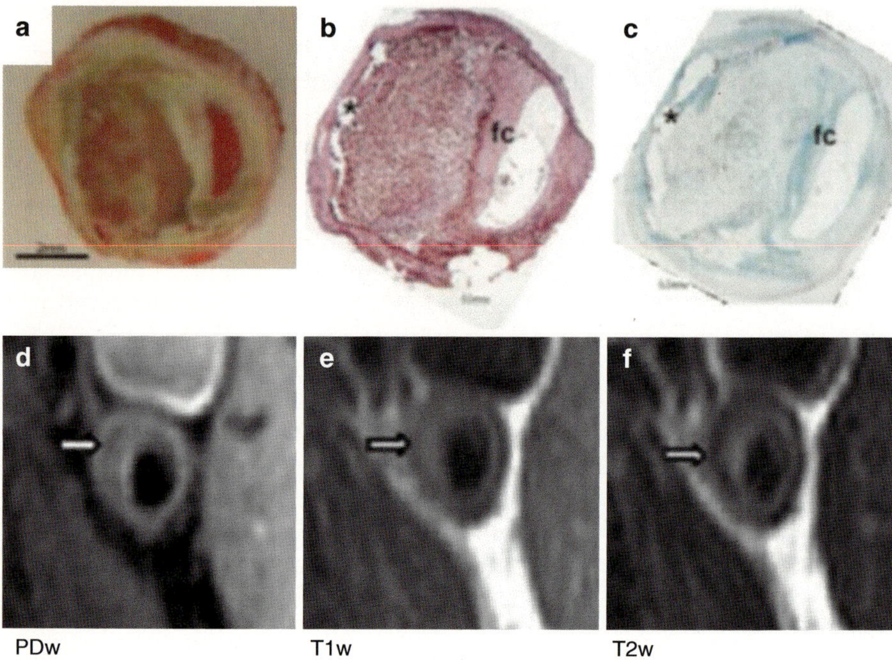

Fig. 8.4 Human carotid plaque: (**a**) macroscopic image, (**b**) macrophage immune staining (CD68) in *dark red*, (**c**) collagen staining (Masson) in *green*. The same plaque assessed in vivo with 3 T MR (**d**) proton density-weighted, (**e**) T1-weighted and (**f**) T2-weighted images. The dark basal rim (*white arrow*) corresponds to calcium marked with * in histology images. *Fc* fibrous cap

purposes in all of these arterial beds. MR allows the identification of fibrous caps on carotid plaques, and their rupture has been related with recent stroke [78]. MR identifies calcium, lipid core, haemorrhage and fibrotic tissue with high sensitivity and specificity [79]. It has also been used to detect inflammation, correlating the transfer of contrast into the extracellular space with macrophages and loose matrix content [80]. Thrombus is a very important component related to plaque rupture or erosion and is sometimes challenging to image. MR has been a good technique to detect not only intraplaque haemorrhage but also juxtaluminal haemorrhage and thrombus [81–83]. Differences between symptomatic and asymptomatic plaques using MR have been found in the same patient [84]. As it is a very reproducible method, MR demands less patients in future clinical trials, being a promising technique to assess VP.

An interesting recent approach with MR has been the non-invasive measurement of temperature of the plaques in vivo, which may reflect plaque inflammatory activation [85]. The technical developments in MR are very fast and exciting including new weightings, new external coils, spectroscopy, targeted molecular imaging (using contrast agents linked to antibodies, peptides or iron oxide compounds, recombinant lipoproteins), higher fields of strength and wall stiffness, just to name a few.

8.3.5 Hybrid Techniques

In the last decades, the wish to combine modalities with good spatial resolution with functional testing has led to the co-registration of images of CT or MR with positron emission tomography (PET). PET detects gamma rays emitted indirectly by a positron-emitting tracer, which is coupled to a biologically active molecule. Lots of molecules could potentially be used, but the most common is fludeoxyglucose (18FDG), an analogue of glucose that is eagerly taken up by metabolically active tissue, in this case, the VP. The VP is rich in inflammatory cells, namely, macrophages. The macrophage uptake of glucose is high because of (a) their high basal glycolytic rate, (b) the further increase in glucose uptake when they are activated and (c) the dependence on an external glucose source because of lack of glycogen storage. Several groups have now shown that carotid plaque inflammation can be imaged with 18FDG-PET and that unstable plaques accumulate more 18FDG than asymptomatic lesions [86, 87]. Even though more challenging, this technique might even be feasible in the coronaries [88]. Some promising studies [89, 90] emphasize a role for CT-PET with 18FDG in the identification of patients that have a higher risk for cardiovascular events.

The combined devices are more expensive as they are actually “two (machines) in one”. The shorter the half-life of the radionuclides, used as tracers, the smaller the radiation dose. On the other hand, the shorter the half-life of the tracers, the closer one has to be to a cyclotron to prepare the tracer on time, which is a logistic and economic burden. Despite CT-PET and MR-PET being non-invasive techniques, their radiation dose is not negligible.

References

1. Lorenz MW, Markus HS, Bots ML, Rosvall M, Sitzer M. Prediction of clinical cardiovascular events with carotid intima-media thickness: a systematic review and meta-analysis. Circulation. 2007;115:459–67.
2. Duivenvoorden R, de Groot E, Elsen BM, et al. In vivo quantification of carotid artery wall dimensions: 3.0-Tesla MRI versus B-mode ultrasound imaging. Circ Cardiovasc Imaging. 2009;2:235–42.
3. Saba L, Tallapally N, Gao H, et al. Semiautomated and automated algorithms for analysis of the carotid artery wall on computed tomography and sonography: a correlation study. J Ultrasound Med. 2013;32:665–74.
4. Goncalves I, Stenström K, Skog G, Mattsson S, Nitulescu M, Nilsson J. Dating components of human atherosclerotic plaques. Circ Res. 2010;106:1174–7.
5. Naghavi M, Libby P, Falk E, et al. From vulnerable plaque to vulnerable patient: a call for new definitions and risk assessment strategies: part I. Circulation. 2003;108:1664–72.
6. Virmani R, Burke AP, Farb A, Kolodgie FD. Pathology of the vulnerable plaque. J Am Coll Cardiol. 2006;47:C13–8.
7. Davies MJ, Richardson PD, Woolf N, Katz DR, Mann J. Risk of thrombosis in human atherosclerotic plaques: role of extracellular lipid, macrophage, and smooth muscle cell content. Br Heart J. 1993;69:377–81.
8. Burke AP, Farb A, Malcom GT, Liang YH, Smialek J, Virmani R. Coronary risk factors and plaque morphology in men with coronary disease who died suddenly. N Engl J Med. 1997;336:1276–82.

9. Falk E, Nakano M, Bentzon JF, Finn AV, Virmani R. Update on acute coronary syndromes: the pathologists' view. Eur Heart J. 2013;34:719–28.
10. Goldstein JA, Demetriou D, Grines CL, Pica M, Shoukfeh M, O'Neill WW. Multiple complex coronary plaques in patients with acute myocardial infarction. N Engl J Med. 2000; 343:915–22.
11. Kolodgie FD, Gold HK, Burke AP, et al. Intraplaque hemorrhage and progression of coronary atheroma. N Engl J Med. 2003;349:2316–25.
12. Hellings WE, Peeters W, Moll FL, et al. Composition of carotid atherosclerotic plaque is associated with cardiovascular outcome: a prognostic study. Circulation. 2010;121:1941–50.
13. Burke AP, Kolodgie FD, Farb A, Weber D, Virmani R. Morphological predictors of arterial remodeling in coronary atherosclerosis. Circulation. 2002;105:297–303.
14. Nissen SE, Nicholls SJ, Sipahi I, et al. Effect of very high-intensity statin therapy on regression of coronary atherosclerosis: the ASTEROID trial. JAMA. 2006;295:1556–65.
15. Bedi U, Singh M, Singh P, Molnar J, Khosla S, Arora R. Effects of statins on progression of coronary artery disease as measured by intravascular ultrasound. J Clin Hypertens. 2011;13:492–6.
16. Puri R, Libby P, Nissen SE, et al. Long-term effects of maximally intensive statin therapy on changes in coronary atheroma composition: insights from SATURN. Eur Heart J Cardiovasc Imaging. 2014;15:380–8.
17. Nissen SE, Tsunoda T, Tuzcu EM, et al. Effect of recombinant ApoA-I Milano on coronary atherosclerosis in patients with acute coronary syndromes: a randomized controlled trial. JAMA. 2003;290:2292–300.
18. Gogas BD, Farooq V, Serruys PW, Garcia-Garcia HM. Assessment of coronary atherosclerosis by IVUS and IVUS-based imaging modalities: progression and regression studies, tissue composition and beyond. Int J Cardiovasc Imaging. 2011;27:225–37.
19. Nicholls SJ, Hsu A, Wolski K, et al. Intravascular ultrasound-derived measures of coronary atherosclerotic plaque burden and clinical outcome. J Am Coll Cardiol. 2010;55:2399–407.
20. Nair A, Kuban BD, Tuzcu EM, Schoenhagen P, Nissen SE, Vince DG. Coronary plaque classification with intravascular ultrasound radiofrequency data analysis. Circulation. 2002;106:2200–6.
21. Nasu K, Tsuchikane E, Katoh O, et al. Accuracy of in vivo coronary plaque morphology assessment: a validation study of in vivo virtual histology compared with in vitro histopathology. J Am Coll Cardiol. 2006;47:2405–12.
22. Murray SW, Stables RH, Garcia-Garcia HM, et al. Construction and validation of a plaque discrimination score from the anatomical and histological differences in coronary atherosclerosis: the Liverpool IVUS-V-HEART (Intra Vascular UltraSound-Virtual-Histology Evaluation of Atherosclerosis Requiring Treatment) study. EuroIntervention. 2014;10:815–23.
23. Thim T, Hagensen MK, Wallace-Bradley D, et al. Unreliable assessment of necrotic core by virtual histology intravascular ultrasound in porcine coronary artery disease. Circ Cardiovasc Imaging. 2010;3:384–91.
24. van der Meer FJ, Faber DJ, Baraznji Sassoon DM, Aalders MC, Pasterkamp G, van Leeuwen TG. Localized measurement of optical attenuation coefficients of atherosclerotic plaque constituents by quantitative optical coherence tomography. IEEE Trans Med Imaging. 2005; 24:1369–76.
25. Meissner OA, Rieber J, Babaryka G, et al. Intravascular optical coherence tomography: comparison with histopathology in atherosclerotic peripheral artery specimens. J Vasc Interv Radiol. 2006;17:343–9.
26. Tearney GJ, Regar E, Akasaka T, et al. Consensus standards for acquisition, measurement, and reporting of intravascular optical coherence tomography studies: a report from the International Working Group for Intravascular Optical Coherence Tomography Standardization and Validation. J Am Coll Cardiol. 2012;59:1058–72.
27. Moreno PR, Lodder RA, Purushothaman KR, Charash WE, O'Connor WN, Muller JE. Detection of lipid pool, thin fibrous cap, and inflammatory cells in human aortic atherosclerotic plaques by near-infrared spectroscopy. Circulation. 2002;105:923–7.

28. Gardner CM, Tan H, Hull EL, et al. Detection of lipid core coronary plaques in autopsy specimens with a novel catheter-based near-infrared spectroscopy system. JACC Cardiovasc Imaging. 2008;1:638–48.
29. Klews PM. Chapter 1. In: Wolf KJ, Fobbe F, editors. Color duplex ultrasonography principles and clinical applications. New York: Thieme Medical Publishers; 1995. p. 2.
30. Gray-Weale AC, Graham JC, Burnett JR, Byrne K, Lusby RJ. Carotid artery atheroma: comparison of preoperative B-mode ultrasound appearance with carotid endarterectomy specimen pathology. J Cardiovasc Surg (Torino). 1988;29:676–81.
31. Elatrozy T, Nicolaides A, Tegos T, Zarka AZ, Griffin M, Sabetai M. The effect of B-mode ultrasonic image standardisation on the echodensity of symptomatic and asymptomatic carotid bifurcation plaques. Int Angiol. 1998;17:179–86.
32. el-Barghouty N, Geroulakos G, Nicolaides A, Androulakis A, Bahal V. Computer-assisted carotid plaque characterisation. Eur J Vasc Endovasc Surg. 1995;9:389–93.
33. El-Barghouty N, Nicoalides A, Bahal V, Geroulakos G, Androulakis A. The identification of the high risk carotid plaque. Eur J Vasc Endovasc Surg. 1996;11:470–8.
34. Gronholdt ML, Nordestgaard BG, Schroeder TV, Vorstrup S, Sillesen H. Ultrasonic echolucent carotid plaques predict future strokes. Circulation. 2001;104:68–73.
35. O'Holleran LW, Kennelly MM, McClurken M, Johnson JM. Natural history of asymptomatic carotid plaque. Five year follow-up study. Am J Surg. 1987;154:659–62.
36. Polak JF, Shemanski L, O'Leary DH, et al. Hypoechoic plaque at US of the carotid artery: an independent risk factor for incident stroke in adults aged 65 years or older. Cardiovascular Health Study. Radiology. 1998;208:649–54.
37. Liapis CD, Kakisis JD, Kostakis AG. Carotid stenosis. Factors affecting symptomatology. Stroke. 2001;32:2782–6.
38. Mathiesen EB, Bonaa KH, Joakimsen O. Echolucent plaques are associated with high risk of ischemic cerebrovascular events in carotid stenosis: the tromso study. Circulation. 2001;103:2171–5.
39. Sterpetti AV, Schultz RD, Feldhaus RJ, et al. Ultrasonographic features of carotid plaque and the risk of subsequent neurologic deficits. Surgery. 1988;104:652–60.
40. Leahy AL, McCollum PT, Feeley TM, et al. Duplex ultrasonography and selection of patients for carotid endarterectomy: plaque morphology or luminal narrowing? J Vasc Surg. 1988;8:558–62.
41. Matalanis G, Lusby RJ. Is there still a place for carotid endarterectomy? Clin Exp Neurol. 1988;25:17–26.
42. Langsfeld M, Gray-Weale AC, Lusby RJ. The role of plaque morphology and diameter reduction in the development of new symptoms in asymptomatic carotid arteries. J Vasc Surg. 1989;9:548–57.
43. Giannoni MF, Speziale F, Faraglia V, et al. Minor asymptomatic carotid stenosis contralateral to carotid endarterectomy (CEA): our experience. Eur J Vasc Surg. 1991;5:237–45.
44. Belcaro G, Laurora G, Cesarone MR, et al. Ultrasonic classification of carotid plaques causing less than 60 % stenosis according to ultrasound morphology and events. J Cardiovasc Surg (Torino). 1993;34:287–94.
45. Rubin JR, Bondi JA, Rhodes RS. Duplex scanning versus conventional arteriography for the evaluation of carotid artery plaque morphology. Surgery. 1987;102:749–55.
46. Comerota AJ, Katz ML, White JV, Grosh JD. The preoperative diagnosis of the ulcerated carotid atheroma. J Vasc Surg. 1990;11:505–10.
47. Bassiouny HS, Sakaguchi Y, Mikucki SA, et al. Juxtalumenal location of plaque necrosis and neoformation in symptomatic carotid stenosis. J Vasc Surg. 1997;26:589–94.
48. Pedro LM, Pedro MM, Goncalves I, et al. Computer-assisted carotid plaque analysis: characteristics of plaques associated with cerebrovascular symptoms and cerebral infarction. Eur J Vasc Endovasc Surg. 2000;19:118–23.
49. Pedro LM, Fernandes e Fernandes J, Pedro MM, et al. Ultrasonographic risk score of carotid plaques. Eur J Vasc Endovasc Surg. 2002;24:492–8.
50. Meairs S, Hennerici M. Four-dimensional ultrasonographic characterization of plaque surface motion in patients with symptomatic and asymptomatic carotid artery stenosis. Stroke. 1999;30:1807–13.

51. Goncalves I, Lindholm MW, Pedro LM, et al. Elastin and calcium rather than collagen or lipid content are associated with echogenicity of human carotid plaques. Stroke. 2004;35:2795–800.
52. Goncalves I, Moses J, Pedro LM, et al. Echolucency of carotid plaques correlates with plaque cellularity. Eur J Vasc Endovasc Surg. 2003;26:32–8.
53. Kardoulas DG, Katsamouris AN, Gallis PT, et al. Ultrasonographic and histologic characteristics of symptom-free and symptomatic carotid plaque. Cardiovasc Surg. 1996;4:580–90.
54. Lammie GA, Wardlaw J, Allan P, Ruckley CV, Peek R, Signorini DF. What pathological components indicate carotid atheroma activity and can these be identified reliably using ultrasound? Eur J Ultrasound. 2000;11:77–86.
55. El-Barghouty NM, Levine T, Ladva S, Flanagan A, Nicolaides A. Histological verification of computerised carotid plaque characterisation. Eur J Vasc Endovasc Surg. 1996;11:414–6.
56. Gronholdt ML, Nordestgaard BG, Bentzon J, et al. Macrophages are associated with lipid-rich carotid artery plaques, echolucency on B-mode imaging, and elevated plasma lipid levels. J Vasc Surg. 2002;35:137–45.
57. Feinstein SB. Contrast ultrasound imaging of the carotid artery vasa vasorum and atherosclerotic plaque neovascularization. J Am Coll Cardiol. 2006;48:236–43.
58. Kadoglou NP, Sailer N, Moumtzouoglou A, Kapelouzou A, Gerasimidis T, Liapis CD. Aggressive lipid-lowering is more effective than moderate lipid-lowering treatment in carotid plaque stabilization. J Vasc Surg. 2010;51:114–21.
59. Yamagami H, Sakaguchi M, Furukado S, et al. Statin therapy increases carotid plaque echogenicity in hypercholesterolemic patients. Ultrasound Med Biol. 2008;34:1353–9.
60. Schmidt C, Fagerberg B, Wikstrand J, Hulthe J. Multiple risk factor intervention reduces cardiovascular risk in hypertensive patients with echolucent plaques in the carotid artery. J Intern Med. 2003;253:430–8.
61. Ostling G, Goncalves I, Wikstrand J, Berglund G, Nilsson J, Hedblad B. Long-term treatment with low-dose metoprolol CR/XL is associated with increased plaque echogenicity: the Beta-blocker Cholesterol-lowering Asymptomatic Plaque Study (BCAPS). Atherosclerosis. 2011;215:440–5.
62. Biasi GM, Froio A, Diethrich EB, et al. Carotid plaque echolucency increases the risk of stroke in carotid stenting: the Imaging in Carotid Angioplasty and Risk of Stroke (ICAROS) study. Circulation. 2004;110:756–62.
63. Sangiorgi G, Rumberger JA, Severson A, et al. Arterial calcification and not lumen stenosis is highly correlated with atherosclerotic plaque burden in humans: a histologic study of 723 coronary artery segments using nondecalcifying methodology. J Am Coll Cardiol. 1998;31:126–33.
64. Agatston AS, Janowitz WR, Hildner FJ, Zusmer NR, Viamonte Jr M, Detrano R. Quantification of coronary artery calcium using ultrafast computed tomography. J Am Coll Cardiol. 1990;15:827–32.
65. Breen JF, Sheedy 2nd PF, Schwartz RS, et al. Coronary artery calcification detected with ultrafast CT as an indication of coronary artery disease. Radiology. 1992;185:435–9.
66. Rixe J, Achenbach S, Ropers D, et al. Assessment of coronary artery stent restenosis by 64-slice multi-detector computed tomography. Eur Heart J. 2006;27:2567–72.
67. Blankstein R, Shturman LD, Rogers IS, et al. Adenosine-induced stress myocardial perfusion imaging using dual-source cardiac computed tomography. J Am Coll Cardiol. 2009;54:1072–84.
68. Min JK, Leipsic J, Pencina MJ, et al. Diagnostic accuracy of fractional flow reserve from anatomic CT angiography. JAMA. 2012;308:1237–45.
69. Becker CR, Nikolaou K, Muders M, et al. Ex vivo coronary atherosclerotic plaque characterization with multi-detector-row CT. Eur Radiol. 2003;13:2094–8.
70. Becker CR, Knez A, Ohnesorge B, Schoepf UJ, Reiser MF. Imaging of noncalcified coronary plaques using helical CT with retrospective ECG gating. AJR Am J Roentgenol. 2000;175:423–4.
71. Gronholdt ML, Wagner A, Wiebe BM, et al. Spiral computed tomographic imaging related to computerized ultrasonographic images of carotid plaque morphology and histology. J Ultrasound Med. 2001;20:451–8.

72. Nandalur KR, Baskurt E, Hagspiel KD, et al. Carotid artery calcification on CT may independently predict stroke risk. AJR Am J Roentgenol. 2006;186:547–52.
73. Nandalur KR, Baskurt E, Hagspiel KD, Phillips CD, Kramer CM. Calcified carotid atherosclerotic plaque is associated less with ischemic symptoms than is noncalcified plaque on MDCT. AJR Am J Roentgenol. 2005;184:295–8.
74. Hoffmann U, Moselewski F, Nieman K, et al. Noninvasive assessment of plaque morphology and composition in culprit and stable lesions in acute coronary syndrome and stable lesions in stable angina by multidetector computed tomography. J Am Coll Cardiol. 2006;47:1655–62.
75. Motoyama S, Sarai M, Harigaya H, et al. Computed tomographic angiography characteristics of atherosclerotic plaques subsequently resulting in acute coronary syndrome. J Am Coll Cardiol. 2009;54:49–57.
76. Seifarth H, Schlett CL, Nakano M, et al. Histopathological correlates of the napkin-ring sign plaque in coronary CT angiography. Atherosclerosis. 2012;224:90–6.
77. Otsuka K, Fukuda S, Tanaka A, et al. Napkin-ring sign on coronary CT angiography for the prediction of acute coronary syndrome. JACC Cardiovasc Imaging. 2013;6:448–57.
78. Yuan C, Zhang SX, Polissar NL, et al. Identification of fibrous cap rupture with magnetic resonance imaging is highly associated with recent transient ischemic attack or stroke. Circulation. 2002;105:181–5.
79. Cappendijk VC, Cleutjens KB, Kessels AG, et al. Assessment of human atherosclerotic carotid plaque components with multisequence MR imaging: initial experience. Radiology. 2005;234:487–92.
80. Kerwin WS, O'Brien KD, Ferguson MS, Polissar N, Hatsukami TS, Yuan C. Inflammation in carotid atherosclerotic plaque: a dynamic contrast-enhanced MR imaging study. Radiology. 2006;241:459–68.
81. Moody AR, Murphy RE, Morgan PS, et al. Characterization of complicated carotid plaque with magnetic resonance direct thrombus imaging in patients with cerebral ischemia. Circulation. 2003;107:3047–52.
82. Cappendijk VC, Cleutjens KB, Heeneman S, et al. In vivo detection of hemorrhage in human atherosclerotic plaques with magnetic resonance imaging. J Magn Reson Imaging. 2004; 20:105–10.
83. Kampschulte A, Ferguson MS, Kerwin WS, et al. Differentiation of intraplaque versus juxtaluminal hemorrhage/thrombus in advanced human carotid atherosclerotic lesions by in vivo magnetic resonance imaging. Circulation. 2004;110:3239–44.
84. Saam T, Cai J, Ma L, et al. Comparison of symptomatic and asymptomatic atherosclerotic carotid plaque features with in vivo MR imaging. Radiology. 2006;240:464–72.
85. Toutouzas K, Grassos C, Drakopoulou M, et al. First in vivo application of microwave radiometry in human carotids: a new noninvasive method for detection of local inflammatory activation. J Am Coll Cardiol. 2012;59:1645–53.
86. Rudd JH, Warburton EA, Fryer TD, et al. Imaging atherosclerotic plaque inflammation with [18F]-fluorodeoxyglucose positron emission tomography. Circulation. 2002;105:2708–11.
87. Tawakol A, Migrino RQ, Bashian GG, et al. In vivo 18F-fluorodeoxyglucose positron emission tomography imaging provides a noninvasive measure of carotid plaque inflammation in patients. J Am Coll Cardiol. 2006;48:1818–24.
88. Rogers IS, Nasir K, Figueroa AL, et al. Feasibility of FDG imaging of the coronary arteries: comparison between acute coronary syndrome and stable angina. JACC Cardiovasc Imaging. 2010;3:388–97.
89. Paulmier B, Duet M, Khayat R, et al. Arterial wall uptake of fluorodeoxyglucose on PET imaging in stable cancer disease patients indicates higher risk for cardiovascular events. J Nucl Cardiol. 2008;15:209–17.
90. Rominger A, Saam T, Wolpers S, et al. 18F-FDG PET/CT identifies patients at risk for future vascular events in an otherwise asymptomatic cohort with neoplastic disease. J Nucl Med. 2009;50:1611–20.

Imaging and Ageing of the Aorta and Large Arteries in the Lower Extremity

9

Nuno V. Dias, Isabel Gonçalves, and Peter M. Nilsson

9.1 Introduction

Imaging of the aorta and lower extremity is highly dependent on the disease to be studied, i.e. aneurysm, dissection or occlusive disease (peripheral artery disease, PAD). Aortic aneurysm imaging has traditionally focused on the assessment of the aneurysm size as a determinant of the rupture risk and, consequently, the indication for elective aneurysm repair. The introduction of endovascular aneurysm repair (EVAR) in the 1990s has led to the need of high-definition 3-D imaging. In these cases, the imaging method of choice is currently contrast-enhanced CT scanning with dedicated post-processing workstations that allow the planning of EVAR. Aortic dissections pose the same imaging requirements as aneurysms, but dynamic information is also very useful. In PAD disease there is the need of obtaining imaging of an extensive area of the peripheral arterial circulation, which poses technical challenges due to varying flow velocities caused by the disease itself.

This chapter will review the different imaging modalities available for imaging of the aortic arch; the descending, thoraco-abdominal and abdominal aorta; and the peripheral circulation in the aorto-iliac segment.

N.V. Dias, MD, PhD
Vascular Center, Skåne University Hospital Malmö, Ruth Lundsskogsgatan 10, 205 02 Malmö, Sweden

I. Gonçalves, MD, PhD
Department of Cardiology, Clinical Sciences Malmö, Lund University, Skåne University Hospital, Malmö, Sweden

P.M. Nilsson, MD, PhD (✉)
Clinical Research Unit, Department of Internal Medicine and Clinical Sciences, Skåne University Hospital, IM Nilssons gata 42, S-205 02 Malmö, Sweden
e-mail: Peter.Nilsson@med.lu.se

E. Agabiti Rosei, G. Mancia (eds.), *Assessment of Preclinical Organ Damage in Hypertension*, DOI 10.1007/978-3-319-15603-3_9

9.2 Plain X-Ray

Plain X-ray was used for the diagnosis of aortic disease when no other methods were available. It relies on indirect signs such as aortic wall calcifications and changes in the mediastinal contour and demands always confirmation by the other imaging methods. Their use has regained importance in the follow-up after EVAR since it allows assessment of the integrity of the stent-graft skeleton, presence of kinks and migration. Standardised X-ray acquisition protocols have been introduced to optimise the evaluation of migration [1, 2], but this becomes unnecessary whenever CT is performed since the same information can be easily obtained from that exam.

9.3 Ultrasound

Ultrasound is a non-invasive method that avoids ionising radiation, is inexpensive and can be rapidly performed at the bedside. It has been the method of choice in aneurysm screening programmes [3] especially in abdominal aortic aneurysms (AAA). Ultrasound does not give the detailed anatomic information required for EVAR and is, therefore, usually completed with other imaging methods in large aneurysms requiring surgical treatment.

The sensitivity and specificity of ultrasound to diagnose and follow aneurysms ≥3 cm exceeds 90 % [4, 5]. However, there is a need for standardised measurement protocols and education to maintain the diagnostic value since ultrasound is observer dependent [6–8]. Moreover, ultrasound underestimates slightly the aneurysm diameter when compared to computed tomography [9–11], but the reproducibility of ultrasound is very high which, combined with its non-invasiveness, makes it the method of choice for the control of dilated aortas that do not reach surgical indication. The frequency of the exams should increase with increasing aortic diameters [12].

Ultrasound can also be used for imaging of the ascending aorta. The inability to perform ultrasound through airfields limits the use of the transthoracic approach in the study of parts of the arch and descending aorta. For these segments, trans-oesophagic ultrasound (TEE) can be used. TEE provides also higher-definition imaging of the ascending aorta making it very useful when there are unclear findings in the ascending aorta on other imaging methods (such as suspected localised type A dissections or intramural haematoma). However, the higher invasiveness of TEE limits its use as a first-line method, and therefore it has been mostly applied for the refinement of the diagnosis or intraoperatively during endovascular repair of type B dissections.

Ultrasound is also increasingly used for the follow-up after EVAR of AAA with different strategies. It has been proposed to be used focusing on diameter measurements with referral to contrast-enhanced CT scans whenever pathological findings are suspected [13]. Other authors use duplex to identify possible endoleaks and flow in target vessels [14, 15]. The diagnostic potential of endoleaks seems to be further potentiated by the use of contrast enhancement [16]. Moreover, ultrasound has also been used to assess aneurysm pulsatility, especially in the follow-up after EVAR, but the value of pulsatile wall motion seems to be limited [17, 18]. More recently 3-D ultrasound imaging has emerged as a promising technique for AAA imaging [19, 20], being even suggested as a means of determining aortic wall strain through speckle-tracking algorithms and finite element analysis [21, 22], and 3-D imaging has also been integrated in robotic models that may have the potential of obtaining imaging from the iliacs down to the popliteal arteries [23].

Ultrasound is widely used for the assessment of PAD. For this application, duplex is very useful since the analysis of the waveform in the femoral artery provides a simple and fast way of excluding and identifying a significant aorto-iliac disease [24–26]. The location, extent and frequent calcifications of the atherosclerotic plaques in the aorta and iliac arteries limit the high-quality ultrasonic analysis, and little is known in this field. This has, however, been done in the femoral segment where there seems to be parallel findings to the carotid arteries with echolucent plaques being associated with higher risk [27, 28].

9.4 Intravascular Ultrasound (IVUS)

As previously described, IVUS relies on the use of an intraluminal high-frequency ultrasound probe mounted on a catheter invasively placed at the point of interest. The technique has been widely used in the coronary arteries with recent developments in the form of virtual histology [29, 30]. IVUS has, however, not gained the same popularity in the PAD and aortic aneurysms mostly due to the costs involved, the complexity of the technique compared and the limited benefit obtained. IVUS-based automated vessel analysis has been used in the preoperative assessment of the sealing zones, but even these have not been widely accepted [31]. On the contrary IVUS has shown some extra value during endovascular repair of type B dissections extending into the abdominal aorta, where it allows a simple and contrast-free assessment of the guide-wire position in the true lumen [32].

9.5 Computer Tomography (CT)

CT is based on the computer creation of 3-D imaging from 2-D X-ray data obtained from rotation around an axis. Initial CT scans gave single axial imaging with poor definition. The development of multidetector-row CT has increased the image resolution and the field of image and made the exam faster [33]. This allows the performance of CT scans also in the acute settings for the diagnosis of aneurysm rupture when the patients are haemodynamically stable [34].

CT is the most commonly used method for the anatomic study of aortic aneurysms, while in occlusive disease, MR has been favoured due to its less dependency on calcium artefacts and the reduced need of time-consuming imaging post-processing. In recent years, the use of dual-energy CT scanning with two X-ray tubes scanning simultaneously at different energy levels (usually 80 and 140 kV) has allowed CT scanning with less interference of calcium [35]. The remaining of this subchapter will focus on aortic aneurysm imaging.

CT of the aorta is usually contrast enhanced, which is done by the peripheral venous injection of a weight-adjusted dose of iodinated contrast medium followed by a saline bolus injection. The scanning is triggered most often by the detection of the contrast column passage at a region of interest (ROI) placed in the ascending or aortic arch when the entire aorta is being studied or at the level of the diaphragm if only the abdominal aorta is going to be studied. In patients with renal insufficiency, the dose of the nephrotoxic iodinated contrast may be reduced by the use of intra-aortic injection through a transfemoral-placed catheter or low-dose CT protocols [36]. Non-contrast-enhanced CT of the aorta has had until recently limited application being done for the diagnosis or follow-up of aneurysms when these were nonaccessible by ultrasound. However, recent preliminary data suggest that the CT texture analysis may reflect the metabolism and be related to aneurysm expansion [37].

9.6 Preoperative Imaging

A preoperative assessment of the aorta should include contrast-enhanced scans in the arterial phase with thin axial reconstructions (≤1 mm) from the skull base to the lesser femoral trochanter. The imaging of the supra-aortic trunks and the circle of Willis is important in deciding the need for revascularisation of the left subclavian artery when the origin of this artery needs to be covered with a thoracic stent graft. Moreover, CTs done for aortic pathology involving the ascending aorta and the arch should be done with EKG-gated scans to avoid movement artefacts, which may also allow triple rule-out diagnostic [38]. Retrospective EKG-gated CT scanning allows also dynamic imaging of the aorta, identifying pulsatile changes in the thoracic and abdominal aorta during the heart cycle [39, 40]. CT imaging with finite element computational analysis has also been used in attempting the refinement of the rupture risk assessment [41]. Another important advancement in recent years in aortic CT imaging is post-processing of the contrast-enhanced images in dedicated workstations. This has become crucial for EVAR planning, especially in more advanced procedures such as branched and fenestrated endografts. The workstation allows simple and fast reconstructions of multiple MPRs (multi-planar reconstructions, Fig. 9.1) and MIPs (maximum intensity projections) with free rotational ability at different angles with assessment of different parts of the anatomy such as aortic branch take-off [42]. Moreover, it enables centre line of flow (CLF) analysis with length measurements and diameters on orthogonal reconstructions without the limitations caused by the tortuosity of the elongated arteries (Fig. 9.2). This is helpful in deciding the length of the endografts [43] and the distance between target vessels in complex cases. The accuracy of the CLF measurements is dependent on the way the graft will follow the CLF upon deployment. This requires sometimes the correction of the CLF in very tortuous cases.

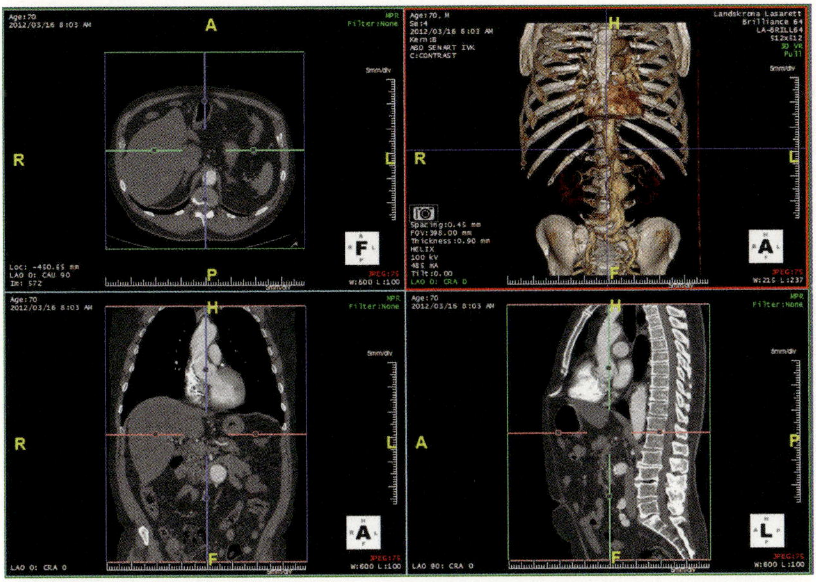

Fig. 9.1 Layout of post-processing of a contrast-enhanced CT with synchronised axial, 3-D rendering imaging, sagittal and coronal multi-planar reconstructions (clockwise)

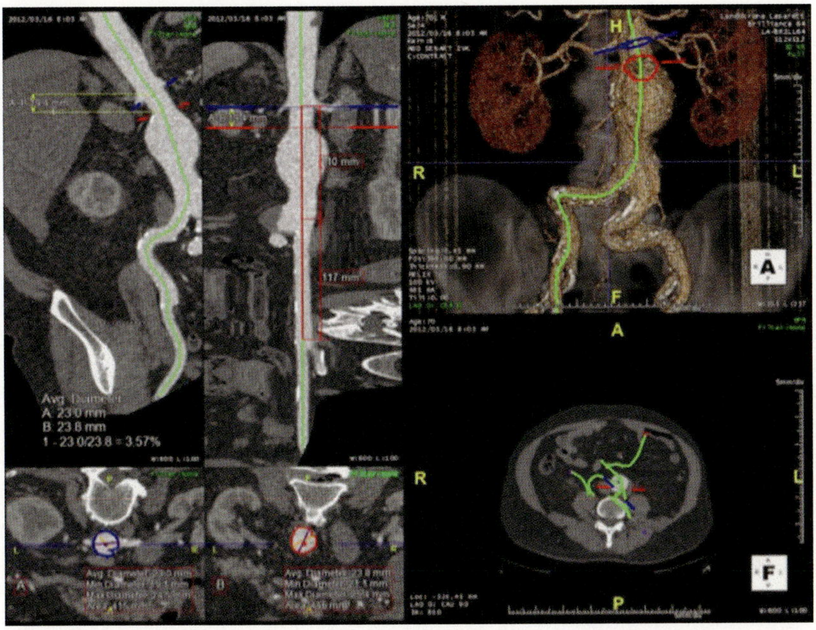

Fig. 9.2 Post-processing of a contrast-enhanced CT scan of a patient with an aortic aneurysm. A centre line of flow is obtained based on the contrast attenuation within the lumen of the aorta (*upper right*). The workstation provides reconstructions orthogonal to the centre line of flow (*bottom left*) and allows length measurements along the centre line (*upper left*)

9.7 Postoperative Imaging

As mentioned before, there has been a trend for replacing CT by ultrasound in the follow-up after standard EVAR of AAA. However, CT is still the golden standard for EVAR postoperative controls, especially in thoracic and more complex EVAR. Postoperative CT aims at measuring aneurysm diameter and identifying endoleaks, migrations, kinks and material fatigue. It should include plain, arterial phase and delayed scans to allow the diagnosis type II endoleaks (from collaterals such as the lumbar arteries) that could otherwise remain unnoticed [44]. Even during follow-up, low-dose and dual-energy CT can be used to reduce radiation, while maintaining the diagnostic outcome [36, 45–48]. Dual-energy CT is also able to produce virtual non-contrast imaging which avoids one scan [49]. Post-processing workstations are also very useful in the follow-up after EVAR allowing the assessment of stent-graft integrity and possible migration [50]. Of particular interest is the fly-through application with virtual angioscopy that provides detailed assessment of the different branches and possible compression or kinking of stents [51]. Moreover, workstations have different methods of measuring the aneurysm size besides the axial diameter. Orthogonal diameters and aneurysm volume seem to increase accuracy in the identification of changes in aneurysm size [11, 52, 53] but demand time-consuming post-processing.

9.8 Magnetic Resonance Imaging (MR)

MR is still used less frequently than CT in the study of aortic aneurysms due to its cost, lower availability and longer time required for scanning. It is however a method widely used for the PAD since it is less susceptible to calcium artefacts and allows imaging of long segments without the same dependency on the varying perfusion as CT (Fig. 9.3) [54, 55]. MR uses magnetic fields and takes advantage of the different relaxation times of the different tissues. Gadolinium contrast agents are commonly used to shorten the T1 (longitudinal) relaxation time and thereby enhance the contrast and shorten the examination time [56]. This contrast agent is also nephrotoxic, but the doses needed for MR angiography are usually below the toxicity levels [57]. On the contrary, gadolinium-based contrast agents have been associated with nephrogenic systemic fibrosis (NSF) in patients with renal insufficiency, and they should be avoided in patients with advanced renal insufficiency [58]. The risks seem nevertheless to be small and should be weighed against the clinical indication for the MR [59]. Unenhanced MR is an upcoming imaging modality that has shown promising results in EVAR planning and diagnosis of PAD [60–64]. This technique may become important in the future for patients with renal insufficiency.

MR angiography images are most commonly analysed as MIP since they are similar to the conventional digital subtraction angiography, i.e. they depict only the lumen. They are nevertheless sensitive to reconstruction artefacts and the raw images should therefore be available. Moreover, raw images enable the identification of the presence of aneurysms and dissections and the measurement of the arterial diameters. Raw images may also identify pathology surrounding the aorta such

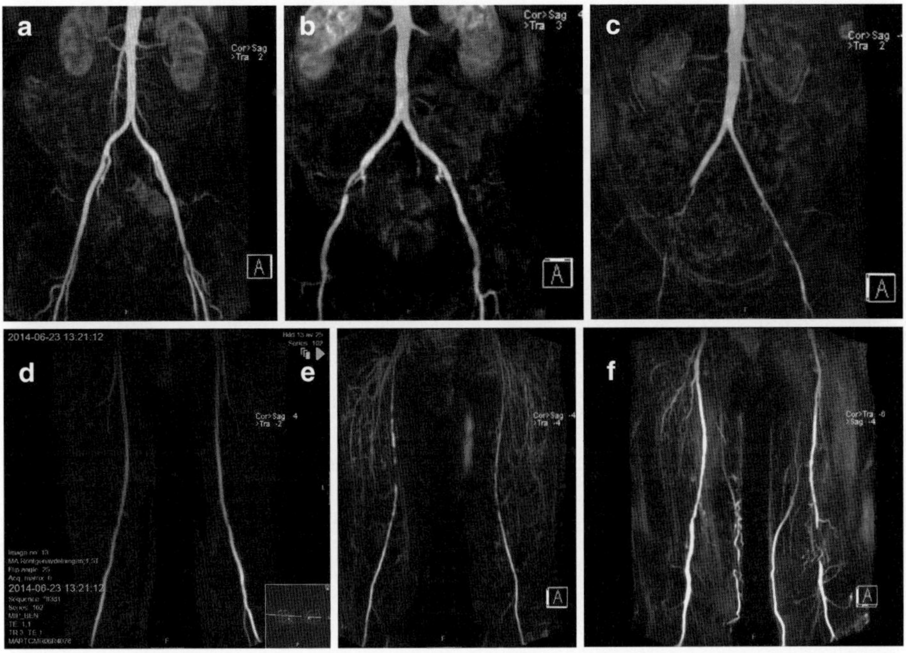

Fig. 9.3 Anterior projections of maximal intensity projections (MIP) of MR angiography for the diagnostic workup of PAD. (**a**) Aorto-iliac arteries without significant stenosis. (**b**) Right-sided external iliac stenosis as opposed to the rest of the aorto-iliac segment that is open without significant stenosis. (**c**) Occluded external iliac artery and significant stenosis in the common femoral artery on the right side. On the left side, there is a distal stenosis of the external iliac artery. (**d**) Femoro-popliteal arteries without significant stenosis bilaterally. (**e**) Bilateral multi-segmental stenosis of the superficial femoral arteries. (**f**) Short occlusion of the left distal superficial femoral artery as opposed the remaining femoro-popliteal arteries

as inflammatory reactions. MR angiography images can also be post-processed in a similar way as described for CT, enabling detailed morphological analysis and planning of EVAR [65]. MR has also good diagnostic accuracy in the follow-up after EVAR, especially for the identification of type II endoleaks [66–68], in particular when blood-pool contrast agents are used [69, 70]. However, MR use is limited when endografts made of stainless steel or having ferromagnetic markers are used since these cause signal void [71]. Dynamic MR has also shown promising diagnostic possibilities in aortic aneurysms [39, 72–75] and dissections, including assessment of flow dynamics and its implications in future aneurysmatic dilatation of the aorta [76, 77] and false lumen thrombosis after endovascular treatment of aortic dissections [78]. Another interesting application of MR imaging is the identification of areas of increased biological activity in the aneurysm wall by the use of ultrasmall superparamagnetic iron oxide contrast agents (USPIO) that are taken up by macrophages [79–82]. These applications together with the possibility of performing MR-guided endovascular procedures can lead to an increased role of MR aortic imaging in the future [83, 84].

9.9 Digital Subtraction Angiography (DSA)

Angiography is the golden standard for the assessment of PAD but is inappropriate for the evaluation of aneurysms since it outlines only the arterial lumen and is insensitive to the aneurysm diameter, especially if the aneurysm is partially affected by thrombosis or the wall is not heavily calcified. DSA was used in the past to complete the preoperative diagnosis of aortic aneurysms concerning the concomitant presence of PAD in the access vessels and aortic branches, to exclude anatomic variations before open surgical repair or to assist in length measurement before EVAR. This has become obsolete with the advent of 3-D dedicated workstations with rapid and detailed volume rendering of CT and MR imaging [85, 86].

Angiography is therefore currently used during endovascular therapeutic procedures. DSA usually requires iodine intra-arterial contrast. This is nephrotoxic as discussed above and modern angiographic equipment allow radiation adjustments in order to be able to limit the amount of contrast used [87]. Moreover, carbon dioxide can also be used as a contrast medium but has limited application when imaging arteries with dorsal origin and should be avoided above the diaphragm [88, 89].

9.10 Rotation Angiography, Cone Beam CT and Fusion

Modern angiographic equipment with flat digital panels has usually the capability of obtaining high-definition volume-rendering imaging. This may be a digitally subtracted rotational angiography that can be used as overlay reference into the fluoroscopy but has limited diagnostic advantages when compared to the high-definition non-invasive methods described above. The other volume-rendering imaging that can be used is a cone beam CT (CB-CT), which has high spatial resolution, but the acquisition volume is limited by the size of the flat detector and centred in its iso-centre. For these reasons, CB-CT is mainly used intraoperatively and has shown good preliminary results in preoperative anatomic evaluation [90–92] and assessment of the final result [92].

Another technical advancement available in modern angiographic systems is the fusion of the preoperative volume-rendering imaging (usually CT) with the intraoperative fluoroscopy. This is achieved by matching the position of the bony structures on the preoperative CT and intraoperatively. The angiographic software can then use the preoperative CT angiography as an overlay reference in the fluoroscopy screen (Fig. 9.4). The initial results of the application of this technique in EVAR are very promising [93–95], and other applications are being developed with similar outcome [96]. Attention should nevertheless be paid to the potential deviation of the anatomy by the stiff wires and introducers in the aorta and movements related to breathing, heart cycle and posture [97]. There is very recent data on the possibility of gating preoperative MR data, which may allow the overcoming movement deviations [98].

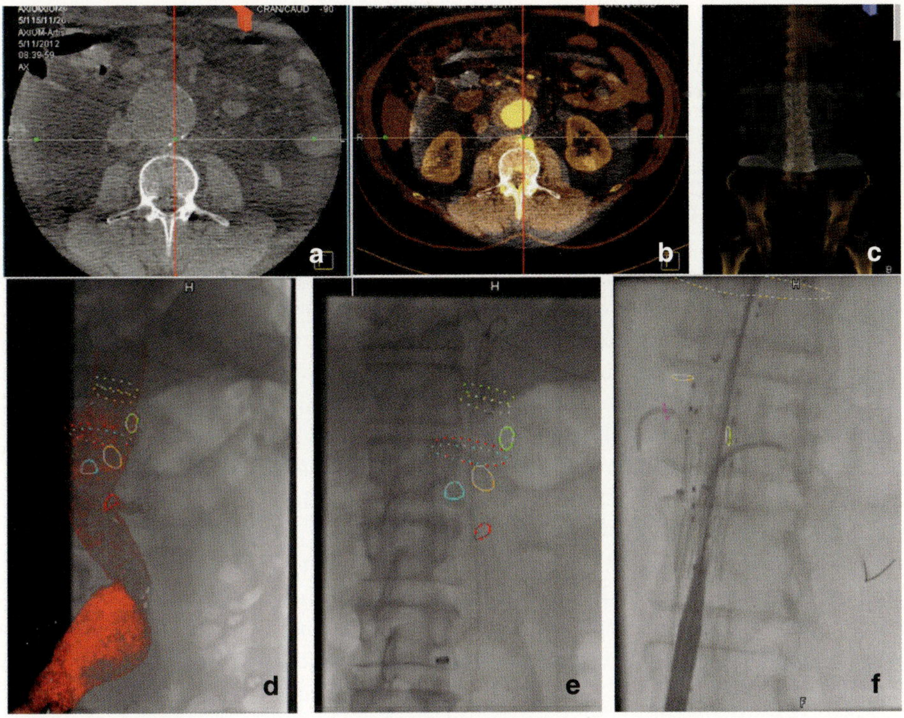

Fig. 9.4 Overlay fusion: (**a**) rudimentary cone beam CT without contrast obtained with the intraoperative angiographic equipment. (**b**) Superimposed cone beam CT (whitish shadow within the small circle) on the preoperative high-definition contrast-enhanced CT scan. (**c**) Superimposed bony reconstructions of the intra- and preoperative CT scans. There is a slight misalignment of the bony structures that will be corrected by the registration process. (**d**) Transparent 3-D reconstruction of the aortic lumen from the preoperative CT scan superimposed in the intraoperative fluoroscopy. The visceral arteries and the positions of interest in the aorta have been marked with colour rings. (**e**) Live overlay of the preoperative 3-D information on the intraoperative fluoroscopy. The 3-D volume has been taken away leaving only the rings marking the positions of interest from the preoperative CT (visceral arteries). (**f**) Example of catheterisation of the renal arteries using only the fusion rings as landmarks and without the need of intraoperative iodine contrast

9.11 Integrated Positron Emission Tomography and Computed Tomography (PET-CT) or Magnetic (MR-PET)

Positron emission tomography (PET) uses fluorine-18 fluorodeoxyglucose (FDG) that is taken up by metabolically active cells such as macrophages in the arterial wall [96, 97] emitting positron and gamma rays upon disintegration that are detected by the camera. CT (and more recently even MR) scanners can be integrated with PET providing, therefore, combined imaging with morphological and functional information. The experiences with PET-CT in pre- and postoperative imaging of aortic aneurysms have been contradictory, and further studies are needed [99–106]. More recent animal studies have shown promising results with the use of PET tracers targeting other components such as integrin, but the value is also awaiting more studies [107].

9.12 Ageing of Arteries: The Role of Arterial Stiffness

Arterial ageing is a process that spans from normal ageing [108] to pathological ageing and the changes described related to *atherosclerosis*.

In recent years, the interest has increased in arterial stiffness and the underlying arteriosclerosis, as a precursor to the more well-known and well-studied atherosclerosis, with its pathology influenced by genetics, high LDL-cholesterol levels, smoking, hypertension, inflammation and overt type 2 diabetes [109]. In many cases, it is believed that early life programming may cause a susceptibility for this increased tendency for arterial stiffening as well as other aspects of vascular tree, for example, the development of capillaries and the microcirculation. As this process is also related to ageing, it has been proposed that a process of early vascular ageing (EVA) is an early sign of arteriosclerosis (in the media) but linked also to early changes in the endothelial function (intima), haemodynamic changes and the influence of abnormal glucose metabolism and increased inflammation [110–112]. The difference between the concept of arterial ageing and EVA is that the latter also encompasses the smaller arteriolae and the microcirculation, based on the cross-talk between the macro- and microcirculation [112]. EVA is now being extensively studied in different population-based cohorts, both in Europe and in Latin America, but still no general definition has been agreed upon. One way to define EVA could be to use the outliers according to the normal range of c-f PWV, i.e. above the two standard deviations (SD) of the normal distribution of c-f PWV in the European reference group [113]. Another way to describe EVA is based on statistical methods when arterial stiffness (c-f PWV), a central aspect of EVA, is used as the dependent variable in multiple regression analyses and a number of risk markers are used as independent variables, based on data from population-based studies. As the influence of haemodynamic changes and sympathetic nervous system (SNS) stimulation on the arterial tone is substantial, the data are normally adjusted for mean arterial pressure (MAP) and heart rate (HR), the latter as a marker of SNS activity. Such investigations in a population-based study in Malmo, Sweden, have revealed that markers of glucose metabolism and dyslipidaemia (elevated triglycerides, low HDL-cholesterol levels), as well as waist circumference (a marker of active abdominal fat tissue with inflammatory action), are significantly associated with arterial stiffness, but not LDL cholesterol, smoking or cystatin C, a marker of impaired renal function [114]. The findings thus point to different clusters of cardiovascular risk factors involved in development of arteriosclerosis and atherosclerosis, respectively.

Still there is a need to better define EVA in different age groups but also in relation to gender and ethnicity, as well as based on genetic studies for improved classification [115]. Some would argue that EVA is just a construct to cover one example of target organ damage (arterial stiffness) in subjects at high cardiovascular or metabolic risk, and primarily influenced by haemodynamic changes and blood pressure levels. However, the modern genetics of hypertension and blood pressure regulation, based on a global study, could not show any marker on chromosome 13 [116], but exactly on this chromosome, a genetic locus (for the *COL4A1* gene, involved in collagen metabolism) was found for arterial stiffness in a study from Sardinia, Italy, with independent replication in another American cohort [117]. This shows that even if arterial stiffness (and EVA) is strongly influenced by the blood pressure load (MAP), HR and SNS activity, there could even exist some other important components (collagen protein synthesis, structure) and vascular risk factors (hyperglycaemia, dyslipidaemia, inflammation) independent of blood pressure regulation. If true, this opens up new possibilities to target these mechanisms of protein/collagen synthesis with new drugs to reduce arterial stiffness.

So far it has been shown that a prolonged control of hypertension will reverse early changes and have a long-term beneficial influence on arterial stiffness with decreasing c-f PWV levels over time, beyond the blood pressure control itself [118]. However, an ongoing randomised controlled study in France (SPARTE) aims to compare a treatment strategy for reduction of arterial stiffness (c-f PWV) by different means, including drugs that specifically influence the renin-angiotensin system, and another treatment strategy (control) to go for implementation of control of the conventional risk factors including blood pressure, as suggested in guidelines [119]. SPARTE is supposed to continue for still a number of years until a sufficient number of cardiovascular endpoints have accumulated to show potential differences in outcomes between the treatment arms. Recruitment is ongoing.

As increased c-f PWV has been documented to be an independent risk marker for future cardiovascular events and total mortality in recent meta-analyses [120, 121], there is a need to target it with multiple risk factor control, aiming for c-f PWV <10 m/s that is the current threshold for increased risk [122].

In summary, the knowledge about morphological changes (imaging) and physiological changes (imaging and haemodynamics) in the arterial wall will make it possible to better understand the double process of arteriosclerosis and atherosclerosis leading to cardiovascular disease manifestations. Current medical and surgical therapies will be expanded in the future for better control of these pathological processes and even for the control of arterial ageing.

References

1. Hodgson R, McWilliams RG, Simpson A, Gould DA, Brennan JA, Gilling-Smith GL, et al. Migration versus apparent migration: importance of errors due to positioning variation in plain radiographic follow-up of aortic stent-grafts. J Endovasc Ther. 2003;10(5):902–10.
2. Murphy M, Hodgson R, Harris PL, McWilliams RG, Hartley DE, Lawrence-Brown MM. Plain radiographic surveillance of abdominal aortic stent-grafts: the Liverpool/Perth protocol. J Endovasc Ther. 2003;10(5):911–2.
3. Wilmink AB, Forshaw M, Quick CR, Hubbard CS, Day NE. Accuracy of serial screening for abdominal aortic aneurysms by ultrasound. J Med Screen. 2002;9(3):125–7.

4. Wilmink AB, Hubbard CS, Quick CR. Quality of the measurement of the infrarenal aortic diameter by ultrasound. J Med Screen. 1997;4(1):49–53.
5. Lindholt JS, Vammen S, Juul S, Henneberg EW, Fasting H. The validity of ultrasonographic scanning as screening method for abdominal aortic aneurysm. Eur J Vasc Endovasc Surg. 1999;17(6):472–5.
6. Beales L, Wolstenhulme S, Evans JA, West R, Scott DJ. Reproducibility of ultrasound measurement of the abdominal aorta. Br J Surg. 2011;98(11):1517–25.
7. Grondal N, Bramsen MB, Thomsen MD, Rasmussen CB, Lindholt JS. The cardiac cycle is a major contributor to variability in size measurements of abdominal aortic aneurysms by ultrasound. Eur J Vasc Endovasc Surg. 2012;43(1):30–3.
8. Hartshorne TC, McCollum CN, Earnshaw JJ, Morris J, Nasim A. Ultrasound measurement of aortic diameter in a national screening programme. Eur J Vasc Endovasc Surg. 2011;42(2):195–9.
9. Sprouse I, Richard L, Meier I, George H, LeSar CJ, DeMasi RJ, Sood J, Parent FN, et al. Comparison of abdominal aortic aneurysm diameter measurements obtained with ultrasound and computed tomography: is there a difference? J Vasc Surg. 2003;38(3):466–71.
10. Lederle FA, Wilson SE, Johnson GR, Reinke DB, Littooy FN, Acher CW, et al. Variability in measurement of abdominal aortic aneurysms. Abdominal Aortic Aneurysm Detection and Management Veterans Administration Cooperative Study Group. J Vasc Surg. 1995;21(6):945–52.
11. Manning BJ, Kristmundsson T, Sonesson B, Resch T. Abdominal aortic aneurysm diameter: a comparison of ultrasound measurements with those from standard and three-dimensional computed tomography reconstruction. J Vasc Surg. 2009;50(2):263–8.
12. Moll FL, Powell JT, Fraedrich G, Verzini F, Haulon S, Waltham M, et al. Management of abdominal aortic aneurysms clinical practice guidelines of the European society for vascular surgery. Eur J Vasc Endovasc Surg. 2011;41 Suppl 1:S1–58.
13. Dias NV, Riva L, Ivancev K, Resch T, Sonesson B, Malina M. Is there a benefit of frequent CT follow-up after EVAR? Eur J Vasc Endovasc Surg. 2009;37(4):425–30.
14. Perini P, Sediri I, Midulla M, Delsart P, Gautier C, Haulon S. Contrast-enhanced ultrasound vs. CT angiography in fenestrated EVAR surveillance: a single-center comparison. J Endovasc Ther. 2012;19(5):648–55.
15. Perini P, Sediri I, Midulla M, Delsart P, Mouton S, Gautier C, et al. Single-centre prospective comparison between contrast-enhanced ultrasound and computed tomography angiography after EVAR. Eur J Vasc Endovasc Surg. 2011;42(6):797–802.
16. Mirza TA, Karthikesalingam A, Jackson D, Walsh SR, Holt PJ, Hayes PD, et al. Duplex ultrasound and contrast-enhanced ultrasound versus computed tomography for the detection of endoleak after EVAR: systematic review and bivariate meta-analysis. Eur J Vasc Endovasc Surg. 2010;39(4):418–28.
17. Malina M, Länne T, Ivancev K, Lindblad B, Brunkwall J. Reduced pulsatile wall motion of abdominal aortic aneurysms after endovascular repair. J Vasc Surg. 1998;27(4):624–31.
18. Lindblad B, Dias N, Malina M, Ivancev K, Resch T, Hansen F, et al. Pulsatile wall motion (PWM) measurements after endovascular abdominal aortic aneurysm exclusion are not useful in the classification of endoleak. Eur J Vasc Endovasc Surg. 2004;28(6):623–8.
19. Long A, Rouet L, Debreuve A, Ardon R, Barbe C, Becquemin JP, et al. Abdominal aortic aneurysm imaging with 3-D ultrasound: 3-D-based maximum diameter measurement and volume quantification. Ultrasound Med Biol. 2013;39(8):1325–36.
20. Bredahl K, Long A, Taudorf M, Lonn L, Rouet L, Ardon R, et al. Volume estimation of the aortic sac after EVAR using 3-D ultrasound – a novel, accurate and promising technique. Eur J Vasc Endovasc Surg. 2013;45(5):450–5; discussion 6.
21. Wittek A, Karatolios K, Bihari P, Schmitz-Rixen T, Moosdorf R, Vogt S, et al. In vivo determination of elastic properties of the human aorta based on 4D ultrasound data. J Mech Behav Biomed Mater. 2013;27:167–83.
22. Karatolios K, Wittek A, Nwe TH, Bihari P, Shelke A, Josef D, et al. Method for aortic wall strain measurement with three-dimensional ultrasound speckle tracking and fitted finite element analysis. Ann Thorac Surg. 2013;96(5):1664–71.

23. Janvier MA, Merouche S, Allard L, Soulez G, Cloutier G. A 3-D ultrasound imaging robotic system to detect and quantify lower limb arterial stenoses: in vivo feasibility. Ultrasound Med Biol. 2014;40(1):232–43.
24. Eiberg JP, Jensen F, Gronvall Rasmussen JB, Schroeder TV. Screening for aortoiliac lesions by visual interpretation of the common femoral Doppler waveform. Eur J Vasc Endovasc Surg. 2001;22(4):331–6.
25. Shaalan WE, French-Sherry E, Castilla M, Lozanski L, Bassiouny HS. Reliability of common femoral artery hemodynamics in assessing the severity of aortoiliac inflow disease. J Vasc Surg. 2003;37(5):960–9.
26. Spronk S, den Hoed PT, de Jonge LC, van Dijk LC, Pattynama PM. Value of the duplex waveform at the common femoral artery for diagnosing obstructive aortoiliac disease. J Vasc Surg. 2005;42(2):236–42; discussion 42.
27. Schiano V, Sirico G, Giugliano G, Laurenzano E, Brevetti L, Perrino C, et al. Femoral plaque echogenicity and cardiovascular risk in claudicants. J Am Coll Cardiol Img. 2012;5(4):348–57.
28. Sirico G, Brevetti G, Lanero S, Laurenzano E, Luciano R, Chiariello M. Echolucent femoral plaques entail higher risk of echolucent carotid plaques and a more severe inflammatory profile in peripheral arterial disease. J Vasc Surg. 2009;49(2):346–51.
29. Kaneda H, Ako J, Terashima M. Intravascular ultrasound imaging for assessing regression and progression in coronary artery disease. Am J Cardiol. 2010;106(12):1735–46.
30. Garcia-Garcia HM, Gogas BD, Serruys PW, Bruining N. IVUS-based imaging modalities for tissue characterization: similarities and differences. Int J Cardiovasc Imaging. 2011;27(2):215–24.
31. van Essen JA, Gussenhoven EJ, Blankensteijn JD, Honkoop J, van Dijk LC, van Sambeek MR, et al. Three-dimensional intravascular ultrasound assessment of abdominal aortic aneurysm necks. J Endovasc Ther. 2000;7(5):380–8.
32. Koschyk DH, Nienaber CA, Knap M, Hofmann T, Kodolitsch YV, Skriabina V, et al. How to guide stent-graft implantation in type B aortic dissection? Comparison of angiography, transesophageal echocardiography, and intravascular ultrasound. Circulation. 2005;112(9 Suppl):I260–4.
33. Rubin GD. MDCT imaging of the aorta and peripheral vessels. Eur J Radiol. 2003;45 Suppl 1:S42–9.
34. Lloyd GM, Bown MJ, Norwood MG, Deb R, Fishwick G, Bell PR, et al. Feasibility of preoperative computer tomography in patients with ruptured abdominal aortic aneurysm: a time-to-death study in patients without operation. J Vasc Surg. 2004;39(4):788–91.
35. Tran DN, Straka M, Roos JE, Napel S, Fleischmann D. Dual-energy CT discrimination of iodine and calcium: experimental results and implications for lower extremity CT angiography. Acad Radiol. 2009;16(2):160–71.
36. Iezzi R, Cotroneo AR, Giammarino A, Spigonardo F, Storto ML. Low-dose multidetector-row CT-angiography of abdominal aortic aneurysm after endovascular repair. Eur J Radiol. 2011;79(1):21–8.
37. Kotze CW, Rudd JH, Ganeshan B, Menezes LJ, Brookes J, Agu O, et al. CT signal heterogeneity of abdominal aortic aneurysm as a possible predictive biomarker for expansion. Atherosclerosis. 2014;233(2):510–7.
38. Shapiro MD. Is the “triple rule-out” study an appropriate indication for cardiovascular CT? J Cardiovasc Comput Tomogr. 2009;3(2):100–3.
39. van Keulen JW, van Prehn J, Prokop M, Moll FL, van Herwaarden JA. Dynamics of the aorta before and after endovascular aneurysm repair: a systematic review. Eur J Vasc Endovasc Surg. 2009;38(5):586–96.
40. Iezzi R, Di Stasi C, Dattesi R, Pirro F, Nestola M, Cina A, et al. Proximal aneurysmal neck: dynamic ECG-gated CT angiography–conformational pulsatile changes with possible consequences for endograft sizing. Radiology. 2011;260(2):591–8.
41. Georgakarakos E, Ioannou CV, Papaharilaou Y, Kostas T, Katsamouris AN. Computational evaluation of aortic aneurysm rupture risk: what have we learned so far? J Endovasc Ther. 2011;18(2):214–25.

42. van Keulen JW, Moll FL, van Herwaarden JA. Tips and techniques for optimal stent graft placement in angulated aneurysm necks. J Vasc Surg. 2010;52(4):1081–6.
43. Higashiura W, Kichikawa K, Sakaguchi S, Tabayashi N, Taniguchi S, Uchida H. Accuracy of centerline of flow measurement for sizing of the Zenith AAA endovascular graft and predictive factor for risk of inadequate sizing. Cardiovasc Intervent Radiol. 2009;32(3):441–8.
44. Rozenblit AM, Patlas M, Rosenbaum AT, Okhi T, Veith FJ, Laks MP, et al. Detection of endoleaks after endovascular repair of abdominal aortic aneurysm: value of unenhanced and delayed helical CT acquisitions. Radiology. 2003;227(2):426–33.
45. Ascenti G, Mazziotti S, Lamberto S, Bottari A, Caloggero S, Racchiusa S, et al. Dual-energy CT for detection of endoleaks after endovascular abdominal aneurysm repair: usefulness of colored iodine overlay. AJR Am J Roentgenol. 2011;196(6):1408–14.
46. Chandarana H, Godoy MC, Vlahos I, Graser A, Babb J, Leidecker C, et al. Abdominal aorta: evaluation with dual-source dual-energy multidetector CT after endovascular repair of aneurysms–initial observations. Radiology. 2008;249(2):692–700.
47. Numburi UD, Schoenhagen P, Flamm SD, Greenberg RK, Primak AN, Saba OI, et al. Feasibility of dual-energy CT in the arterial phase: imaging after endovascular aortic repair. AJR Am J Roentgenol. 2010;195(2):486–93.
48. Stolzmann P, Frauenfelder T, Pfammatter T, Peter N, Scheffel H, Lachat M, et al. Endoleaks after endovascular abdominal aortic aneurysm repair: detection with dual-energy dual-source CT. Radiology. 2008;249(2):682–91.
49. Sommer WH, Graser A, Becker CR, Clevert DA, Reiser MF, Nikolaou K, et al. Image quality of virtual noncontrast images derived from dual-energy CT angiography after endovascular aneurysm repair. J Vasc Interv Radiol. 2010;21(3):315–21.
50. O'Neill S, Greenberg RK, Resch T, Bathurst S, Fleming D, Kashyap V, et al. An evaluation of centerline of flow measurement techniques to assess migration after thoracic endovascular aneurysm repair. J Vasc Surg. 2006;43(6):1103–10.
51. Louis N, Bruguiere E, Kobeiter H, Desgranges P, Allaire E, Kirsch M, et al. Virtual angioscopy and 3D navigation: a new technique for analysis of the aortic arch after vascular surgery. Eur J Vasc Endovasc Surg. 2010;40(3):340–7.
52. Lee JT, Aziz IN, Haukoos JS, Donayre CE, Walot I, Kopchok GE, et al. Volume regression of abdominal aortic aneurysms and its relation to successful endoluminal exclusion. J Vasc Surg. 2003;38(6):1254–63.
53. Wever JJ, Blankensteijn JD, Th M Mali WP, Eikelboom BC. Maximal aneurysm diameter follow-up is inadequate after endovascular abdominal aortic aneurysm repair. Eur J Vasc Endovasc Surg. 2000;20(2):177–82.
54. Leung DA, Debatin JF. Three-dimensional contrast-enhanced magnetic resonance angiography of the thoracic vasculature. Eur Radiol. 1997;7(7):981–9.
55. Leung DA, Hany TF, Debatin JF. Three-dimensional contrast-enhanced magnetic resonance angiography of the abdominal arterial system. Cardiovasc Intervent Radiol. 1998;21:1–10.
56. Zhang Z, Nair SA, McMurry TJ. Gadolinium meets medicinal chemistry: MRI contrast agent development. Curr Med Chem. 2005;12(7):751–78.
57. Elmstahl B, Nyman U, Leander P, Chai CM, Golman K, Bjork J, et al. Gadolinium contrast media are more nephrotoxic than iodine media. The importance of osmolality in direct renal artery injections. Eur Radiol. 2006;16(12):2712–20.
58. Sadowski EA, Bennett LK, Chan MR, Wentland AL, Garrett AL, Garrett RW, et al. Nephrogenic systemic fibrosis: risk factors and incidence estimation. Radiology. 2007;243(1):148–57.
59. Abu-Alfa AK. Nephrogenic systemic fibrosis and gadolinium-based contrast agents. Adv Chronic Kidney Dis. 2011;18(3):188–98.
60. Saida T, Mori K, Sato F, Shindo M, Takahashi H, Takahashi N, et al. Prospective intraindividual comparison of unenhanced magnetic resonance imaging vs contrast-enhanced computed tomography for the planning of endovascular abdominal aortic aneurysm repair. J Vasc Surg. 2012;55(3):679–87.
61. Krishnam MS, Tomasian A, Malik S, Desphande V, Laub G, Ruehm SG. Image quality and diagnostic accuracy of unenhanced SSFP MR angiography compared with conventional

contrast-enhanced MR angiography for the assessment of thoracic aortic diseases. Eur Radiol. 2010;20(6):1311–20.
62. Thierfelder KM, Meimarakis G, Nikolaou K, Sommer WH, Schmitt P, Kazmierczak PM, et al. Non-contrast-enhanced MR angiography at 3 Tesla in patients with advanced peripheral arterial occlusive disease. PLoS One. 2014;9(3):e91078.
63. Knobloch G, Gielen M, Lauff MT, Romano VC, Schmitt P, Rick M, et al. ECG-gated quiescent-interval single-shot MR angiography of the lower extremities: initial experience at 3 T. Clin Radiol. 2014;69:485–91.
64. Francois CJ, Tuite D, Deshpande V, Jerecic R, Weale P, Carr JC. Unenhanced MR angiography of the thoracic aorta: initial clinical evaluation. AJR Am J Roentgenol. 2008;190(4):902–6.
65. Ludman CN, Yusuf SW, Whitaker SC, Gregson RH, Walker S, Hopkinson BR. Feasibility of using dynamic contrast-enhanced magnetic resonance angiography as the sole imaging modality prior to endovascular repair of abdominal aortic aneurysms. Eur J Vasc Endovasc Surg. 2000;19(5):524–30.
66. Haulon S, Lions C, McFadden EP, Koussa M, Gaxotte V, Halna P, et al. Prospective evaluation of magnetic resonance imaging after endovascular treatment of infrarenal aortic aneurysms. Eur J Vasc Endovasc Surg. 2001;22(1):62–9.
67. Alerci M, Oberson M, Fogliata A, Gallino A, Vock P, Wyttenbach R. Prospective, intraindividual comparison of MRI versus MDCT for endoleak detection after endovascular repair of abdominal aortic aneurysms. Eur Radiol. 2009;19(5):1223–31.
68. van der Laan MJ, Bartels LW, Viergever MA, Blankensteijn JD. Computed tomography versus magnetic resonance imaging of endoleaks after EVAR. Eur J Vasc Endovasc Surg. 2006;32(4):361–5.
69. Cornelissen SA, Prokop M, Verhagen HJ, Adriaensen ME, Moll FL, Bartels LW. Detection of occult endoleaks after endovascular treatment of abdominal aortic aneurysm using magnetic resonance imaging with a blood pool contrast agent: preliminary observations. Invest Radiol. 2010;45(9):548–53.
70. Ersoy H, Jacobs P, Kent CK, Prince MR. Blood pool MR angiography of aortic stent-graft endoleak. AJR Am J Roentgenol. 2004;182(5):1181–6.
71. van der Laan MJ, Bartels LW, Bakker CJ, Viergever MA, Blankensteijn JD. Suitability of 7 aortic stent-graft models for MRI-based surveillance. J Endovasc Ther. 2004;11(4):366–71.
72. Merkx MA, van 't Veer M, Speelman L, Breeuwer M, Buth J, van de Vosse FN. Importance of initial stress for abdominal aortic aneurysm wall motion: dynamic MRI validated finite element analysis. J Biomech. 2009;42(14):2369–73.
73. van der Laan MJ, Bakker CJ, Blankensteijn JD, Bartels LW. Dynamic CE-MRA for endoleak classification after endovascular aneurysm repair. Eur J Vasc Endovasc Surg. 2006;31(2):130–5.
74. van Herwaarden JA, Bartels LW, Muhs BE, Vincken KL, Lindeboom MY, Teutelink A, et al. Dynamic magnetic resonance angiography of the aneurysm neck: conformational changes during the cardiac cycle with possible consequences for endograft sizing and future design. J Vasc Surg. 2006;44(1):22–8.
75. van Prehn J, Vincken KL, Sprinkhuizen SM, Viergever MA, van Keulen JW, van Herwaarden JA, et al. Aortic pulsatile distention in young healthy volunteers is asymmetric: analysis with ECG-gated MRI. Eur J Vasc Endovasc Surg. 2009;37(2):168–74.
76. Clough RE, Waltham M, Giese D, Taylor PR, Schaeffter T. A new imaging method for assessment of aortic dissection using four-dimensional phase contrast magnetic resonance imaging. J Vasc Surg. 2012;55(4):914–23.
77. Francois CJ, Markl M, Schiebler ML, Niespodzany E, Landgraf BR, Schlensak C, et al. Four-dimensional, flow-sensitive magnetic resonance imaging of blood flow patterns in thoracic aortic dissections. J Thorac Cardiovasc Surg. 2013;145(5):1359–66.
78. Clough RE, Hussain T, Uribe S, Greil GF, Razavi R, Taylor PR, et al. A new method for quantification of false lumen thrombosis in aortic dissection using magnetic resonance imaging and a blood pool contrast agent. J Vasc Surg. 2011;54(5):1251–8.

79. Howarth SP, Tang TY, Graves MJ, U-King-Im JM, Li ZY, Walsh SR, et al. Non-invasive MR imaging of inflammation in a patient with both asymptomatic carotid atheroma and an abdominal aortic aneurysm: a case report. Ann Surg Innov Res. 2007;1:4.
80. Richards JM, Semple SI, MacGillivray TJ, Gray C, Langrish JP, Williams M, et al. Abdominal aortic aneurysm growth predicted by uptake of ultrasmall superparamagnetic particles of iron oxide: a pilot study. Circ Cardiovasc Imaging. 2011;4(3):274–81.
81. Sadat U, Taviani V, Patterson AJ, Young VE, Graves MJ, Teng Z, et al. Ultrasmall superparamagnetic iron oxide-enhanced magnetic resonance imaging of abdominal aortic aneurysms–a feasibility study. Eur J Vasc Endovasc Surg. 2011;41(2):167–74.
82. Truijers M, Futterer JJ, Takahashi S, Heesakkers RA, Blankensteijn JD, Barentsz JO. In vivo imaging of the aneurysm wall with MRI and a macrophage-specific contrast agent. AJR Am J Roentgenol. 2009;193(5):W437–41.
83. Eggebrecht H, Kuhl H, Kaiser GM, Aker S, Zenge MO, Stock F, et al. Feasibility of real-time magnetic resonance-guided stent-graft placement in a swine model of descending aortic dissection. Eur Heart J. 2006;27(5):613–20.
84. Raman VK, Karmarkar PV, Guttman MA, Dick AJ, Peters DC, Ozturk C, et al. Real-time magnetic resonance-guided endovascular repair of experimental abdominal aortic aneurysm in swine. J Am Coll Cardiol. 2005;45(12):2069–77.
85. Wyers MC, Fillinger MF, Schermerhorn ML, Powell RJ, Rzucidlo EM, Walsh DB, et al. Endovascular repair of abdominal aortic aneurysm without preoperative arteriography. J Vasc Surg. 2003;38(4):730–8.
86. Beebe HG, Kritpracha B, Serres S, Pigott JP, Price CI, Williams DM. Endograft planning without preoperative arteriography: a clinical feasibility study. J Endovasc Ther. 2000;7(1):8–15.
87. Walker TG, Kalva SP, Ganguli S, Oklu R, Salazar GM, Waltman AC, et al. Image optimization during endovascular aneurysm repair. AJR Am J Roentgenol. 2012;198(1):200–6.
88. Criado E, Upchurch Jr GR, Young K, Rectenwald JE, Coleman DM, Eliason JL, et al. Endovascular aortic aneurysm repair with carbon dioxide-guided angiography in patients with renal insufficiency. J Vasc Surg. 2012;55:1570–5.
89. Lee AD, Hall RG. An evaluation of the use of carbon dioxide angiography in endovascular aortic aneurysm repair. Vasc Endovascular Surg. 2010;44(5):341–4.
90. Eide KR, Odegard A, Myhre HO, Hatlinghus S, Haraldseth O. DynaCT in pre-treatment evaluation of aortic aneurysm before EVAR. Eur J Vasc Endovasc Surg. 2011;42(3):332–9.
91. Eide KR, Odegard A, Myhre HO, Lydersen S, Hatlinghus S, Haraldseth O. DynaCT during EVAR–a comparison with multidetector CT. Eur J Vasc Endovasc Surg. 2009;37(1):23–30.
92. Nordon IM, Hinchliffe RJ, Malkawi AH, Taylor J, Holt PJ, Morgan R, et al. Validation of DynaCT in the morphological assessment of abdominal aortic aneurysm for endovascular repair. J Endovasc Ther. 2010;17(2):183–9.
93. Dijkstra ML, Eagleton MJ, Greenberg RK, Mastracci T, Hernandez A. Intraoperative C-arm cone-beam computed tomography in fenestrated/branched aortic endografting. J Vasc Surg. 2011;53(3):583–90.
94. Sailer AM, de Haan MW, Peppelenbosch AG, Jacobs MJ, Wildberger JE, Schurink GW. CTA with fluoroscopy image fusion guidance in endovascular complex aortic aneurysm repair. Eur J Vasc Endovasc Surg. 2014;47(4):349–56.
95. Tacher V, Lin M, Desgranges P, Deux JF, Grunhagen T, Becquemin JP, et al. Image guidance for endovascular repair of complex aortic aneurysms: comparison of two-dimensional and three-dimensional angiography and image fusion. J Vasc Interv Radiol. 2013;24(11):1698–706.
96. Carrell TWG, Modarai B, Brown JRI, Penney GP. Feasibility and limitations of an automated 2D-3D rigid image registration system for complex endovascular aortic procedures. J Endovasc Ther. 2010;17(4):527–33.

97. Maurel B, Hertault A, Gonzalez TM, Sobocinski J, Le Roux M, Delaplace J, et al. Evaluation of visceral artery displacement by endograft delivery system insertion. J Endovasc Ther. 2014;21(2):339–47.
98. Faranesh AZ, Kellman P, Ratnayaka K, Lederman RJ. Integration of cardiac and respiratory motion into MRI roadmaps fused with x-ray. Med Phys. 2013;40(3):032302.
99. Kotze CW, Groves AM, Menezes LJ, Harvey R, Endozo R, Kayani IA, et al. What is the relationship between (1)F-FDG aortic aneurysm uptake on PET/CT and future growth rate? Eur J Nucl Med Mol Imaging. 2011;38(8):1493–9.
100. Kotze CW, Menezes LJ, Endozo R, Groves AM, Ell PJ, Yusuf SW. Increased metabolic activity in abdominal aortic aneurysm detected by 18F-fluorodeoxyglucose (18F-FDG) positron emission tomography/computed tomography (PET/CT). Eur J Vasc Endovasc Surg. 2009;38(1):93–9.
101. Palombo D, Morbelli S, Spinella G, Pane B, Marini C, Rousas N, et al. A positron emission tomography/computed tomography (PET/CT) evaluation of asymptomatic abdominal aortic aneurysms: another point of view. Ann Vasc Surg. 2012;26:491–9.
102. Reeps C, Essler M, Pelisek J, Seidl S, Eckstein HH, Krause BJ. Increased 18F-fluorodeoxyglucose uptake in abdominal aortic aneurysms in positron emission/computed tomography is associated with inflammation, aortic wall instability, and acute symptoms. J Vasc Surg. 2008;48(2):417–23; discussion 24.
103. Truijers M, Kurvers HA, Bredie SJ, Oyen WJ, Blankensteijn JD. In vivo imaging of abdominal aortic aneurysms: increased FDG uptake suggests inflammation in the aneurysm wall. J Endovasc Ther. 2008;15(4):462–7.
104. Wasselius J, Malmstedt J, Kalin B, Larsson S, Sundin A, Hedin U, et al. High 18F-FDG uptake in synthetic aortic vascular grafts on PET/CT in symptomatic and asymptomatic patients. J Nucl Med. 2008;49(10):1601–5.
105. Xu XY, Borghi A, Nchimi A, Leung J, Gomez P, Cheng Z, et al. High levels of 18F-FDG uptake in aortic aneurysm wall are associated with high wall stress. Eur J Vasc Endovasc Surg. 2010;39(3):295–301.
106. Cavalcanti Filho JL, de Souza Leao Lima R, de Souza Machado Neto L, Kayat Bittencourt L, Domingues RC, da Fonseca LM. PET/CT and vascular disease: current concepts. Eur J Radiol. 2011;80(1):60–7.
107. Kitagawa T, Kosuge H, Chang E, James ML, Yamamoto T, Shen B, et al. Integrin-targeted molecular imaging of experimental abdominal aortic aneurysms by (18)F-labeled Arg-Gly-Asp positron-emission tomography. Circ Cardiovasc Imaging. 2013;6(6):950–6.
108. Najjar SS, Scuteri A, Lakatta EG. Arterial aging: is it an immutable cardiovascular risk factor? Hypertension. 2005;46:454–62.
109. Hansson GK. Inflammation, atherosclerosis, and coronary artery disease. N Engl J Med. 2005;352:1685–95.
110. Nilsson PM, Lurbe E, Laurent S. The early life origins of vascular ageing and cardiovascular risk: the EVA syndrome (review). J Hypertens. 2008;26:1049–57.
111. Nilsson PM, Boutouyrie P, Laurent S. Vascular aging: a tale of EVA and ADAM in cardiovascular risk assessment and prevention. Hypertension. 2009;54:3–10.
112. Nilsson PM, Boutouyrie P, Cunha P, Kotsis V, Narkiewicz K, Parati G, et al. Early vascular ageing in translation: from laboratory investigations to clinical applications in cardiovascular prevention. J Hypertens. 2013;8:1517–26.
113. Reference Values for Arterial Stiffness' Collaboration. Determinants of pulse wave velocity in healthy people and in the presence of cardiovascular risk factors: 'establishing normal and reference values'. Eur Heart J. 2010;31:2338–50.
114. Gottsäter M, Östling G, Persson M, Engström G, Melander O, Nilsson PM. Non-hemodynamic predictors of arterial stiffness after 17 years of follow-up: the Malmö Diet and Cancer study. J Hypertens. 2015 Jan 28. [Epub ahead of print] PubMed PMID: 25634451.

115. Nilsson PM. Genetic and environmental determinants of early vascular ageing (EVA). Curr Vasc Pharmacol. 2012;10:700–1.
116. International Consortium for Blood Pressure Genome-Wide Association Studies, Ehret GB, Munroe PB, Rice KM, Bochud M, Johnson AD, Chasman DI, Smith AV, et al. Genetic variants in novel pathways influence blood pressure and cardiovascular disease risk. Nature. 2011;478:103–9.
117. Tarasov KV, Sanna S, Scuteri A, Strait JB, Orrù M, Parsa A, et al. COL4A1 is associated with arterial stiffness by genome-wide association scan. Circ Cardiovasc Genet. 2009;2:151–8.
118. Ong KT, Delerme S, Pannier B, Safar ME, Benetos A, Laurent S, Boutouyrie P; investigators. Aortic stiffness is reduced beyond blood pressure lowering by short-term and long-term antihypertensive treatment: a meta-analysis of individual data in 294 patients. J Hypertens 2011;29:1034–42.
119. Laurent S, Mousseaux E, Boutouyrie P. Arterial stiffness as an imaging biomarker: are all pathways equal? Hypertension. 2013;62:10–2.
120. Vlachopoulos C, Aznaouridis K, Stefanadis C. Prediction of cardiovascular events and all-cause mortality with arterial stiffness: a systematic review and meta-analysis. J Am Coll Cardiol. 2010;55:1318–27.
121. Ben-Shlomo Y, Spears M, Boustred C, May M, Anderson SG, Benjamin EJ, et al. Aortic pulse wave velocity improves cardiovascular event prediction: an individual participant meta-analysis of prospective observational data from 17,635 subjects. J Am Coll Cardiol. 2014;63:636–46.
122. Van Bortel LM, Laurent S, Boutouyrie P, Chowienczyk P, Cruickshank JK, De Backer T, Artery Society, European Society of Hypertension Working Group on Vascular Structure and Function, European Network for Non-invasive Investigation of Large Arteries, et al. Expert consensus document on the measurement of aortic stiffness in daily practice using carotid-femoral pulse wave velocity. J Hypertens. 2012;30:445–8.

Part III

Small Arteries

Micromyography

10

Enrico Agabiti Rosei and Damiano Rizzoni

10.1 Introduction

The microcirculation represents the district of the vascular bed in which the major part of energy dissipation in order to overcome resistance occurs; it includes small arteries (diameter ranging from 100 to 300 μm), arterioles (diameter less than 100 μm) and the capillary network (diameter around 7 μm) [1] (Fig. 10.1). Small arteries probably contribute for about 30–50 % of pre-capillary blood pressure drop, while an additional 30 % drop occurs at the arteriolar level (50–100 μm) with a distribution of resistance that varies among different vascular beds and between species [2]. Figure 10.1 represents a typical but generic example of blood pressure drop in the vascular system, since pressure-diameter curves might differ in various tissues/organs.

In the different forms of experimental hypertension, an increased resistance to flow was actually observed at the microcirculatory level [3]. Structural, mechanical and functional changes in small vessels may determine a reduction of the internal lumen and, therefore, an increase in vascular resistance. This may directly induce an increase of systemic blood pressure. There is general agreement on the fact that essential hypertension is associated with the presence of structural alterations in the microcirculation [1–5]. An increase in the vascular wall thickness, together with a reduction in the internal diameter, may play a major role in the increased peripheral resistance, being also a possible adaptive mechanism to the increased blood pressure load.

E. Agabiti Rosei (✉) • D. Rizzoni
Department of Clinical and Experimental Sciences, Clinica Medica, University of Brescia, Piazzale Spedali Civili 1, Brescia 25121, Italy
e-mail: enrico.agabitirosei@unibs.it

E. Agabiti Rosei, G. Mancia (eds.), *Assessment of Preclinical Organ Damage in Hypertension*, DOI 10.1007/978-3-319-15603-3_10

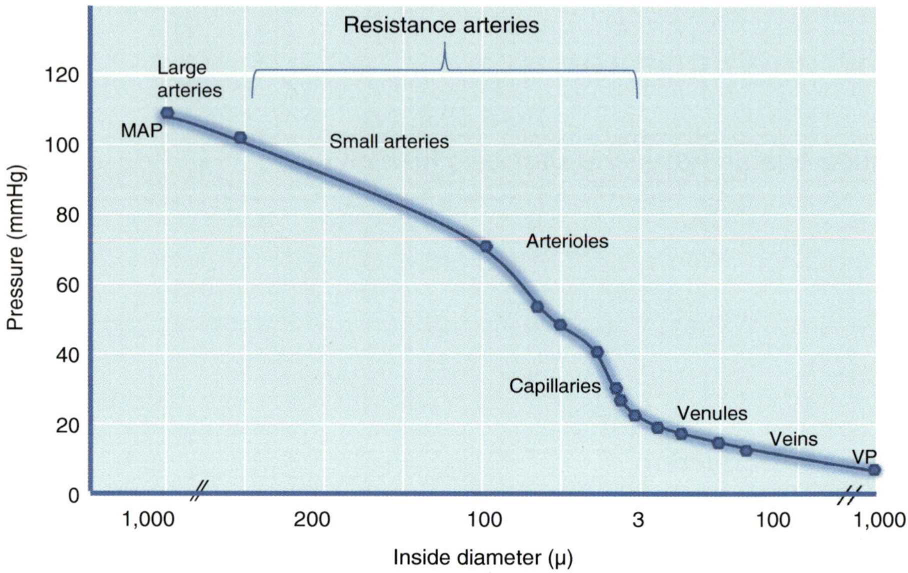

Fig. 10.1 Blood pressure drop in the vascular bed, from large, conductance arteries to veins (Redrawn from Ref. [1]). *MAP* mean arterial pressure, *VP* venous pressure

The mechanisms underlying the development of microvascular structural alterations are only partially elucidated [6–9]. However, if we recognise that structural alterations might have hemodynamic consequences, then their evaluation represents an important target, also in terms of cardiovascular risk stratification [8, 10].

10.2 Methods of Evaluation of Vascular Structural Alterations

The methods for the evaluation of microvascular structural alterations available in humans are relatively few (Table 10.1).

Histological approaches are charged with substantial pitfalls, due to the artefacts introduced by fixation, staining and dehydration with possible coarctation of the samples [1] (Table 10.1).

The methodological approach that has the widest application is represented by the wire or pressure micromyography that allows a reliable evaluation of structural changes within the vascular wall and of functional aspects as well (Table 10.1).

Wire micromyography (Fig. 10.2) was developed by Mulvany and Halpern [11, 12] in the 1970s, and it was subsequently applied to vascular segments (mesenteric, cerebral, coronary, renal, femoral, etc.) obtained from several animal models of hypertension. Interestingly enough, the wire micromyography technique was also

Table 10.1 Advantages and disadvantages of the commonly used techniques for assessment of functional and remodelling of small arteries

Technique	Advantage	Disadvantage
Histology	Easy to analyse; sample can be stored; inexpensive	Microinvasive; artefacts introduced by fixation, staining and dehydration; possible coarctation of the samples
Plethysmography	Easy access; inexpensive; evaluation of minimum vascular resistance in the forearm; drug challenge	Challenging to have good performance; need for standardisation, personnel training and setup
Wire and pressure micromyography	Well-standardised technique, evaluation of vascular morphology and function; evaluation of parameters with prognostic significance (media to lumen ratio) with high sensibility, specificity and accuracy; reliable and reproducible functional data (better evaluation with pressure micromyography) and morphological data (more precise with wire micromyography)	Microinvasive; well-trained personnel; bias related to mechanical damage of the vessel
Scanning laser Doppler flowmetry (retinal district)	Non-invasive; easy access to vascular district; correlates with parameters obtained with micromyography	Not extensively used; further validation and standardisation of the technique needed

used for the evaluation of morphology and function of small arteries obtained from biopsies of the subcutaneous tissue from the gluteal or anterior abdominal region, in normotensive subjects as well as in hypertensive patients [13, 14].

For this technique, small artery segments, diameter ranging from 100 to 300 μm, few millimetres long are obtained by dissection and made free of periadventitial fat tissue. Then the vessels are cannulated with stainless steel wires (40 micron of diameter), resulting in a ring preparation that is mounted on a micromyograph. A mechanical stretch may be applied through a micrometric screw while a force transducer records the passive tension developed, or the vessel may be maintained to a constant stretch and stimulated to contract by adding various substances to the organ bath, such as norepinephrine, potassium, serotonin, etc., thus allowing the measurements of the active tension developed. It is mandatory that the vessel is not damaged during dissection, cannulation and mounting procedures, inasmuch even minimum damage to the vessel's wall may translate into alterations in the contractile responses and in errors in the morphological evaluations as well.

Subsequently, the vessel, in a relaxed condition, is transferred on the stage of an immersion lens microscope, and through a micrometric ocular (magnitude about 600×), the total wall thickness as well as the relative thicknesses of the adventitia, media and intima tunica and the internal diameter are evaluated. Also cross-sectional areas and volumes may be calculated, together with the thicknesses of the different

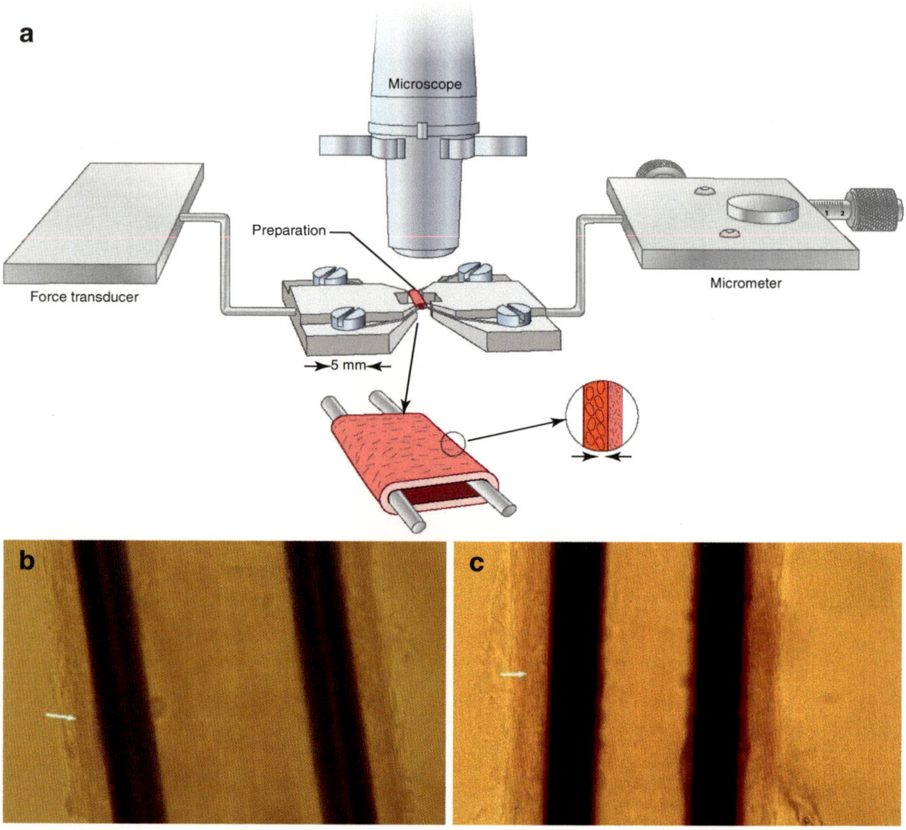

Fig. 10.2 Wire micromyography: drawing (**a**) and photo of subcutaneous small resistance arteries mounted on a wire micromyograph as a ring preparation (Mulvany's technique) (**b**, **c**). (**c**) Small artery of a normotensive subject. (**b**) Small artery of a hypertensive patient; the internal lumen is smaller and the media thickness slightly greater. The arrow indicates the boundary between the tunica media and the tunica adventitia. Vertical black areas: stainless steel wires used for cannulation

tunicae in normalised conditions; that is to say these thicknesses would be present in vivo with the vessels distended by a transmural pressure slightly less than 100 mmHg. It is therefore possible to obtain reliable and reproducible morphological data, overcoming many of the limitations related to histomorphological approaches [1].

The most relevant and useful parameter obtained with micromyographic approaches is represented by the tunica media to internal lumen ratio, since it appears independent from the vessel's dimensions [15, 16].

On the contrary, media thickness and internal diameters are obviously dependent on the dimensions of the vascular segment [15]; therefore comparisons between such parameters examined in different experiments may be problematic in the absence of a rigorous selection of the sampling site, which is not feasible in humans and sometimes difficult also in experimental animals.

Possibly, small mesenteric arteries of the rats represent the vascular district where it is possible to obtain vascular segments from anatomically well-defined positions: here the branching pattern allows an easy identification of small arteries of 1st, 2nd, 3rd and 4th level, until they enter the intestinal wall as arterioles with diameters of around 80 μm.

A possible alternative to the wire micromyography is represented by perfusion-pressure micromyography (Fig. 10.3). With this approach, isolated vessels are mounted in a pressurised myograph chamber and slipped into two glass microcannulae, connected to a perfusion system that allows a constant intraluminal pressure of 60 mmHg [17]. Morphology of the vessels is evaluated by computer-assisted video analysers. In a previous study, no difference was observed between wire or pressure micromyography in terms of morphological evaluations, provided that the vessels are analysed in comparable conditions [15, 18–20]. Vessels may be analysed at constant pressure or constant flow. It is likely that, when compared with wire micromyography, pressure micromyography allows a better evaluation of functional responses, while the precision of the morphological assessment could be slightly lower [15].

In a group of normotensive subjects and hypertensive patients, a close correlation between media to lumen ratio of subcutaneous small arteries, measured by wire micromyography, and forearm minimum vascular resistance, measured by plethysmography [14], was observed (see dedicated chapter). Thus, although the two methods seem to possess different characteristics (a direct, invasive in vitro ex vivo approach and an indirect, non-invasive in vivo technique), results obtained are in reasonable agreement. In summary, micromyographic in vitro studies have the advantage to allow a precise and accurate measurement of morphological features of small vessels, without the fixation artefacts related to histological studies, but have also the limitation of the relative invasiveness of the procedure. In fact, dissection and mounting of the single vessel on the pressure or wire micromyograph require the availability of adequate tissue (in humans usually obtained during a surgical procedure or by a biopsy of the subcutaneous fat tissue) [13, 14]. These subcutaneous or skin biopsies are small, ethically acceptable interventions which are tolerated well by patients and have been employed already for some time to study the structure of small arteries from hypertensive patients [18]. Biopsies of the gluteal region have been performed in two essentially equivalent ways [18]. After local anaesthesia has been administered, the classical way to perform these biopsies is to obtain a segment of skin from the upper external quadrant together with subcutaneous fat (Fig. 10.4). This allows vessels to be visualised from the inside of the skin, isolated from the subcutis as well as from the underlying subcutaneous fat [18]. An advantage is that the vessel diameter can be grossly evaluated and essentially equivalent vessels may be isolated from different patients, facilitating comparison of parameters since the arteries obtained are from essentially the same level of the vasculature. Another technique, used by Schiffrin and coll. [18], is simply to cut a horizontal incision 1 cm in length in the upper external gluteal quadrant. The superficial subcutaneous tissue and immediately underlying fat are excised carefully with a scalpel. No skin is removed, facilitating repeat procedures and rendering the intervention a smaller, less invasive and better tolerated one, with very little

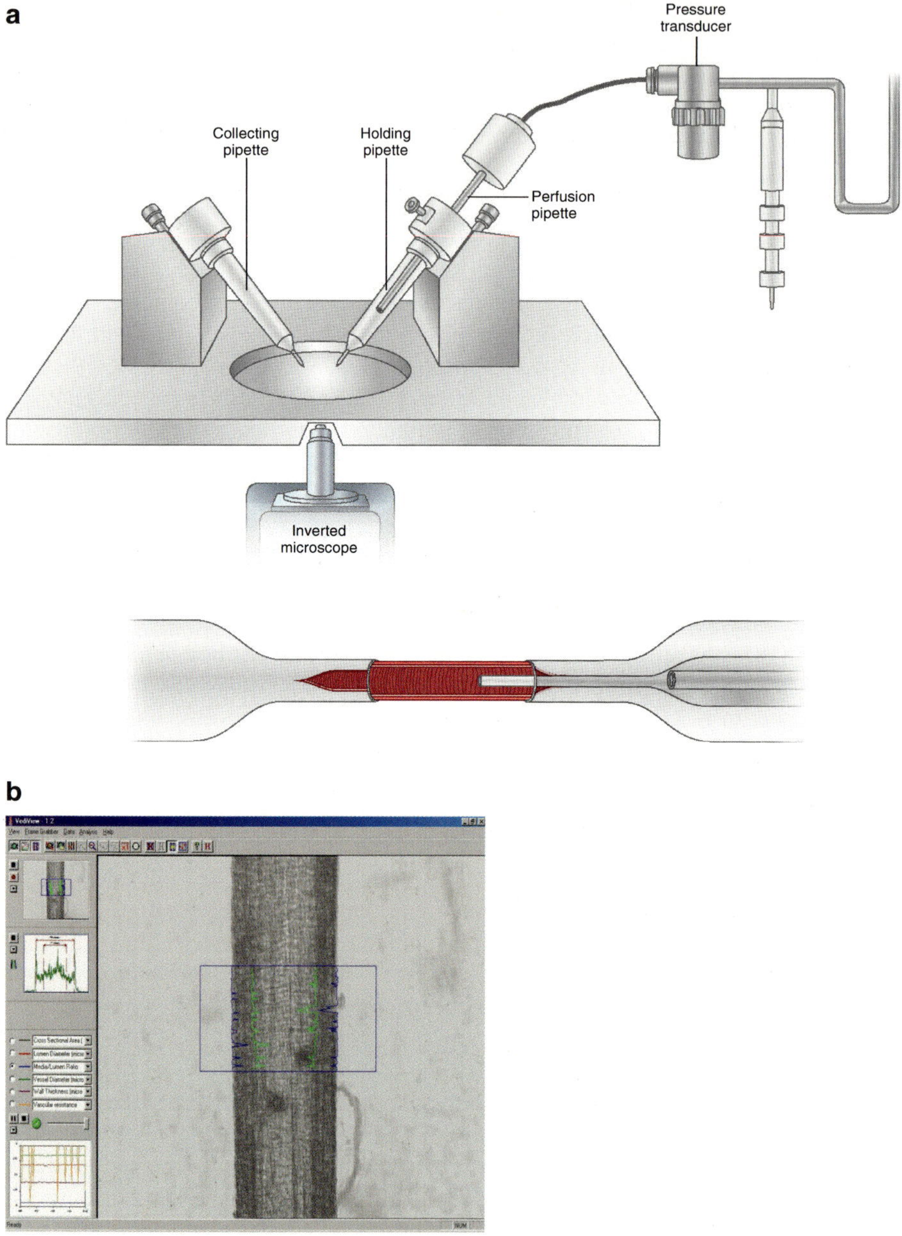

Fig. 10.3 Pressure micromyography: drawing (**a**) and image of a mounted vessel during measurement of vessel wall thickness (**b**)

residual discomfort and practically no opportunity for complication [18]. A disadvantage of this approach is that it is not known whether exactly comparable vessels have been dissected [18].

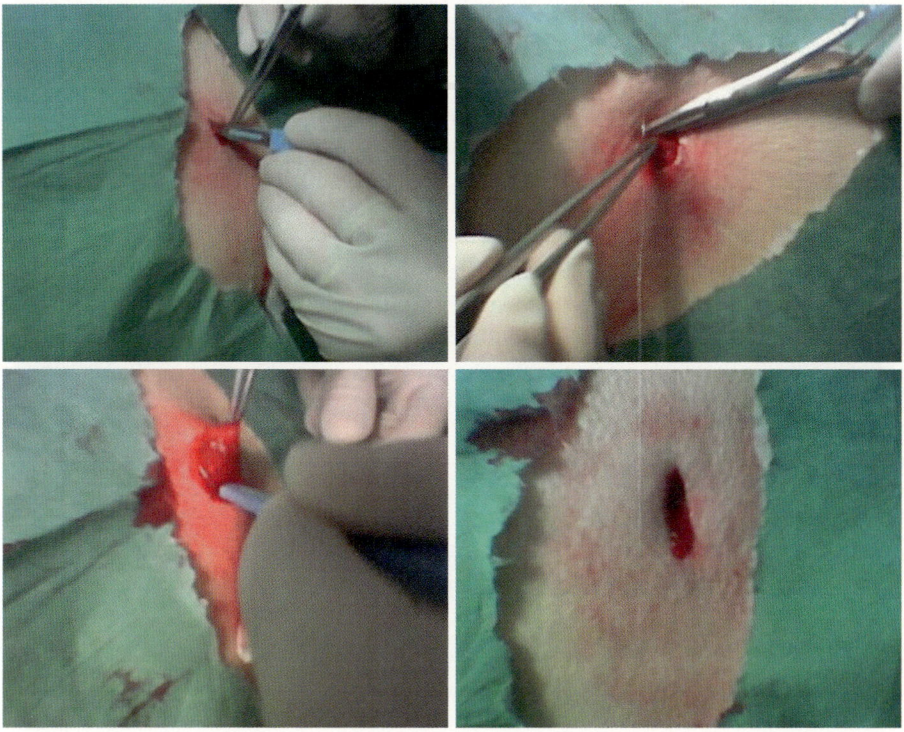

Fig. 10.4 Biopsy of subcutaneous fat obtained from the gluteal region: surgical approach

In summary, no method of evaluation of microvascular structure is ideal under all aspects (see also chapters on capillaroscopy and other methodological approaches). As previously mentioned, in contrast to animal studies, in which vessels can be chosen from equivalent levels of the vascular tree, in humans studies using subcutaneous biopsies, arteries may be sampled at slightly different levels of the vasculature [15]. This results in dissection of vessels showing random variations in external and luminal diameters, which challenges a reliable comparison of these parameters. However, if the measurement is restricted to the ratio between wall thickness and lumen (or media thickness/lumen), there is general agreement that the ratio is increased in hypertension, and this is the best available index of small resistance artery structure, being, in large part, as previously mentioned, independent from the vessels' dimensions [15, 18], highly reproducible and stable; it presents little drift over time, allowing reliable comparisons within subjects and between subjects [15, 18, 21]. Therefore, the wire or pressure micromyographic measurement of the media to lumen ratio is presently considered, due to sensitivity, specificity and accuracy, the gold standard for the evaluation of structural alterations of small resistance arteries in humans [18, 22, 23] (Table 10.1).

10.3 Vascular Structural Alterations as Evaluated by Micromyography, Organ Damage and Prognosis

An important consequence of the presence of an increased media to lumen ratio may be an impairment of vasodilator reserve. In fact, remodelling of small resistance arteries is characterised by a narrowing of the lumen, which leads to an increase of flow resistance even at full dilatation, i.e. in the absence of vascular tone. A significant correlation between coronary flow reserve and subcutaneous small resistance artery remodelling has been detected in hypertensive patients [24], suggesting that structural alterations in small resistance arteries may be present at the same time in different vascular districts, thus reflecting even clinically more important alterations in other vascular beds, including the coronary circulation. Therefore, alterations in the microcirculation may play an important role in the development of organ damage in hypertension.

The extent of structural alterations in subcutaneous small resistance arteries is particularly pronounced in hypertensive patients with type 2 diabetes mellitus [25] or obesity [17, 26, 27]. In particular, the administration of a selective angiotensin receptor blocker, in addition to other antihypertensive medications, results in an improvement of resistance artery remodelling in diabetic hypertensive patients but not in a full normalisation [28].

It seems therefore that the association of several cardiovascular risk factors may have a synergistic, deleterious effect on the microcirculation. Until a decade ago, no direct demonstration of a prognostic role of microvascular structural alterations, independently of blood pressure values, was available.

In a population of 150 normotensive subjects and hypertensive patients, some of them with concomitant diabetes mellitus, an assessment of subcutaneous small artery morphology by wire micromyography was performed [29]. The subjects were subdivided according to the presence of a media to lumen ratio of small arteries greater or smaller than the mean and median value observed in the whole population. After an average follow-up time of 6 years, a significant difference in event-free survival was observed between the subgroups, being the incidence of cardiovascular events greater in patients with greater media to lumen ratio. In fact, Cox's proportional hazard model, considering all known cardiovascular risk factors, indicated that only pulse pressure and media to lumen ratio were significantly associated to the occurrence of cardiovascular events [29]. These results strongly indicate a relevant prognostic significance of small resistance artery structural alterations in a high-risk population.

The results were confirmed in a larger population at lower global cardiovascular risk (more than 300 subjects and patients) [30], and similar data were also obtained by Mathiassen and coll. in a population of essential hypertensive patients [31].

More recently, Buus et al. [32] have demonstrated a prognostic role of changes of small resistance artery structure during antihypertensive treatment. This demonstration of the prognostic role of changes in microvascular structure during treatment, independently of the extent of blood pressure reduction, could substantially support the idea to consider microvascular structure as an intermediate end point in the evaluation of the benefits of antihypertensive treatment [32, 33].

References

1. Mulvany MJ, Aalkjaer C. Structure and function of small arteries. Physiol Rev. 1990;70:921–71.
2. Christensen KL, Mulvany MJ. Location of resistance arteries. J Vasc Res. 2001;38:1–12.
3. Folkow B. Physiological aspects of primary hypertension. Physiol Rev. 1982;62:347–504.
4. Schiffrin EL. Remodeling of resistance arteries in essential hypertension and effects of antihypertensive treatment. Am J Hypertens. 2004;17(12 Pt 1):1192–200.
5. De Ciuceis C, Rizzoni D, Agabiti Rosei C, Porteri E, Boari GEM, Agabiti RE. Remodelling of small resistance arteries in essential hypertension. High Blood Press. 2006;13:1–6.
6. Savoia C, Schiffrin EL. Inflammation in hypertension. Curr Opin Nephrol Hypertens. 2006;15:152–8.
7. Savoia C, Schiffrin EL. Vascular inflammation in hypertension and diabetes: molecular mechanisms and therapeutic interventions. Clin Sci (Lond). 2007;112(7):375–84.
8. Mulvany MJ. Structural abnormalities of the resistance vasculature in hypertension. J Vasc Res. 2003;40:558–60.
9. Callera G, Tostes R, Savoia C, Muscara MN, Touyz RM. Vasoactive peptides in cardiovascular (patho)physiology. Expert Rev Cardiovasc Ther. 2007;5(3):531–52.
10. Mulvany MJ. Small artery remodeling and significance in the development of hypertension. News Physiol Sci. 2002;17:105–9.
11. Mulvany MJ, Halpern W. Contractile properties of small resistance vessels in spontaneously hypertensive and normotensive rats. Circ Res. 1977;41(1):19–26.
12. Mulvany MJ, Hansen PK, Aalkjaer C. Direct evidence that the greater contractility of resistance vessels in spontaneously hypertensive rats is associated with a narrowed lumen, a thickened media, and an increased number of smooth muscle cell layers. Circ Res. 1978;43(6):854–64.
13. Aalkjaer C, Eiskjaer H, Mulvany MJ, Jespersen B, Kjaer T, Sorensen SS, Pedersen EB. Abnormal structure and function of isolated subcutaneous resistance vessels from essential hypertensive patients despite antihypertensive treatment. J Hypertens. 1989;7:305–10.
14. Agabiti-Rosei E, Rizzoni D, Castellano M, Porteri E, Zulli R, Muiesan ML, Bettoni G, Salvetti M, Muiesan P, Giulini SM. Media:lumen ratio in human small resistance arteries is related to forearm minimal vascular resistance. J Hypertens. 1995;13:341–7.
15. Schiffrin EL, Deng LY. Structure and function of resistance arteries of hypertensive patients treated with a beta-blocker or a calcium channel antagonist. J Hypertens. 1996;14:1247–55.
16. Endemann DH, Pu Q, De Ciuceis C, Savoia C, Virdis A, Neves MF, Touyz RM, Schiffrin EL. Persistent remodeling of resistance arteries in type 2 diabetic patients on antihypertensive treatment. Hypertension. 2004;43:399–404.
17. De Ciuceis C, Porteri E, Rizzoni D, Corbellini C, La Boria E, Boari GEM, Pilu A, Mittempergher F, Di Betta E, Casella C, Nascimbeni R, Agabiti Rosei C, Ruggeri G, Caimi L, Agabiti RE. Effects of weight loss on structural and functional alterations of subcutaneous small arteries in obese patients. Hypertension. 2011;58:29–36.
18. Schiffrin EL, Hayoz D. How to assess vascular remodelling in small and medium-sized muscular arteries in humans. J Hypertens. 1997;15:571–84.
19. Lew MJ. Wall stress and wall to lumen ratios differ between pressurised and myograph-mounted arteries. In: Mulvany MJ, Aalkjaer C, Heagerty AM, Nyborg NCB, Strandgaard S, editors. Resistance arteries: structure and function, Excerpta Medica. 1991. p. 353–6.
20. Falloon BJ, Stephens N, Tulip JR, Heagerty AM. Comparison of small artery sensitivity and morphology in pressurized and wire-mounted preparations. Am J Physiol. 1995;268(2 Pt 2):H670–8.
21. Schiffrin EL, Deng LY, Larochelle P. Effects of a beta-blocker or a converting enzyme inhibitor on resistance arteries in essential hypertension. Hypertension. 1994;23:83–91.
22. Rizzoni D, Aalkjaer C, De Ciuceis C, Porteri E, Rossini C, Rosei CA, Sarkar A, Agabiti RE. How to assess microvascular structure in humans. High Blood Press Cardiovasc Prev. 2011;18:169–77.

23. Rizzoni D, Agabiti-Rosei E. Structural abnormalities of small resistance arteries in essential hypertension. Intern Emerg Med. 2012;7:205–12.
24. Rizzoni D, Palombo C, Porteri E, Muiesan ML, Kozàkovà M, La Canna G, Nardi M, Guelfi D, Salvetti M, Morizzo C, Vittone F, Agabiti RE. Relationships between coronary vasodilator capacity and small artery remodeling in hypertensive patients. J Hypertens. 2003;21:625–32.
25. Rizzoni D, Porteri E, Guelfi D, Muiesan ML, Valentini U, Cimino A, Girelli A, Rodella L, Bianchi R, Sleiman I, Agabiti RE. Structural alterations in subcutaneous small arteries of normotensive and hypertensive patients with non insulin dependent diabetes mellitus. Circulation. 2001;103:1238–44.
26. Grassi G, Seravalle G, Scopelliti F, Dell'Oro R, Fattori L, Quarti-Trevano F, Brambilla G, Schiffrin EL, Mancia G. Structural and functional alterations of subcutaneous small resistance arteries in severe human obesity. Obesity (Silver Spring). 2010;18:92–8.
27. Grassi G, Seravalle G, Brambilla G, Facchetti R, Bolla G, Mozzi E, Mancia G. Impact of the metabolic syndrome on subcutaneous microcirculation in obese patients. J Hypertens. 2010;28:1708–14.
28. Savoia C, Touyz RM, Endemann DH, Pu Q, Ko EA, De Ciuceis C, Schiffrin EL. Angiotensin receptor blocker added to previous antihypertensive agents on arteries of diabetic hypertensive patients. Hypertension. 2006;48(2):271–7.
29. Rizzoni D, Porteri E, Boari GEM, De Ciuceis C, Sleiman I, Muiesan ML, Castellano M, Miclini M, Agabiti-Rosei E. Prognostic significance of small artery structure in hypertension. Circulation. 2003;108:2230–5.
30. De Ciuceis C, Porteri E, Rizzoni D, Rizzardi N, Paiardi S, Boari GEM, Miclini M, Zani F, Muiesan ML, Donato F, Salvetti M, Castellano M, Tiberio GAM, Giulini SM, Agabiti RE. Structural alterations of subcutaneous small arteries may predict major cardiovascular events in hypertensive patients. Am J Hypertens. 2007;20:846–52.
31. Mathiassen ON, Buus NH, Sihm I, Thybo NK, Mørn B, Schroeder AP, Thygesen K, Aalkjaer C, Lederballe O, Mulvany MJ, Christensen KL. Small artery structure is an independent predictor of cardiovascular events in essential hypertension. J Hypertens. 2007;25:1021–6.
32. Buus NH, Mathiassen ON, Fenger-Grøn M, Præstholm MN, Sihm I, Thybo NK, Schroeder AP, Thygesen K, Aalkjær C, Pedersen OL, Mulvany MJ, Christensen KL. Small artery structure during antihypertensive therapy is an independent predictor of cardiovascular events in essential hypertension. J Hypertens. 2013;31:791–7.
33. Mulvany MJ. Small artery remodelling in hypertension. Basic Clin Pharmacol Toxicol. 2012;110:49–55.

Damage of Retinal Arterioles in Hypertension

11

Christian Ott and Roland E. Schmieder

Hypertension causes alterations in vascular structure and function. Structural changes in small arterioles can be diverged to two different patterns: first eutrophic remodeling characterized by a rearrangement of the smooth muscle cells around a narrowed lumen but without growth response (meaning that media cross-sectional area remains unchanged) and second hypertrophic remodeling, a growth response with increment of media cross-sectional area observed in patients with long-standing and/or severe hypertension [1]. Regardless of the pattern, both are characterized by an increased wall-to-lumen ratio (WLR).

The analysis of retinal vessels offers the exceptional opportunity to assess directly and noninvasively human microvasculature in vivo. In the last years several methods have been introduced for the assessment of retinal changes. Since this book is proposed as a practical approach guiding the reader in the assessment, the focus is on the most established methods, namely, funduscopy and scanning laser Doppler flowmetry (SLDF).

11.1 Assessment of the Retinal Arterioles

For a long time, direct ophthalmoscopic examination using the traditional four-grade classification system with increasing severity (Table 11.1, Fig. 11.1) introduced by Keith, Wagener, and Barker [1], modified by Scheie [3], was regarded as part of standard evaluation of patients suffering from hypertension [4]. Nowadays, its clinical usefulness in current clinical practice has been questioned due to its

C. Ott • R.E. Schmieder (✉)
Department of Nephrology and Hypertension, University Hospital of the Friedrich-Alexander, University Erlangen-Nürnberg, Ulmenweg 18, Erlangen 91054, Germany
e-mail: christian.ott@uk-erlangen.de; roland.schmieder@uk-erlangen.de

E. Agabiti Rosei, G. Mancia (eds.), *Assessment of Preclinical Organ Damage in Hypertension*, DOI 10.1007/978-3-319-15603-3_11

Table 11.1 Keith-Wagener-Barker classification

Grade	Features
1	Mild generalized retinal arteriolar narrowing
2	Definite focal narrowing and arteriovenous nipping
3	Signs of grade 2 retinopathy plus retinal hemorrhages, exudates, and cotton wool spots
4	Severe grade 3 retinopathy plus papilledema

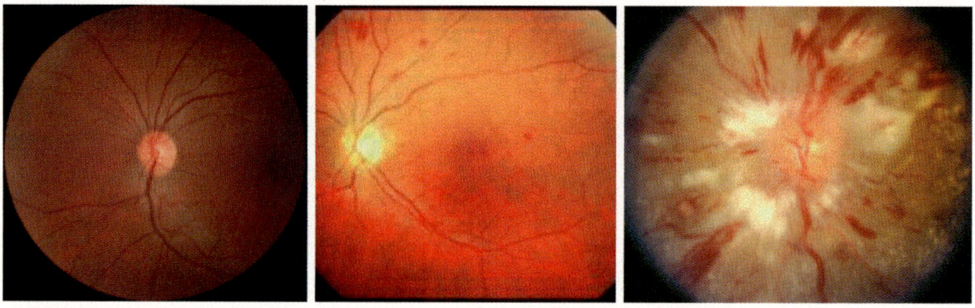

Fig. 11.1 Funduscopic changes (e.g., cotton wool) (Republished from Ott and Schmieder [2])

unreliable reproducibility [5], and hence routine funduscopic examination is no longer recommended [6]. Reliable assessment was only shown for advanced alterations like hemorrhages and exudates referring to at least grade 3 [7].

11.1.1 Funduscopy

In the last decade several approaches have been developed, assessing more sensitive and quantitative alterations of retinal microvascular changes. Although protocols may differ in some minor points, the principles are similar. According to standardized protocols, one (e.g., 45°) nonstereoscopic color retinal photograph centered between the optic disk and the macula and approximately two disk diameters nasal to the optic disk has to be done in a darkened room. Hence, due to dark adaption, mydriatic agents are no longer necessary. However, in some studies (e.g., Rotterdam Study), pharmacological mydriasis was routinely done. For quantitative assessment of retinal vessels, the photographs have to be converted to digital pictures and analyzed by specific imaging software, e.g., the "Interactive Vessels Analysis" (IVAN) (University of Wisconsin, Madison, WI, USA). This software analysis provides semiautomated measurement of retinal arterioles and venules. Using formulas (e.g., Parr and Spears [8] or Knudtson et al. [9]), a single "central retinal artery equivalent (CRAE)" and a "central retinal vein equivalent (CRVE)" are calculated. Subsequently, arteriole-to-venule ratio (AVR) can be computed; for details see Hubbard et al. [10]. However, by this method, it is not possible to evaluate the retinal vascular wall thickness or vessel diameter directly.

11.1.2 Scanning Laser Doppler Flowmetry

SLDF, introduced by our study group about 10 years ago, allows the dynamic assessment of both functional (i.e., vascular tone) and structural parameters (i.e., wall and lumen diameter). In brief, SLDF is performed in the juxtapapillary area of the right eye, 2–3 mm temporal superior of the optic nerve at 670 nm (Heidelberg Retina Flowmeter, Heidelberg Engineering, Germany). A retinal sample of $2.56 \times 0.64 \times 0.30$ nm is scanned within 2 s (at least one full systolic and one diastolic phase) and measured every 10 μm of this specific length of the retinal arteriole (80–140 μm). The confocal technique of the device ensures that only capillary flow of the superficial layer of 300 μm is measured. No pupil dilation is necessary (i.e., no constriction of patient daily routine) [11].

For assessment of functional parameters, mean retinal capillary flow (RCF) is assessed in the area of interest, and for further dynamic analysis, non pharmacological and pharmacological tools can be applied. Flicker light increases RCF at least in part via a nitric oxide (NO)-dependent mechanism and represents a non pharmacological tool to investigate vasodilatory capacity of retinal arterioles. It is noteworthy to mention that flicker light exposure has no effects on systemic blood pressure (BP), thereby minimizing potential systemic hemodynamic influences on RCF. Moreover, basal NO activity can be assessed by administration of the NO synthase inhibitor N^G-monomethyl-L-arginine (L-NMMA).

For assessment of structural parameters, the outer arteriole diameter (AD) is measured by reflection images, and the lumen diameter (LD) is measured by perfusion images. From the raw parameters, wall thickness (WT, [AD–LD]/2), WLR ([AD–LD]/LD) (Fig. 11.2), and wall cross-sectional area (WCSA, $\pi/4 \times [AD^2 - LD^2]$) can be calculated.

Importantly, also individual pulsatile pattern of functional (RCF) and structural (e.g., WT) parameters of retinal arterioles in systole and diastole can be reliably assessed (Fig. 11.2).

All analyses are performed offline with automatic full-field perfusion imaging analysis (AFFPIA) (SLDF Version 4.0 by Welzenbach with improved resolution) [11].

11.2 Prevalence and Incidence (General Population, Hypertension)

11.2.1 Funduscopy

Several population-based studies have provided data on prevalence of retinal signs using standardized funduscopic photographs in the general population, partly with subsequent categorization according to (among others) hypertension status. In general, retinal signs are common in people aged 40 years or older, even in those without arterial hypertension. However, these findings can only be respected with caution, since different definitions of arterial hypertension have been used.

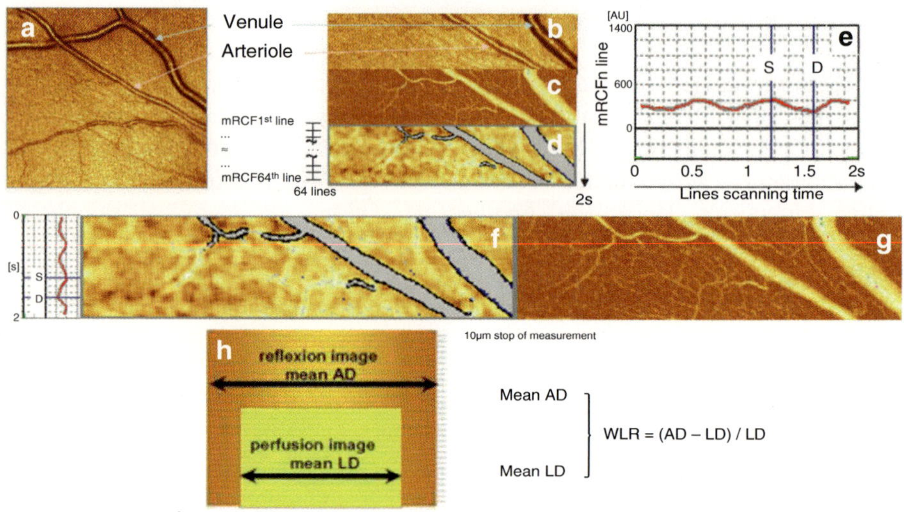

Fig. 11.2 Scanning laser Doppler flowmetry (SLDF) (Republished from Ott and Schmieder [2]). (**a**) Differentiation between retinal arteriole and venule (SLDF live image before measurement). (**b**) Scanned area – reflection image. (**c**) Scanned area – perfusion image. (**d**) Scanned area – corrected and analyzed flow image. (**e**) Pulse curve run as mean retinal capillary flow (*RCF*) and time plot. (**f**) Localization of systolic and diastolic RCF on the image (**d**). (**g**) Localization of systolic and diastolic RCF on the image (**c**). (**h**) Calculation of wall-to-lumen ratio

Moreover, the reported prevalence of retinal signs depends also largely on the assessed parameter, e.g., retinopathy per se, AV nicking, or focal/generalized arteriolar narrowing (for details see Table 11.2).

In the Cardiovascular Health Study (CHS) (aged ≥65 years), 16.6 % (men 19.7 %; women 14.3 %) of normotensive participants and 25.4 % (men 30.0 %; women 23.0 %) of hypertensive patients (defined as BP ≥140/90 mmHg or history of hypertension with use of antihypertensive drugs) were reported to have generalized arteriolar narrowing (defined as the lowest twentieth percentile of AVR). In contrast, retinopathy was by far less frequently documented in this study, i.e., in 5.6 % (men 4.7 %; women 6.3 %) of normotensive participants and in 10.4 % (men 7.5 %; women 11.9 %) of hypertensive patients [16]. Confirmatory results were found in the Beijing study (aged ≥ 40 years), which also used the accepted criteria of hypertension (BP ≥140/90 mmHg or history of hypertension with use of antihypertensive drugs) [19]. Moreover, in the former study another important point was found, namely, differences in the prevalence of retinal signs according gender [16].

Other influencing factors are age and ethnicity. In the Blue Mountains Eye Study (BMES) [14] and the Atherosclerosis Risk in Communities (ARIC) Study [20], the prevalence of retinopathy increased with advancing age, whereas in the CHS only some retinal signs revealed an age-dependent relationship [16]. Regarding ethnicity, an enhanced prevalence of retinopathy was suggested in Afro-Caribbeans compared to Europeans, but in this study the use of standardized protocols was not clearly

Table 11.2 Prevalence/incidence of retinal signs in normotensive and hypertensive populations using funduscopy

Study	Ref.	Ethnicity	Year	Sample	Age	FU	BP definition	Retinal signs	Prevalence	Incidence normo-/hypertensive people
London, England	[12]	White (Afro-Caribbean)	1995	1,164	40–64	–	≥160/95 mmHg or use of drugs	Keith classification	8 (13)/32 (31) (men)	
									8 (20)/18 (28) (women)	
Beaver Dam Eye Study (BDES)	[13]	White	1997	3,115	43–86	5	≥160/95 mmHg or use of drugs	Focal art. narrowing		7.7/15.2
								Retinopathy[a]		4.6/9.2
Blue Mountains Eye Study (BMES)	[14]	White	1998	3,275	≥49	–	≥160/95 mmHg or use of drugs	Retinopathy[a]	8.6/12.5 (men)	
									7.4/12.6 (women)	
	[15]		2006	1,725		5	≥140/90 mmHg or use of drugs	Retinopathy[a]		8.2/10.4
Cardiovascular Health Study (CHS)	[16]	White, black	2003	2,050	≥65	–	≥140/90 mmHg or use of drugs	Retinopathy[a]	4.7/7.5 (men)	
									6.3/11.9 (women)	
								Focal art. narrowing	5.3/7.2 (men)	
									6.7/15.0 (women)	
								AV nicking	5.8/8.0 (men)	
									6.0/9.6 (women)	
								General. art. narrowing	19.7/30.0 (men)	
								(Lowest 20 % of AVR)	14.3 /23.0 (women)	
Atherosclerosis Risk in Communities (ARIC) Study	[17]	White, black	2003	9,734	51–72	–	≥140/90 mmHg or use of drugs	Retinopathy[a]	3.6/5.3 (whites)	
									5.9/9.1 (blacks)	
Hoorn Study	[18]	White	2003	176	50–74	9.4	≥160/95 mmHg or use of drugs	Retinopathy[a]		6.1/20.0
Beijing Eye Study	[19]	Chinese	2009	3,322	≥40	–	≥140/90 mmHg or use of drugs	Focal art. narrowing	6.2/12.1	
								AV nicking	6.1/12.3	
								General. art. narrowing (lowest 25 % of AVR)	14.6/25.4	

[a](Among others) presence of microaneurysm, hemorrhage, or hard exudate or occurred in combination of cotton wool exudates, venous banding, intraretinal microvascular abnormalities

outlined [12]. In the ARIC study higher prevalence of retinopathy has been documented in blacks compared to whites [17]; however this difference was largely explained by the severity of hypertension.

Much less data are available addressing the frequency of new retinal signs. In the Beaver Dam Eye Study (BDES), the 5-year incidence of focal arteriolar narrowing was 7.7 % and of retinopathy 4.6 %, respectively, in normotensive (BP <160/95 mmHg) participants. Both incidences were about doubled in hypertensive patients [13]. In contrast, in the BMES the 5-year incidence for retinopathy was numerically higher in normotensive (BP <140/90 mmHg) subjects (8.2 %) but not clearly increased in hypertensive subjects (10.4 %) [15]. On the other hand, there is good evidence from several epidemiological studies that retinal alterations (i.e., generalized arteriolar narrowing) precedes the development of hypertension (Table 11.3), as a preclinical marker of hypertension.

11.2.2 Scanning Laser Doppler Flowmetry

Large epidemiological studies addressing prevalence and incidence of functional and structural microvascular alterations assessed with SLDF are lacking. Regarding RCF, similar values were found in young hypertensive patients compared to normotensive controls, which was confirmed by findings of an unaltered RCF between middle-aged patients with and without hypertension [49, 50]. Moreover, mean RCF was found to be similar in patients with hypertension stage 1–2 compared to patients with advanced stage of hypertensive disease, e.g., patients with treatment-resistant hypertension (TRH). However, by analyzing the individual pulsatile pattern of RCF in latter both groups, we were able to demonstrate a different pattern. RCF in systole was higher, whereas RCF in diastole was lower, and hence an exaggerated pulsed RCF (difference in RCF between systole and diastole) in patients with TRH was observed compared to patients with hypertension stage 1–2 [51].

Regarding structural parameters, small (monocentric) studies point toward similar findings as seen with funduscopy, namely, an increment of retinal alterations (e.g., WLR) with increased BP [52]. Moreover, a pooled analysis comprising ≥500 patients suggests an increased WLR with aging (Schmieder RE, Ott C, unpublished data). Prevalence and incidence rates of retinal alterations assessed by SLDF are difficult to describe since no thresholds values for the parameters are yet established.

11.3 Change with Treatment (Criteria for Significant Change, Incidence During Treatment)

11.3.1 Funduscopy

It was repeatedly shown that initiating effective antihypertensive therapy resulted in disappearance of severe (grade III and IV) hypertensive retinopathy [53, 54]. In a case report of a 34-year-old woman with a short history of hypertension, headache,

Table 11.3 Large-scale, population-based studies (in alphabetical order) assessing associations between retinal vascular caliber (based on retinal photography) and blood pressure, target-organ damage, and cardiovascular risk (in chronological order)

Study	Ref.	Country	Ethnicity	Year	Sample size	Retinal vascular	Finding
Atherosclerosis Risk in Communities (ARIC) Study	[21]	USA	White, black	1999	9,300	AVR ↓	Past and current blood pressure
	[22]			2001	10,358	AVR ↓	Incident stroke
	[23]			2002	9,648	AVR ↓	Incident CHD, acute MI (only in women)
	[24]			2004	5,628	AVR ↓	Incident hypertension
	[25]		(Only) black	2008	1,439	CRAE ↓	Left ventricular hypertrophy
						AVR ↓	Left ventricular hypertrophy
	[26]		White, black	2010	10,496	CRAE ↓	Incident lacunar stroke
						CRVE ↑	Incident lacunar stroke
Beaver Dam Eye Study (BDES)	[27]	USA	White	2003	1,611	AVR ↓	CV mortality (43–74 years)
	[28]			2003	4,926	CRAE ↓	Current blood pressure
						AVR ↓	Current blood pressure
	[29]			2004	2,451	AVR ↓	Incident hypertension
	[30]			2007	4,926	CRAE ↓	CHD death
						CRVE ↑	CHD death

(continued)

Table 11.3 (continued)

Study	Ref.	Country	Ethnicity	Year	Sample size	Retinal vascular	Finding
Blue Mountains Eye Study (BMES)	[31]	Australia	White	2003	3,654	CRAE ↓	Current blood pressure
						CRVE ↓	Current blood pressure
						AVR ↓	Current blood pressure
	[32]			2004	2,335	CRAE ↓	Past and current systolic/diastolic blood pressure
						AVR ↓	Past diastolic and current systolic/diastolic blood pressure
	[33]			2004	1,319	CRAE ↓	Incident severe hypertension
						AVR ↓	Incident severe hypertension
	[34]			2006	3,654	CRVE ↑	CHD death (men and women, 49–75 years)
						CRAE ↓	CHD death (women, 49–75 years)
						AVR ↓	CHD death (women, 49–75 years)
Cardiovascular Health Study (CHS)	[35]	USA	White, black	2002	2,405	CRAE ↓	Past and current blood pressure
						AVR ↓	Current blood pressure
	[36]			2006	1,992	CRAE ↓	Incident CHD
						CRVE ↑	Incident CHD and stroke
						AVR ↓	Incident CHD
Multi-Ethnic Study of Atherosclerosis, (MESA)	[37]	USA	White, Hispanics, black, Chinese	2006	5,979	CRAE ↓	Current blood pressure
	[38]			2009	2,583	CRAE ↓	Incident hypertension
						CRVE ↑	Incident hypertension
	[39]			2011	4,594	CRAE ↓	Incident CKD stage 3 (only whites)

Rotterdam Study	[40]	Netherlands	White	2004	5,674	CRAE ↓	Current blood pressure
						CRVE ↓	Current blood pressure
						AVR ↓	Current blood pressure
	[41]			2006	1,900	CRAE ↓	Incident hypertension
						CRVE ↓	Incident hypertension
						AVR ↓	Incident hypertension
	[42]			2006	5,540	CRVE ↑	Incident stroke, cerebral infarction
	[43]			2010	5,518	CRVE ↑	Incident stroke, cerebral infarction, intracerebral hemorrhage
Singapore Malay Eye Study (SiMES)	[44]	Singapore	Malay	2008	3,019	CRAE ↓	Current blood pressure
	[45]			2009	2,581	CRAE ↓	Prevalent CKD and micro-/macroalbuminuria
Singapore Prospective Study Program (SP2)	[46]	Singapore	Chinese, Malay, Indian	2009	3,749	CRAE ↓	Current blood pressure
						CRVE ↑	Current blood pressure
						AVR ↓	Current blood pressure
	[47]			2009	3,602	CRAE ↓	Prevalent CKD
Sydney Childhood Eye Study	[48]	Australia	White, Chinese, and others	2007	1,572	CRAE ↓	Current blood pressure

Republished from Ott and Schmieder [2]

AVR arteriole-to-venule ratio, ratio of the summary indexes of the averaged arteriolar and venular width, *CRAE* central retinal artery equivalent, summary index of the averaged arteriolar width, *CRVE* central retinal vein equivalent, summary index of the averaged venular width and blurred vision, all indicative of malignant hypertension (her BP was 240/150 mmHg), funduscopic examination found swelling of the optic disk, widespread hemorrhages, and soft and hard exudates, consistent with grade IV or malignant hypertensive retinopathy, respectively. Antihypertensive treatment was initiated, and 10 months follow-up revealed a good BP control (110/70 mmHg). In accordance, funduscopy demonstrated an improvement of hypertensive retinopathy [55]. In a small cohort ($n = 28$), comprising previously untreated men with hypertension stage 1–2, scored (0–4) funduscopic changes were evaluated before and after 26 weeks of treatment with enalapril or hydrochlorothiazide, respectively. Both treatments resulted in a significant BP reduction but numerically higher after enalapril (−14.3 vs. −7.1 mmHg) compared to hydrochlorothiazide without reaching significant difference. Treatment with enalapril reduced numerically but nonsignificantly the frequency of arteriolar narrowing and arteriovenous crossing, whereas no changes were seen after treatment with hydrochlorothiazide [56].

Whether these observed changes are associated with improved cardiovascular (CV) and cerebrovascular prognosis remains to be determined. Indirect evidence comes from epidemiological studies. For example, in the BMES prevalence of hemorrhages and/or microaneurysm was comparable between normotensive and controlled (BP <160/95 mmHg) hypertensive men but not in women [14]. A subsequent sub-analysis of BMES revealed that prevalence of focal arteriolar narrowing was similar between normotensive (4.6 %) and controlled (BP <160/95 mmHg) hypertensive subjects (6.5 %), whereas its prevalence was more than doubled in treated uncontrolled (14.5 %) and untreated (15.3 %) hypertensive patients. In contrast, generalized arteriolar narrowing (narrowest quintile of AVR) was similarly prevalent in treated and controlled (22.0 %), treated and uncontrolled (22.5 %), and untreated hypertensive (27.2 %) patients but significantly greater compared to normotensive subjects (17.0 %) [57].

Thus, in contrast to data on improvement or even disappearance of qualitative hypertensive retinal abnormalities (e.g., papilledema, exudates), data are much less clear for quantitative retinal signs (e.g., arteriolar narrowing). On the other hand, generalized retinal arteriolar narrowing and AV nicking appear to be (irreversible) markers of mild to moderate hypertension, related not only to current and past BP levels but to cerebrovascular diseases as well [58].

11.3.2 Scanning Laser Doppler Flowmetry

Again data are limited with SLDF compared to funduscopy and are based on small studies only. Data with SLDF revealed that endothelial function (basal NO activity) was impaired in young hypertensive patients and improved after treatment with the angiotensin receptor blocker (ARB) candesartan [49], whereas no improvement was demonstrated in elderly hypertensive men after treatment with ARB valsartan [59]. Whether this discrepancy is related to the different ARB, different duration of therapy, or a potential irreversibility of vascular changes in the elderly patients is subject of ongoing investigations. Moreover, we were able to demonstrate that vasodilatory capacity (magnitude of vasodilation to flicker light) was lower in untreated hypertensive patients compared to normotensive controls, and systolic BP was inversely related to the percent increase of RCF due to flicker light exposure, independently of other CV risk factors [60]. Another study of our group suggests that BP and hence pulse pressure (PP) changes have an impact on pulsed RCF. In hypertensive patients with TRH, we observed a decrease of systolic and pulsed RCF 6 and 12 months after renal denervation (RDN), in parallel to decreases of BP and heart rate (HR). The reduction of pulsed RCF after RDN transfers into less shear stress on the vascular wall and, thereby, suggests an improvement of retinal (and potentially cerebral) microcirculation [61].

In a cross-sectional study, we observed that in treated hypertensive patients with BP control <140/90 mmHg, WLR was at the same level as observed in normotensive subjects but significantly lower than in treated hypertensive subjects with BP >140/90 mmHg [62]. Previously, two small prospective studies assessed the effect of antihypertensive treatment on retinal structural parameters using SLDF. In one study, hypertensive patients with non-insulin-dependent diabetes mellitus were treated with either aliskiren ($n=9$) or ramipril ($n=7$) for one year. To achieve equivalent BP control, open-label hydrochlorothiazide could be added, and hence only one patient in each group had BP ≥140/90 mmHg. Both treatment regimes resulted in a significant regression of retinal WLR after 1-year treatment without a difference between the groups [63]. In a second small unblinded study, hypertensive patients were treated with lercanidipine for 4 weeks and thereafter randomized to additional antihypertensive therapy with either enalapril ($n=10$) or hydrochlorothiazide ($n=10$) for 24 weeks. There was an improvement of WLR already after 4 weeks of treatment with lercanidipine alone, and only enalapril on top further reduced WLR (but not hydrochlorothiazide) [64]. Of note, both studies had small sample sizes, and surprisingly high values of WLR (>0.5) at baseline were reported. The reduction of WLR of about 50 % in both studies is very high in comparison to changes observed after treatment in analyses relying on the assessment in vascular remodeling of subcutaneous small arteries [65]. In a double-blind randomized study comprising in total of 40 patients with mild to moderate hypertension, treatment with manidipine or amlodipine for 4 weeks resulted not in any significant changes in WLR compared to baseline values (Ott et al., unpublished data). Overall data are sparse, and to clarify the effects of various antihypertensive agents on reversal of WLR, multicenter double-blind randomized studies with large number of patients are required.

11.4 Prognostic Value of Change

11.4.1 Funduscopy

No data are available whether treatment-induced regression of retinal alterations is related with reduction of other target-organ damages (e.g., left ventricular hypertrophy) or incident CV outcomes. So far, only epidemiological studies uniformly found that qualitative retinal signs of hypertensive retinopathy are related with incidence of CV disease. In accordance, quantitative retinal vascular caliber was associated with BP, target-organ damage, and CV disease (Table 11.2). Cross-sectional studies also indicated that the prevalence in retinal signs differs between normotensive, treated and controlled, treated and uncontrolled, and never-treated hypertensive patients. Thus, in addition to our pathophysiological understanding of vascular remodeling and its consequences, there seems to be a strong rationale that treatment-induced changes may also result in an improved CV outcome.

11.4.2 Scanning Laser Doppler Flowmetry

No prospective study analyzing the effects of treatment changes of retinal alterations assessed by SLDF, and hence its prognostic significance, is available. Again, at least indirect evidence exists that is based on findings of media-to-lumen ratio of subcutaneous small arterioles (measured with a myograph ex vivo) and cross-sectional studies.

In an Italian study ($n = 126$) with an averaged follow-up of 5.4 years including both patients with primary and secondary hypertension (e.g., pheochromocytoma) as well as normotensive subjects, an increment of subcutaneous media-to-lumen ratio was predictive of a diminished event-free survival [66]. Subsequent analysis, with an increased study population ($n = 303$) and a mean follow-up of 6.9 years, revealed that increased media-to-lumen ratio was of prognostic significance with regard to adverse CV and cerebrovascular outcome [67]. Accordingly, a Danish study comprising 159 patients with primary hypertension and moderate CV risk reported that media-to-lumen ratio was an independent predictor for the incidence of CV outcome even after adjustment of the Heart Score level over the follow-up of 4.6 years [68]. Recently, it was shown in a long-term follow-up survey (comprising 124 hypertensive patients) that after 9–12 months of antihypertensive treatment, SBP was reduced from 164 ± 15 to 134 ± 14 mmHg, which was accompanied by an regression of media-to-lumen ratio of subcutaneous small arteries (0.084 ± 0.03 vs. 0.075 ± 0.02, $p < 0.01$). Importantly, in the subsequent follow-up period of 15 years, the extent of the reduction in the media-to-lumen ratio of subcutaneous small arteries was demonstrated to be an independent predictor of CV events [69].

The relevance of these data on subcutaneous small arteries for retinal arteriolar changes comes from the nowadays recognized concept that changes seen in the small subcutaneous small arterioles are reflecting alterations seen also in other vascular beds. Indeed, Rizzoni et al. have previously demonstrated that WLR assessed by SLDF (retinal arterioles in vivo) and media-to-lumen ratio measured with myograph (subcutaneous small arteries taken from a biopsy) showed close correlation in hypertensive subjects ($r = 0.80$, $p < 0.001$), suggesting that SLDF may provide similar information about microcirculation alterations compared to subcutaneous small arteries [68].

References

1. Keith NM, Wagener HP, Barker NW. Some different types of essential hypertension: their course and prognosis. Am J Med Sci. 1939;197:332–43.
2. Ott C, Schmieder RE. Retinal circulation in arterial disease. In: Berbari A, Mancia G, editors. Arterial disorders. Springer; 2015.
3. Scheie HG. Evaluation of ophthalmoscopic changes of hypertension and arteriolar sclerosis. AMA Archiv Ophthalmol. 1953;49:117–38.
4. Guidelines Subcommittee. 1999 World Health Organization-International Society of Hypertension guidelines for the management of hypertension. J Hypertens. 1999;17:151–83.
5. Dimmitt SB, West JN, Eames SM, Gibson JM, Gosling P, Littler WA. Usefulness of ophthalmoscopy in mild to moderate hypertension. Lancet. 1989;1:1103–6.
6. Mancia G, Fagard R, Narkiewicz K, et al. 2013 ESH/ESC Guidelines for the management of arterial hypertension: the Task Force for the management of arterial hypertension of the European Society of Hypertension (ESH) and of the European Society of Cardiology (ESC). J Hypertens. 2013;31:1281–357.
7. van den Born BJ, Hulsman CA, Hoekstra JB, Schlingemann RO, van Montfrans GA. Value of routine funduscopy in patients with hypertension: systematic review. BMJ. 2005;331:73.
8. Parr JC, Spears GF. General caliber of the retinal arteries expressed as the equivalent width of the central retinal artery. Am J Ophthalmol. 1974;77:472–7.
9. Knudtson MD, Lee KE, Hubbard LD, Wong TY, Klein R, Klein BE. Revised formulas for summarizing retinal vessel diameters. Curr Eye Res. 2003;27:143–9.
10. Hubbard LD, Brothers RJ, King WN, et al. Methods for evaluation of retinal microvascular abnormalities associated with hypertension/sclerosis in the Atherosclerosis Risk in Communities Study. Ophthalmology. 1999;106:2269–80.
11. Harazny JM, Raff U, Welzenbach J, et al. New software analyses increase the reliability of measurements of retinal arterioles morphology by scanning laser Doppler flowmetry in humans. J Hypertens. 2011;29:777–82.
12. Sharp PS, Chaturvedi N, Wormald R, McKeigue PM, Marmot MG, Young SM. Hypertensive retinopathy in Afro-Caribbeans and Europeans. Prevalence and risk factor relationships. Hypertension. 1995;25:1322–5.
13. Klein R, Klein BE, Moss SE. The relation of systemic hypertension to changes in the retinal vasculature: the Beaver Dam Eye Study. Trans Am Ophthalmol Soc. 1997;95:329–48; discussion 348–50.
14. Yu T, Mitchell P, Berry G, Li W, Wang JJ. Retinopathy in older persons without diabetes and its relationship to hypertension. Arch Ophthalmol. 1998;116:83–9.
15. Cugati S, Cikamatana L, Wang JJ, Kifley A, Liew G, Mitchell P. Five-year incidence and progression of vascular retinopathy in persons without diabetes: the Blue Mountains Eye Study. Eye. 2006;20:1239–45.
16. Wong TY, Klein R, Sharrett AR, et al. The prevalence and risk factors of retinal microvascular abnormalities in older persons: The Cardiovascular Health Study. Ophthalmology. 2003;110:658–66.
17. Wong TY, Klein R, Duncan BB, et al. Racial differences in the prevalence of hypertensive retinopathy. Hypertension. 2003;41:1086–91.
18. van Leiden HA, Dekker JM, Moll AC, et al. Risk factors for incident retinopathy in a diabetic and nondiabetic population: the Hoorn study. Arch Ophthalmol. 2003;121:245–51.
19. Wang S, Xu L, Jonas JB, et al. Major eye diseases and risk factors associated with systemic hypertension in an adult Chinese population: the Beijing Eye Study. Ophthalmology. 2009;116:2373–80.
20. Klein R, Sharrett AR, Klein BE, et al. Are retinal arteriolar abnormalities related to atherosclerosis?: The Atherosclerosis Risk in Communities Study. Arterioscler Thromb Vasc Biol. 2000;20:1644–50.

21. Sharrett AR, Hubbard LD, Cooper LS, et al. Retinal arteriolar diameters and elevated blood pressure: the Atherosclerosis Risk in Communities Study. Am J Epidemiol. 1999;150:263–70.
22. Wong TY, Klein R, Couper DJ, et al. Retinal microvascular abnormalities and incident stroke: the Atherosclerosis Risk in Communities Study. Lancet. 2001;358:1134–40.
23. Wong TY, Klein R, Sharrett AR, et al. Retinal arteriolar narrowing and risk of coronary heart disease in men and women. The Atherosclerosis Risk in Communities Study. JAMA. 2002;287:1153–9.
24. Wong TY, Klein R, Sharrett AR, et al. Retinal arteriolar diameter and risk for hypertension. Ann Intern Med. 2004;140:248–55.
25. Tikellis G, Arnett DK, Skelton TN, et al. Retinal arteriolar narrowing and left ventricular hypertrophy in African Americans. The Atherosclerosis Risk in Communities (ARIC) study. Am J Hypertens. 2008;21:352–9.
26. Yatsuya H, Folsom AR, Wong TY, et al. Retinal microvascular abnormalities and risk of lacunar stroke: Atherosclerosis Risk in Communities Study. Stroke J Cerebral Circ. 2010;41:1349–55.
27. Wong TY, Klein R, Nieto FJ, et al. Retinal microvascular abnormalities and 10-year cardiovascular mortality: a population-based case-control study. Ophthalmology. 2003;110:933–40.
28. Wong TY, Klein R, Klein BE, Meuer SM, Hubbard LD. Retinal vessel diameters and their associations with age and blood pressure. Invest Ophthalmol Vis Sci. 2003;44:4644–50.
29. Wong TY, Shankar A, Klein R, Klein BE, Hubbard LD. Prospective cohort study of retinal vessel diameters and risk of hypertension. BMJ. 2004;329:79.
30. Wang JJ, Liew G, Klein R, et al. Retinal vessel diameter and cardiovascular mortality: pooled data analysis from two older populations. Eur Heart J. 2007;28:1984–92.
31. Leung H, Wang JJ, Rochtchina E, et al. Relationships between age, blood pressure, and retinal vessel diameters in an older population. Invest Ophthalmol Vis Sci. 2003;44:2900–4.
32. Leung H, Wang JJ, Rochtchina E, Wong TY, Klein R, Mitchell P. Impact of current and past blood pressure on retinal arteriolar diameter in an older population. J Hypertens. 2004;22:1543–9.
33. Smith W, Wang JJ, Wong TY, et al. Retinal arteriolar narrowing is associated with 5-year incident severe hypertension: the Blue Mountains Eye Study. Hypertension. 2004;44:442–7.
34. Wang JJ, Liew G, Wong TY, et al. Retinal vascular calibre and the risk of coronary heart disease-related death. Heart. 2006;92:1583–7.
35. Wong TY, Hubbard LD, Klein R, et al. Retinal microvascular abnormalities and blood pressure in older people: the Cardiovascular Health Study. Br J Ophthalmol. 2002;86:1007–13.
36. Wong TY, Kamineni A, Klein R, et al. Quantitative retinal venular caliber and risk of cardiovascular disease in older persons: the cardiovascular health study. Arch Intern Med. 2006;166:2388–94.
37. Wong TY, Islam FM, Klein R, et al. Retinal vascular caliber, cardiovascular risk factors, and inflammation: the multi-ethnic study of atherosclerosis (MESA). Invest Ophthalmol Vis Sci. 2006;47:2341–50.
38. Kawasaki R, Cheung N, Wang JJ, et al. Retinal vessel diameters and risk of hypertension: the Multiethnic Study of Atherosclerosis. J Hypertens. 2009;27:2386–93.
39. Yau JW, Xie J, Kawasaki R, et al. Retinal arteriolar narrowing and subsequent development of CKD Stage 3: the Multi-Ethnic Study of Atherosclerosis (MESA). Am J Kidney Dis Off J Nat Kidney Found. 2011;58:39–46.
40. Ikram MK, de Jong FJ, Vingerling JR, et al. Are retinal arteriolar or venular diameters associated with markers for cardiovascular disorders? The Rotterdam Study. Invest Ophthalmol Vis Sci. 2004;45:2129–34.
41. Ikram MK, Witteman JC, Vingerling JR, Breteler MM, Hofman A, de Jong PT. Retinal vessel diameters and risk of hypertension: the Rotterdam Study. Hypertension. 2006;47:189–94.
42. Ikram MK, de Jong FJ, Bos MJ, et al. Retinal vessel diameters and risk of stroke: the Rotterdam Study. Neurology. 2006;66:1339–43.

43. Wieberdink RG, Ikram MK, Koudstaal PJ, Hofman A, Vingerling JR, Breteler MM. Retinal vascular calibers and the risk of intracerebral hemorrhage and cerebral infarction: the Rotterdam Study. Stroke J Cerebral Circ. 2010;41:2757–61.
44. Sun C, Liew G, Wang JJ, et al. Retinal vascular caliber, blood pressure, and cardiovascular risk factors in an Asian population: the Singapore Malay Eye Study. Invest Ophthalmol Vis Sci. 2008;49:1784–90.
45. Sabanayagam C, Shankar A, Koh D, et al. Retinal microvascular caliber and chronic kidney disease in an Asian population. Am J Epidemiol. 2009;169:625–32.
46. Jeganathan VS, Sabanayagam C, Tai ES, et al. Effect of blood pressure on the retinal vasculature in a multi-ethnic Asian population. Hypertension Res Off J Jpn Soc Hypertens. 2009;32:975–82.
47. Sabanayagam C, Tai ES, Shankar A, Lee J, Sun C, Wong TY. Retinal arteriolar narrowing increases the likelihood of chronic kidney disease in hypertension. J Hypertens. 2009;27:2209–17.
48. Mitchell P, Cheung N, de Haseth K, et al. Blood pressure and retinal arteriolar narrowing in children. Hypertension. 2007;49:1156–62.
49. Delles C, Michelson G, Harazny J, Oehmer S, Hilgers KF, Schmieder RE. Impaired endothelial function of the retinal vasculature in hypertensive patients. Stroke J Cerebral Circ. 2004;35:1289–93.
50. Ritt M, Harazny JM, Ott C, et al. Analysis of retinal arteriolar structure in never-treated patients with essential hypertension. J Hypertens. 2008;26:1427–34.
51. Harazny JM, Ott C, Raff U, et al. First experience in analysing pulsatile retinal capillary flow and arteriolar structural parameters measured noninvasively in hypertensive patients. J Hypertens. 2014;32:2246–52; discussion 2252.
52. Ott C, Raff U, Harazny JM, Michelson G, Schmieder RE. Central pulse pressure is an independent determinant of vascular remodeling in the retinal circulation. Hypertension. 2013;61:1340–5.
53. Kirkendall WM, Armstrong ML. Vascular changes in the eye of the treated and untreated patient with essential hypertension. Am J Cardiol. 1962;9:663–8.
54. Bock KD. Regression of retinal vascular changes by antihypertensive therapy. Hypertension. 1984;6:III158–62.
55. Strachan MW, McKnight JA. Images in clinical medicine. Improvement in hypertensive retinopathy after treatment of hypertension. New Engl J Med. 2005;352:e17.
56. Dahlof B, Stenkula S, Hansson L. Hypertensive retinal vascular changes: relationship to left ventricular hypertrophy and arteriolar changes before and after treatment. Blood Press. 1992;1:35–44.
57. Wang JJ, Mitchell P, Leung H, Rochtchina E, Wong TY, Klein R. Hypertensive retinal vessel wall signs in a general older population: the Blue Mountains Eye Study. Hypertension. 2003;42:534–41.
58. Wong TY, Klein R, Klein BE, Tielsch JM, Hubbard L, Nieto FJ. Retinal microvascular abnormalities and their relationship with hypertension, cardiovascular disease, and mortality. Surv Ophthalmol. 2001;46:59–80.
59. Oehmer S, Harazny J, Delles C, et al. Valsartan and retinal endothelial function in elderly hypertensive patients. Blood Press. 2006;15:185–91.
60. Ritt M, Harazny JM, Ott C, et al. Impaired increase of retinal capillary blood flow to flicker light exposure in arterial hypertension. Hypertension. 2012;60:871–6.
61. Ott C, Harazny JM, Schmid A, et al. Retinal microperfusion after renal denervation in treatment resistant hypertensive patients. Clin Res Cardiol. submitted.
62. Harazny JM, Ritt M, Baleanu D, et al. Increased wall:lumen ratio of retinal arterioles in male patients with a history of a cerebrovascular event. Hypertension. 2007;50:623–9.
63. De Ciuceis C, Savoia C, Arrabito E, et al. Effects of a long-term treatment with aliskiren or ramipril on structural alterations of subcutaneous small-resistance arteries of diabetic hypertensive patients. Hypertension. 2014;64:717–24.
64. De Ciuceis C, Salvetti M, Rossini C, et al. Effect of antihypertensive treatment on microvascular structure, central blood pressure and oxidative stress in patients with mild essential hypertension. J Hypertens. 2014;32:565–74.

65. Agabiti-Rosei E, Heagerty AM, Rizzoni D. Effects of antihypertensive treatment on small artery remodelling. J Hypertens. 2009;27:1107–14.
66. Rizzoni D, Porteri E, Boari GE, et al. Prognostic significance of small-artery structure in hypertension. Circulation. 2003;108:2230–5.
67. De Ciuceis C, Porteri E, Rizzoni D, et al. Structural alterations of subcutaneous small-resistance arteries may predict major cardiovascular events in patients with hypertension. Am J Hypertens. 2007;20:846–52.
68. Rizzoni D, Porteri E, Duse S, et al. Relationship between media-to-lumen ratio of subcutaneous small arteries and wall-to-lumen ratio of retinal arterioles evaluated noninvasively by scanning laser Doppler flowmetry. J Hypertens. 2012;30:1169–75.
69. Buus NH, Mathiassen ON, Fenger-Gron M, et al. Small artery structure during antihypertensive therapy is an independent predictor of cardiovascular events in essential hypertension. J Hypertens. 2013;31:791–7.

Capillaroscopy

12

Enrico Agabiti Rosei, Carolina De Ciuceis, and Damiano Rizzoni

Capillaroscopy or intravital videomicroscopy is a noninvasive imaging technique that is used for in vivo assessment of the microcirculation [1] providing a 2-D projection of a 3-D capillary network. It generates high-contrast images, videotapes, or photographs of skin capillaries by means of television, video, and/or informatic systems. It allows the assessment of capillary morphology and capillary density (traditional capillaroscopy), capillary flow velocity (dynamic capillaroscopy), and capillary red cell column width [2]. It can also be employed in combination with sophisticated methods in order to measure red blood cell velocity, capillary pressure (i.e., cannulated capillaries using micropipettes and micropressure devices) [2, 3], and transcapillary diffusion (capillary permeability) in combination with intravenous administration of fluorescent dyes, such as sodium fluorescein or indocyanine green (fluorescence videomicroscopy or fluorescence angiography) in order to evaluate the heterogeneity of capillary flow distribution or to disclose structures that cannot be seen with traditional capillaroscopy (such as capillary aneurisms) [2], thus allowing comprehensive physiological and pharmacological studies in humans.

12.1 How to Perform

Capillaroscopy is often applied to the nail fold area of the fingers, where the capillaries run parallel to the skin surface and can be evaluated in their entire architecture; different microscope design may be used to study other areas of the body,

E. Agabiti Rosei (✉) • D. Rizzoni
Department of Clinical and Experimental Sciences, Clinica Medica, University of Brescia, Piazzale Spedali Civili 1, Brescia 25121, Italy
e-mail: enrico.agabitirosei@unibs.it

C. De Ciuceis
Department of Clinical and Experimental Sciences, University of Brescia, Piazzale Spedali Civili 1, Brescia 25121, Italy

E. Agabiti Rosei, G. Mancia (eds.), *Assessment of Preclinical Organ Damage in Hypertension*, DOI 10.1007/978-3-319-15603-3_12

including lips, tongue, and mouth [4]. Depending on the underlying investigated area, the capillaries will appear as black (or red in color imaging systems) dots (if they are perpendicular to the surface), lines (if the capillaries are lying on an oblique surface), or both. Red blood cells look black in capillaroscopy as the emission spectrum of the mercury lamp is similar to the absorption spectrum of hemoglobin (i.e., 370–450 nm) [2].

Capillaroscopy can be performed with various optical instruments, and it needs the correct magnification lens (usually from 40× to 300×) to enable wide or narrow field views. In clinical practice, skin capillaries are generally observed through an incident light microscope or videocapillaroscopic microcamera [5] (Fig. 12.1). Immersion oil is needed for better visibility of the capillaries. Once captured, images can be post-processed to enhance quality, quantitatively analyzed to calculate loop size and density, printed in a patient report, and archived.

It is performed at room temperature after 15–20 min of acclimatization of the patient in a sitting position on both hands from the second to the fifth finger [5]. The best examination conditions are usually found on the fourth finger. The nail folds at the toes can also be studied, albeit it does not provide equivalent diagnostic information compared to the other fingers [4].

From a structural point of view, the most interesting parameter to be analyzed by capillaroscopy is capillary density. Capillary density is defined as the number of capillaries per unit of skin area. It is measured recording images from the capillary microscope and counting the capillaries in a known skin area.

12.2 Clinical Application of Capillaroscopy

Capillaroscopy is conceptually a simple technique, but nevertheless it can provide valuable diagnostic information in the clinical microvascular setting. Indeed, capillaries play a critical role in cardiovascular function being responsible for nutrients and waste products exchange between the tissues and circulation [2]. Understanding their structure and physiology in health and disease is therefore very important.

The physiologic pattern of finger capillaries consists of homogeneous distribution of hairpin-like, parallel capillary loops with a mean length of 200–300 μm and a density of 9–14 capillaries/mm (average 10) [5]. However, capillaroscopic pattern in

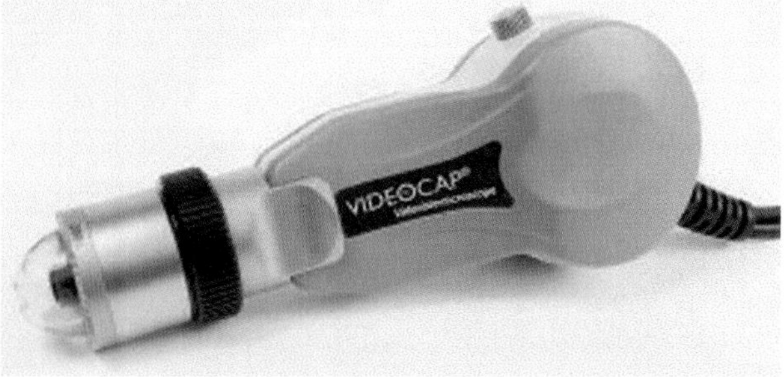

Fig. 12.1 Representative image of videocapillaroscope (Courtesy of DS Medica)

healthy subjects is characterized by a great inter- and intra-variability of findings [5, 6]. Irregularity in their capillary morphology and lower loop density than in adults have been observed in children, whereas old adults can progressively develop mild, nonspecific morphological changes including tortuosity and microaneurysms [7].

The main clinical application of capillaroscopy is in the rheumatologic field where it is of outstanding importance in patients with Raynaud's phenomenon and connective tissue diseases as well as in the early diagnosis and monitoring of systemic sclerosis. Systemic sclerosis is a multi-organ disease characterized by tissue fibrosis and immune/microvascular abnormalities. The most specific finding in this pathological condition is the so-called scleroderma pattern, characterized by the presence of dilated capillaries, hemorrhages, avascular areas, and neoangiogenesis [8]. In particular, the presence of giant capillaries and micro-hemorrhages on nail fold capillaries is sufficient to identify the "early" scleroderma pattern, and an increase in these features along with the progressive loss of capillaries (active pattern) is followed by neoangiogenesis, fibrosis, and "desertification" (late pattern) [5]. These different stages reflect the development of the disease processes and correlate with visceral involvement [9, 10]. In addition, capillaroscopy has been suggested to possess prognostic value in evaluation of the risk of developing systemic sclerosis in patients with Raynaud's phenomenon or digital ulcers in patients with systemic sclerosis [11].

Significant microangiopathy is also often present in patients with dermatomyositis, Sjogren's syndrome, systemic lupus erythematosus, and undifferentiated connective tissue disease, albeit the changes observed are often not specific [11].

Apart from rheumatologic diseases, changes in nail fold capillary morphology, including microaneurysms, apical dilatations, branching, and hemorrhagic extravasations, may be detected also in diabetes mellitus. The presence of a dilatation at the apex of loops is quite commonly observed in diabetes, but these changes do not seem to be related to disease duration [11].

Nonspecific nail fold microangiopathy has been also identified in several other conditions such as glaucoma, wound healing, including venous ulcer healing and critical limb ischemia [11].

In essential hypertension, many abnormalities are known to occur in the capillary circulation. These include capillary hypertension, increased looping, increased transcapillary filtration, and reduced capillary density [12–15]. Particularly, decreased capillary density, or rarefaction, is a consistent finding in patients with essential hypertension [15–18].

12.3 Microvascular Rarefaction in Hypertension

Vascular rarefaction may be defined either as a functional rarefaction, when the vessels are temporarily not perfused or "recruited," or an anatomical rarefaction, when vessels are actually missing. Many studies have reported microvascular rarefaction in some, but not all vascular beds in hypertensive animals; data available for humans are relatively scanty. A reduction of arteriolar (vessels smaller than

100 μm) and capillary number in skeletal muscle and other vascular beds of spontaneously hypertensive rats has been observed, together with a rarefaction of small vessels in the cremasteric muscle of renal hypertensive rats [19, 20]. A reduction of arteriolar and capillary density in conjunctival microcirculation of hypertensive patients has been also detected by direct visualization in vivo [14]. Similarly, a 20 % reduction of capillary density in the nail fold capillaries using capillary microscopy was observed [16].

Using the same technique, Antonios and other groups [15, 21–23] have demonstrated the presence of capillary rarefaction in the skin of fingers of patients with essential hypertension or borderline hypertension and also of normotensive offspring of patients with essential hypertension, suggesting that structural rarefaction seems to be due to a primary abnormality that antedates the onset of sustained hypertension, rather than being secondary to the elevation of blood pressure.

From a pathophysiological point of view, microvascular rarefaction increases peripheral vascular resistance, thereby increasing blood pressure and aggravating blood pressure-related target organ damage [24]. Indeed, not only the diameter of individual vessels but also the absolute number of perfused vessels contributes to total vascular resistance. A rarefaction of about 42 % of third order arterioles would increase tissue flow resistance by 21 % [25]. Moreover, a reduction in the microvascular network may decrease tissue perfusion [26] inducing a nonuniform distribution of microvascular flow among exchange vessels [25] and alterations of skeletal muscle perfusion and metabolism (i.e., oxygen uptake and insulin-mediated glucose uptake) [27].

In the last decades, direct intravital videomicroscopy has been widely used to investigate whether capillary rarefaction in essential hypertension is caused by a structural (anatomic) absence of capillaries or by functional non-perfusion secondary to severe vasoconstriction upstream [15]. As the visualization of capillaries, without using specific dyes, depends on the presence of red blood cells inside, standard capillaroscopy cannot directly show capillaries that are not perfused at resting conditions. Indeed, different methods have been assessed, such as venous congestion and postocclusive reactive hyperemia, in order to maximize the number of visible perfused capillaries during intravital capillary microscopy [15, 17, 28, 29].

In venous congestion, a miniature blood pressure cuff is applied to the base of the fourth finger of the nondominant hand, and the cuff is then inflated and maintained at 60 mmHg for 2 min. The consequent increase in venous back pressure allows to passively open up, and therefore to visualize, non-perfused and intermittently perfused capillaries. In reactive hyperemia, arterial blood flow in the forearm and hand is stopped for 3 min by inflating a sphygmomanometer cuff applied to the upper arm at 200 mmHg. The cuff is then deflated abruptly, and subsequent capillaroscopic images are obtained continuously usually for 15 s (up to 2 min). Differently from venous congestion, reactive hyperemia induces a vasodilator response possibly mediated by both myogenic and/or local chemical factors [30, 31]. Therefore, capillary density during venous congestion depends mainly on the anatomic number of capillaries [15, 29], whereas postocclusive reactive hyperemia may detect functional recruitment of initially non-perfused capillaries (microvascular reactivity) [28, 29, 32], thus reflecting both functional and structural factors [33]. In particular, it has been suggested [15, 23] that venous congestion allows to visualize a greater number of capillaries compared to postocclusive reactive hyperemia, making this technique probably the best method to maximize capillary number [29].

A reduction of capillary density at rest and after venous congestion [15] has been shown in hypertensive patients suggesting that much of the reduction in capillary density in these patients is due to the structural (anatomical) absence of capillaries, rather than to functional non-perfusion. However, no differences in capillary density at rest between normotensive and hypertensive subjects have been observed in other studies [17, 28]. In addition, hypertensive patients, as compared to normotensive subjects, show a decreased capillary recruitment after arterial occlusion [28] albeit this is not confirmed by all the studies [17]. Discrepancy of findings from different studies may be possibly due by the different definitions of capillary density in the resting condition and during postocclusive reactive hyperemia (capillary recruitment) depending on different periods for acquisition of images used in these studies [33].

Importantly, structural capillary rarefaction in the nail fold may suggest a generalized microvascular abnormality that may play a role in the pathogenesis of cardiovascular diseases. Indeed, patients with anginal chest pain and normal coronary arteriograms have significantly lower skin capillary density both at baseline and after maximization with venous congestion than matched healthy volunteers, independently on the presence of hypertension [34]. Accordingly, Pedrinelli and other groups [35–38] have demonstrated a significant higher minimal forearm vascular resistance during maximal postischemic vasodilation in patients with syndrome X compared to controls, indicating structural vasodilatory abnormalities. However, the pathophysiological importance of capillary rarefaction in these patients remains still unknown since a similar reduction of capillary density is present also in asymptomatic hypertensive patients.

Interestingly, also obese subjects show structural and functional alterations in skin microcirculation that are proportional to the degree of global and central obesity [39]. In addition, in obese subjects with metabolic syndrome, the cutaneous capillaries at rest are already maximally recruited, indicating an absence of functional capillary reserve. This may be related to the insulin resistance observed in obese individuals with metabolic syndrome [39]. Recently, the presence of microvascular rarefaction has been also detected in obese patients with or without concomitant increase of blood pressure values [40].

It is not presently known whether capillary rarefaction may possess a prognostic significance. Since a preliminary study suggests that microvascular rarefaction might be correlated with media/lumen ratio of small arteries [41], it is also possible that vascular changes at a more distal level might contribute to the higher incidence of cardiovascular events observed in hypertensive and/or diabetic patients.

References

1. Bollinger A, Fagrell B, editors. Clinical capillaroscopy: a guide to its use in clinical research and practice. Stuttgart: Hofgrefe & Huber Publishers; 1990.
2. Shore AC. Capillaroscopy and the measurement of capillary pressure. Br J Clin Pharmacol. 2000;50:501–13.
3. Morris SJ, Shore AC, Tooke JE. Responses of the skin microcirculation to acetylcholine and sodium nitroprusside in patients with NIDDM. Diabetologia. 1995;38:1337–44.
4. Allen J, Howell K. Microvascular imaging: techniques and opportunities for clinical physiological measurements. Physiol Meas. 2014;35:R91–141.
5. Cutolo M, Sulli A, Smith V. How to perform and interpret capillaroscopy. Best Pract Res Clin Rheumatol. 2013;27(2):237–48.
6. Ingegnoli F, Gualtierotti R, Lubatti C, Bertolazzi C, Gutierrez M, Boracchi P, Fornili M, De Angelis R. Nailfold capillary patterns in healthy subjects: a real issue in capillaroscopy. Microvasc Res. 2013;90:90–5.
7. Dolezalova P, Young SP, Bacon PA, Southwood TR. Nailfold capillary microscopy in healthy children and in childhood rheumatic diseases: a prospective single blind observational study. Ann Rheum Dis. 2003;62(5):444–9.
8. Lambova SN, Müller-Ladner U. The specificity of capillaroscopic pattern in connective autoimmune diseases. A comparison with microvascular changes in diseases of social importance: arterial hypertension and diabetes mellitus. Mod Rheumatol. 2009;19(6):600–5.
9. Chen ZY, Silver RM, Ainsworth SK, Dobson RL, Rust P, Maricq HR. Association between fluorescent antinuclear antibodies, capillary patterns, and clinical features in scleroderma spectrum disorders. Am J Med. 1984;77(5):812–22.
10. Cutolo M, Sulli A, Smith V. Assessing microvascular changes in systemic sclerosis diagnosis and management. Nat Rev Rheumatol. 2010;6(10):578–87.
11. Jung P, Trautinger F. Capillaroscopy. Minireview. J German Soc Dermatol. 2013;–:731–6.
12. Lack A. Biomicroscopy of conjunctival vessels in hypertension. Am Heart J. 1949;38:654–64.
13. Williams SA, Boolell M, MacGregor GA, Smaje LH, Wasserman SM, Tooke JE. Capillary hypertension and abnormal pressure dynamics in patients with essential hypertension. Clin Sci. 1990;79:5–8.
14. Harper RN, Moore MA, Marr MC, Watts LE, Hutchins PM. Arteriolar rarefaction in the conjunctiva of human essential hypertensives. Microvasc Res. 1978;16:369–72.
15. Antonios TFT, Singer DRJ, Markandu ND, Mortimer PS, MacGregor GA. Structural skin capillary rarefaction in essential hypertension. Hypertension. 1999;33:998–1001.
16. Gasser P, Buhler FR. Nailfold microcirculation in normotensive and essential hypertensive subjects, as assessed by video-microscopy. J Hypertens. 1992;10:83–6.
17. Draaijer P, de Leeuw PW, van Hooff JP, Leunissen KM. Nailfold capillary density in salt- sensitive and salt-resistant borderline hypertension. J Hypertens. 1993;11:1195–8.
18. Prasad A, Dunnill GS, Mortimer PS, MacGregor GA. Capillary rarefaction in the forearm skin in essential hypertension. J Hypertens. 1995;13:265–8.
19. Schiffrin EL. Reactivity of small blood vessels in hypertension: relation with structural changes. State of the art lecture. Hypertension. 1992;19(Suppl II):II1–9.
20. Struijker-Boudier HA, Agabiti Rosei E, Bruneval P, Camici PG, Christ F, Henrion D, Lévy BI, Pries A, Vanoverschelde JL. Evaluation of the microcirculation in hypertension and cardiovascular disease. Eur Heart J. 2007;28:2834–40.
21. Antonios TF, Singer DR, Markandu ND, Mortimer PS, MacGregor GA. Rarefaction of skin capillaries in borderline essential hypertension suggests an early structural abnormality. Hypertension. 1999;34(4 Pt 1):655–8.
22. Antonios TF, Rattray FM, Singer DR, Markandu ND, Mortimer PS, MacGregor GA. Rarefaction of skin capillaries in normotensive offspring of individuals with essential hypertension. Heart. 2003;89(2):175–8.
23. Noon JP, Walker BR, Webb DJ, Shore AC, Holton DW, Edwards HV, Watt GCM. Impaired microvascular dilatation and capillary rarefaction in young adults with a predisposition to high blood pressure. J Clin Invest. 1997;99:1873–9.

24. Humar R, Zimmerli L, Battegay E. Angiogenesis and hypertension: an update. J Hum Hypertens. 2009;23:773–82.
25. Greene AS, Tonellato PJ, Lui J, Lombard JH, Cowley Jr AW. Microvascular rarefaction and tissue vascular resistance in hypertension. Am J Physiol. 1989;256:H126–31.
26. Levy BI, Schiffrin EL, Mourad JJ, Agostini D, Vicaut E, Safar ME, Struijker-Boudier HA. Impaired tissue perfusion: a pathology common to hypertension, obesity, and diabetes mellitus. Circulation. 2008;118:968–76.
27. Clark MG, Colquhoun EQ, Rattigan S, Dora KA, Eldershaw TP, Hall JL, Ye J. Vascular and endocrine control of muscle metabolism. Am J Physiol. 1995;268:E797–812.
28. Serné EH, Gans ROB, Ter Maaten JC, Ter Wee PM, Donker AJM, Stehouwer CDA. Capillary recruitment is impaired in essential hypertension and relates to insulin's metabolic and vascular actions. Cardiovasc Res. 2001;49:161–8.
29. Antonios TFT, Rattray FE, Singer DRJ, Markandu ND, Mortimer PS, MacGregor GA. Maximization of skin capillaries during intravital video-microscopy in essential hypertension: comparison between venous congestion, reactive hyperaemia and core heat load test. Clin Sci. 1999;97:523–8.
30. Schubert R, Mulvany MJ. The myogenic response: established facts and attractive hypotheses. Clin Sci. 1999;96:313–26.
31. Johnson PC, Burton KS, Henrich H, Henrich U. Effect of occlusion duration on reactive hyperemia in sartorius muscle capillaries. Am J Physiol. 1976;230:715–9.
32. Serné EH, Stehouwer CDA, Ter Maaten JC, Ter Wee PM, Rauwerda JA, Donker AJM, Gans ROB. Microvascular function relates to insulin sensitivity and blood pressure in normal subjects. Circulation. 1999;99:896–902.
33. Serné EH, Gans RO, ter Maaten JC, Tangelder GJ, Donker AJ, Stehouwer CD. Impaired skin capillary recruitment in essential hypertension is caused by both functional and structural capillary rarefaction. Hypertension. 2001;38(2):238–42.
34. Antonios TF, Kaski JC, Hasan KM, Brown SJ, Singer DR. Rarefaction of skin capillaries in patients with anginal chest pain and normal coronary arteriograms. Eur Heart J. 2001;22(13):1144–8.
35. Pedrinelli R, Spessot M, Lorenzoni R, Marraccini P, L'Abbate A, Salvetti A, Camici P. Forearm vasodilatory capacity in patients with syndrome X: a comparison with normal and hypertensive subjects. J Hypertens Suppl. 1989;7(6):S92–3.
36. Sax FL, Cannon 3rd RO, Hanson C, Epstein SE. Impaired forearm vasodilator reserve in patients with microvascular angina. Evidence of a generalized disorder of vascular function? N Engl J Med. 1987;317(22):1366–70.
37. Buus NH, Bøttcher M, Bøttker HE, Sørensen KE, Nielsen TT, Mulvany MJ. Reduced vasodilator capacity in syndrome X related to structure and function of resistance arteries. Am J Cardiol. 1999;83(2):149–54.
38. Bøtker HE, Sonne HS, Sørensen KE. Frequency of systemic microvascular dysfunction in syndrome X and in variant angina. Am J Cardiol. 1996;78(2):182–6.
39. Francischetti EA, Tibirica E, da Silva EG, Rodrigues E, Celoria BM, de Abreu VG. Skin capillary density and microvascular reactivity in obese subjects with and without metabolic syndrome. Microvasc Res. 2011;81(3):325–30.
40. De Ciuceis C, Rossini C, Porteri E, La Boria E, Corbellini C, Mittempergher F, Di Betta E, Petroboni B, Sarkar A, Agabiti-Rosei C, Casella C, Nascimbeni R, Rezzani R, Rodella LF, Bonomini F, Agabiti-Rosei E, Rizzoni D. Circulating endothelial progenitor cells, microvascular density and fibrosis in obesity before and after bariatric surgery. Blood Press. 2013;22:165–72.
41. Paiardi S, Rodella LF, De Ciuceis C, Porteri E, Boari GEM, Rezzani R, Rizzardi N, Plato C, Tiberio GAM, Giulini SM, Rizzoni D, Agabiti Rosei E. Immunohistochemical evaluation of microvascular rarefaction in hypertensive humans and in spontaneously hypertensive rats. Clin Hemorheol Microcirc. 2009;42:259–68.

Other Techniques for the Assessment of Small Artery Damage in Hypertension

13

Damiano Rizzoni and Claudia Agabiti Rosei

13.1 Plethysmography

The evaluation of minimum vascular resistance in the forearm with a plethysmographic technique is one of the earliest methods employed for the assessment of the microcirculation. Maximum postischemic flow is indeed correlated with the ratio between wall thickness and internal lumen in resistance arterioles [1]. For such an evaluation, it is therefore mandatory that the vascular district investigated is at a real maximum vasodilatation. In humans, this may be obtained by a combination of ischemia, muscular effort and, possibly, heat. It is not possible to obtain maximal flow with pharmacological approaches, such as the administration of acetylcholine, isoproterenol, adenosine, or sodium nitroprusside [2, 3]. From the maximum postischemic blood flow, it is possible to calculate minimum vascular resistance, which represents an indirect index of microvascular structural alterations, with the additional advantage of an in vivo evaluation [2, 3]. The plethysmographic technique requires the occlusion of the brachial artery of the dominant arm, through the inflation of a sphygmomanometric bladder up to 300 mmHg for 13 min and then a dynamic exercise (20–30 handgrips against the resistance offered by a rubber ball). The arterial occlusion is rapidly removed, while venous occlusion is maintained (around 60 mmHg of pressure in the sphygmomanometric bladder). Arterial flow is measured every 10 s for 3 min by a mercury strain gauge, which evaluates the increased volume of the forearm. In the absence of venous backward flow, the increased forearm volume is proportional to the arterial flow. The mean blood pressure, evaluated with an invasive or noninvasive method, divided by maximum arterial flow, allows the calculation of minimum vascular resistance.

D. Rizzoni (✉) • C. Agabiti Rosei
Department of Clinical and Experimental Sciences, Clinica Medica,
University of Brescia, Piazzale Spedali Civili 1, Brescia 25121, Italy
e-mail: damiano.rizzoni@unibs.it

E. Agabiti Rosei, G. Mancia (eds.), *Assessment of Preclinical Organ Damage in Hypertension*, DOI 10.1007/978-3-319-15603-3_13

13.2 New Techniques of Evaluation of Microcirculation

Although the prognostic value of structural alterations in small subcutaneous arteries has been confirmed by two independent studies [4–6], according to the guidelines for the management of arterial hypertension of the European Society of Hypertension and of the European Society of Cardiology, "an increase in the wall-lumen ratio of small arteries can be measured in subcutaneous tissues obtained through gluteal biopsies. These measurements can demonstrate early alterations in diabetes and hypertension and have a predictive value for CV morbidity and mortality, but the invasiveness of the method makes this approach unsuitable for general use" [7].

Therefore, the development of new, noninvasive approaches for the evaluation of microvascular damage is needed. The interest of researchers was focused, in the last decade, on the retinal vascular district, since it represents the only microvascular bed that may be directly viewed with relatively simple approaches, such as an ophthalmoscope or a slit lamp [8]. Cerebral and retinal circulation share anatomic, physiological, and embryological features [9]. The same kind of structural alterations previously observed in subcutaneous small resistance arteries are also present in cerebral small arteries of hypertensive patients [10].

One of the first attempt to precisely quantify structural alterations of retinal microcirculation was made by Wong et al. [11]. By means of an automated computerized method, the authors have calculated the ratio between the arteriolar and venular external diameters (arteriolar to venular ratio (AVR)) in circular segments of the retina. Such a ratio resulted smaller in hypertensive patients compared with normotensive controls [11].

However, the prognostic significance of AVR is still controversial, since a correlation between AVR and incidence of cardiovascular events was detected only in women [11]. Furthermore, some studies have challenged the ability of the AVR to correctly stratify hypertensive patients according to the extent of target organ damage. Indeed, no relationship between quartiles of AVR and left ventricular mass, carotid artery intima-media thickness, or urinary albumin excretion was observed [12, 13].

An additional approach was proposed by Hughes et al. [14]. They demonstrated the possibility to quantify morphological changes in retinal vascular architecture by means of a dedicated software. In their study, essential hypertension was associated with an increase in the arteriolar length-to-diameter ratio [14]. There were also alterations in arteriolar morphology indicative of rarefaction, including a marked reduction in the number of terminal branches in essential hypertensive patients compared with normotensive subjects. These changes in the arteriolar network were exaggerated in patients with malignant hypertension [14]. The authors' conclusion was that "hypertension is associated with marked topological alterations in the retinal vasculature, and quantification of these changes may be a useful novel approach to the assessment of target organ damage in hypertension" [14]. The same authors have demonstrated that antihypertensive drugs might beneficially affect some of these parameters [15]. Presently, however, there are no data about relationships between these topological parameters and target organ damage or with structural

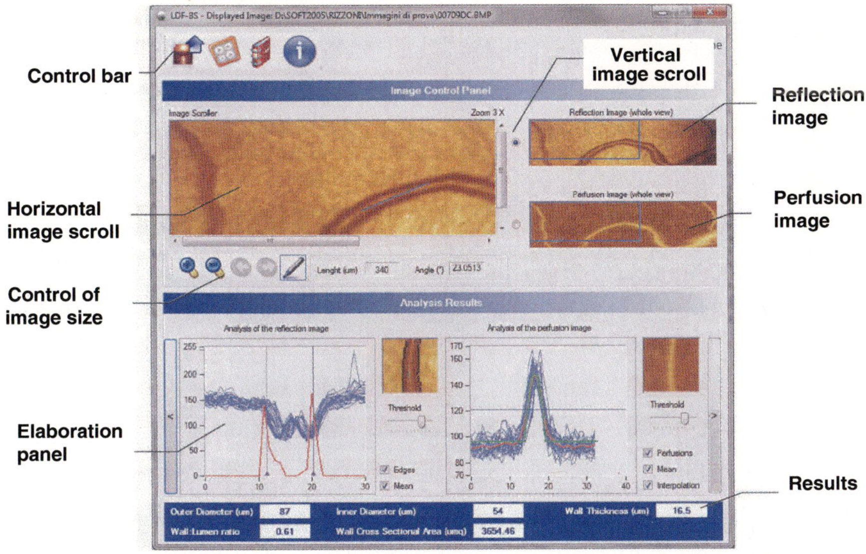

Fig. 13.1 Evaluation of small retinal artery morphology by scanning laser Doppler flowmetry and automatic full-field perfusion imaging analysis: example of the program output (Clinica Medica, University of Brescia; Reproduced from Rizzoni et al. [21], with permission)

alterations in other vascular beds; thus this approach, although stimulating and promising, needs further application and confirm.

More recently, Harazny et al. proposed a further, interesting and promising approach [16]. The method is based on the association between a confocal measurement of the external diameter of retinal arteriole and an evaluation of the internal diameter with a laser Doppler technique. The comparison between the two images, defined as "reflection image" and "perfusion image," is made by a dedicated software [16] (Fig. 13.1). From these two measurements, it is relatively easy to calculate the ratio between wall thickness and internal lumen (WL) [16]. The same authors, using this approach, based on a scanning laser Doppler flowmetry (Heidelberg Retinal Flowmeter, Heidelberg Engineering, Germany), could observe that WL is increased in untreated essential hypertensive patients compared with normotensive controls [17] and that an even more marked increase is present in hypertensive patients with a history of cerebrovascular event [16]. WL of retinal arterioles was closely related with blood pressure values [16], included those recorded on treatment [17]. Finally, a close relationship was observed between WL and urinary albumin excretion, a marker of the microvascular damage at the kidney level [18]. When WL and AVR of retinal vessels were evaluated in the same patients, only the first parameter was progressively higher comparing normotensives, treated hypertensives, and hypertensives with a history of a cerebrovascular event, and these differences closely paralleled those observed for carotid artery intima-media thickness [19]. Intraobserver and interobserved variation coefficients were quite satisfactory, being below 10 % [20].

A recent study compared in the same subjects WL of retinal arterioles evaluated with scanning laser Doppler flowmetry and media/lumen ratio of subcutaneous small resistance arteries evaluated by wire micromyography, which is commonly considered the reference approach for the measurement of structural alterations in the small vessels. A rather good agreement between the two techniques, with a Pearson's correlation index above 0.76, was observed [21].

Recent evidence, obtained by both micromyographic approaches [22], as well as by the evaluation of retinal arteriolar morphology by scanning laser Doppler flowmetry [23, 24], suggests that presence of structural alterations of small resistance arteries may be associated with the increase in large arteries stiffness and possibly contribute to an increase in central pressure by increasing the magnitude of wave reflections.

Conclusions

In experimental hypertension, the increase in peripheral resistance occurs at the microvascular level. It was clearly demonstrated that wall thickness is increased in relation to internal lumen and that this alteration contributes to peripheral resistance. The increased media/lumen ratio may impair organ flow reserve [25]. This may be important in the maintenance and, probably, also in the progressive worsening of hypertensive disease. The evaluation of microvascular structure is not an easy task. The techniques with highest accuracy, such as wire or pressure micromyography, have the limitation of requiring biological samples, obtained by surgical approaches (e.g., gluteal biopsies). However, the presence of structural alterations evaluated by such approaches represents a prognostically relevant factor, in terms of development of target organ damage or cardiovascular events, thus allowing the prediction of hypertension complications [26, 27].

New, noninvasive techniques are needed before suggesting extensive application of the evaluation of microvascular morphology for the cardiovascular risk stratification in hypertensive patients. Some new techniques for evaluation of microvascular morphology in the retina, presently under clinical investigation, seem to represent a promising and interesting future perspective.

Presently, we may safely state that the evaluation of microvascular structure is progressively moving from bench to bedside [28], and it could represent, in the immediate future, an evaluation to be performed in all hypertensive patients, in order to obtain a better stratification of cardiovascular risk, and perhaps, it might be considered as an intermediate end point in the evaluation of the effects of antihypertensive therapy [29, 30].

References

1. Agabiti-Rosei E, Rizzoni D, Castellano M, Porteri E, Zulli R, Muiesan ML, Bettoni G, Salvetti M, Muiesan P, Giulini SM. Media: lumen ratio in human small resistance arteries is related to forearm minimal vascular resistance. J Hypertens. 1995;13:341–7.
2. Pedrinelli R, Taddei S, Spessot M, Salvetti A. Maximal postischemic forearm vasodilation in human hypertension: a reassessment of the method. J Hypertens. 1987;5 Suppl 5:S431–3.

3. Pedrinelli R, Spessot M, Salvetti A. Reactive hyperemia during short-term blood flow and pressure changes in the hypertensive forearm. J Hypertens. 1990;8:467–71.
4. Rizzoni D, Porteri E, Boari GEM, De Ciuceis C, Sleiman I, Muiesan ML, Castellano M, Miclini M, Agabiti-Rosei E. Prognostic significance of small artery structure in hypertension. Circulation. 2003;108:2230–5.
5. De Ciuceis C, Porteri E, Rizzoni D, Rizzardi N, Paiardi S, Boari GEM, Miclini M, Zani F, Muiesan ML, Donato F, Salvetti M, Castellano M, Tiberio GAM, Giulini SM, Agabiti RE. Structural alterations of subcutaneous small arteries may predict major cardiovascular events in hypertensive patients. Am J Hypertens. 2007;20:846–52.
6. Mathiassen ON, Buus NH, Sihm I, Thybo NK, Mørn B, Schroeder AP, Thygesen K, Aalkjaer C, Lederballe O, Mulvany MJ, Christensen KL. Small artery structure is an independent predictor of cardiovascular events in essential hypertension. J Hypertens. 2007;25:1021–6.
7. Mancia G, Fagard R, Narkiewicz K, Redón J, Zanchetti A, Böhm M, Christiaens T, Cifkova R, De Backer G, Dominiczak A, Galderisi M, Grobbee DE, Jaarsma T, Kirchhof P, Kjeldsen SE, Laurent S, Manolis AJ, Nilsson PM, Ruilope LM, Schmieder RE, Sirnes PA, Sleight P, Viigimaa M, Waeber B, Zannad F, Task Force Members. 2013 ESH/ESC Guidelines for the management of arterial hypertension: the Task Force for the management of arterial hypertension of the European Society of Hypertension (ESH) and of the European Society of Cardiology (ESC). J Hypertens. 2013;31:1281–357.
8. Flammer J, Konieczka K, Bruno RM, Virdis A, Flammer AJ, Taddei S. The eye and the heart. Eur Heart J. 2013;34:1270–8.
9. Wong TY, Mitchell P. Hypertensive retinopathy. N Engl J Med. 2004;351:2310–7.
10. Rizzoni D, De Ciuceis C, Porteri E, Paiardi S, Boari GE, Mortini P, Cornali C, Cenzato M, Rodella LF, Borsani E, Rizzardi N, Platto C, Rezzani R, Agabiti RE. Altered structure of small cerebral arteries in patients with essential hypertension. J Hypertens. 2009;27:838–45.
11. Wong TY, Klein R, Sharrett AR, Duncan BB, Couper DJ, Tielsch JM, Klein BE, Hubbard LD. Retinal arteriolar narrowing and risk of coronary heart disease in men and women. The Atherosclerosis Risk in Communities Study. JAMA. 2002;287:1153–9.
12. Masaidi M, Cuspidi C, Giudici V, Negri F, Sala C, Zanchetti A, Grassi G, Mancia G. Is retinal arteriolar-venular ratio associated with cardiac and extracardiac organ damage in essential hypertension ? J Hypertens. 2009;27:1277–83.
13. Rizzoni D, Muiesan ML. Retinal vascular caliber and the development of hypertension: a meta-analysis of individual participant data. J Hypertens. 2014;32:225–7.
14. Hughes AD, Martinez-Perez E, Jabbar AS, Hassan A, Witt NW, Mistry PD, Chapman N, Stanton AV, Beevers G, Pedrinelli R, Parker KH, Thom SA. Quantification of topological changes in retinal vascular architecture in essential and malignant hypertension. J Hypertens. 2006;24:889–94.
15. Hughes AD, Stanton AV, Jabbar AS, Chapman N, Martinez-Perez ME, McG Thom SA. Effect of antihypertensive treatment on retinal microvascular changes in hypertension. J Hypertens. 2008;26:1703–7.
16. Harazny JM, Ritt M, Baleanu D, Ott C, Heckmann J, Schlaich MP, Michelson G, Schmieder RE. Increased wall:lumen ratio of retinal arterioles in male patients with a history of a cerebrovascular event. Hypertension. 2007;50(4):623–829.
17. Ritt M, Harazny JM, Ott C, Schlaich MP, Schneider MP, Michelson G, Schmieder RE. Analysis of retinal arteriolar structure in never-treated patients with essential hypertension. J Hypertens. 2008;26(7):1427–34.
18. Ritt M, Harazny JM, Ott C, Schneider MP, Schlaich MP, Michelson G, Schmieder RE. Wall-to-lumen ratio of retinal arterioles is related with urinary albumin excretion and altered vascular reactivity to infusion of the nitric oxide synthase inhibitor N-monomethyl-L-arginine. J Hypertens. 2009;27:2201–18.
19. Baleanu D, Ritt M, Harazny J, Heckmann J, Schmieder RE, Michelson G. Wall-to-lumen ratio of retinal arterioles and arteriole-to-venule ratio of retinal vessels in patients with cerebrovascular damage. Invest Ophthalmol Vis Sci. 2009;50:4351–9.
20. Harazny JM, Raff U, Welzenbach J, Ott C, Ritt M, Lehmann M, Michelson G, Schmieder RE. New software analyses increase the reliability of measurements of retinal arterioles morphology by scanning laser Doppler flowmetry in humans. J Hypertens. 2011;29:777–82.

21. Rizzoni D, Porteri E, Duse S, De Ciuceis C, Agabiti Rosei C, La Boria E, Semeraro F, Costagliola C, Sebastiani A, Danzi P, Tiberio GAM, Giulini SM, Docchio F, Sansoni G, Sarkar A, Agabiti RE. Relationship between media to lumen ratio of subcutaneous small arteries and wall to lumen ratio of retinal arterioles evaluated non-invasively by scanning laser Doppler flowmetry. J Hypertens. 2012;30:1169–75.
22. Muiesan ML, Salvetti M, Rizzoni D, Paini A, Agabiti-Rosei C, Aggiusti C, Bertacchini F, Stassaldi D, Gavazzi A, Porteri E, De Ciuceis C, Agabiti-Rosei E. Pulsatile hemodynamics and microcirculation: evidence for a close relationship in hypertensive patients. Hypertension. 2013;61:130–6.
23. Ott C, Raff U, Harazny JM, Michelson G, Schmieder RE. Central pulse pressure is an independent determinant of vascular remodeling in the retinal circulation. Hypertension. 2013;61:1340–5.
24. Salvetti M, Agabiti Rosei C, Paini A, Aggiusti C, Cancarini A, Duse S, Semeraro F, Rizzoni D, Agabiti Rosei E, Muiesan ML. Relationship of wall-to-lumen ratio of retinal arterioles with clinic and 24-hour blood pressure. Hypertension. 2014;63:1110–5.
25. Rizzoni D, Palombo C, Porteri E, Muiesan ML, Kozàkovà M, La Canna G, Nardi M, Guelfi D, Salvetti M, Morizzo C, Vittone F, Agabiti RE. Relationships between coronary vasodilator capacity and small artery remodeling in hypertensive patients. J Hypertens. 2003;21:625–32.
26. Izzard AS, Rizzoni D, Agabiti-Rosei E, Heagerty AM. Small artery structure and hypertension: adaptive changes and target organ damage. J Hypertens. 2005;23:247–50.
27. Heagerty AM. Predicting hypertension complications from small artery structure. J Hypertens. 2007;25:939–40.
28. Schiffrin EL, Touyz RM. From bedside to bench to bedside: role of renin-angiotensin-aldosterone system in remodeling of resistance arteries in hypertension. Am J Physiol Heart Circ Physiol. 2004;287:H435–46.
29. Mulvany MJ. Small artery structure: time to take note? Am J Hypertens. 2007;20:853–4.
30. Rizzoni D, Aalkjaer C, De Ciuceis C, Porteri E, Rossini C, Rosei CA, Sarkar A, Agabiti RE. How to assess microvascular structure in humans. High Blood Press Cardiovasc Prev. 2011;18:169–77.

Part IV

Kidney

14 Proteinuria-Microalbuminuria in Renal Damage

Josep Redon, Gernot Pichler, and Fernando Martinez

14.1 Introduction

Proteinuria (P) usually results from an insult in the glomerular and/or tubular structures of the kidney. It has been considered a marker of risk not only to develop renal insufficiency but also to suffer cardiovascular events, based on prospective studies carried out in the general population as well as in diabetic and hypertensive patients [1]. In fact, proteinuria has been considered a strong marker of risk and an intermediate endpoint during treatment [2, 3].

Proteinuria, however, is a blend of molecules that are excreted in the urine with different origins and also from different mechanisms [4]. The large fraction of urine protein is albumin, a molecule with a size of around 60 kd. Loss in the permselectivity of the glomerular barrier largely increases its presence in urine. Although partially reabsorbed in the proximal tubule by a mechanism that involves specific carriers, megalin and cubilin, a significant increment in urinary albumin excretion depends mainly on abnormal filtration. If the permselectivity loss is greater, other molecules with a larger size are also filtered and excreted, such as immunoglobulins. In cases with an important component of interstitial and tubular damage, tubular proteinuria can be present. "Tubular proteinuria" is due to a failure in protein reabsorption by the

J. Redon (✉)
Hypertension Unit, Internal Medicine, Hospital Clinico, INCLIVA Research Institute, University of Valencia, Valencia, Spain

CIBERObn, Health Institute Carlos III, Madrid, Spain

Hypertension Clinic, Hospital Clinico, Avda Blasco Ibañez, 17, 46010 Valencia, Spain
e-mail: josep.redon@uv.es

G. Pichler • F. Martinez
Hypertension Unit, Internal Medicine, Hospital Clinico, INCLIVA Research Institute, University of Valencia, Valencia, Spain
e-mail: gernotpichler@gmx.at; fernandoctor@hotmail.com

E. Agabiti Rosei, G. Mancia (eds.), *Assessment of Preclinical Organ Damage in Hypertension*, DOI 10.1007/978-3-319-15603-3_14

proximal tubule and is characterized by increased excretion of several low molecular weight (LMW) proteins, as well as albumin and β_2-glycoprotein I (molecular weight 50 kd). These LMW proteins include β_2-microglobulin, α_1-microglobulin, retinol-binding protein, neutrophil gelatinase-associated lipocalin (NGAL), and liver-type fatty-acid-binding protein (L-FABP) [5, 6].

In the following section, we will focus on P and on urinary albumin excretion (UAE), since tubular proteinuria is less relevant in the assessment of cardiovascular and renal risk.

14.2 How to Assess

At the time to assess P and/or UAE, some main issues should be considered to properly assess the excretion and to reduce intraindividual variability, especially relevant for UAE since quantification requires more precision.

14.2.1 Urine Sample

In this regard the ideal would be 24-h collection with simultaneous assessment of total creatinine excretion to be sure that the collection is well performed. This is not practical due to the difficulties when collecting the urine, and alternative methods are more frequently used such as spot urine measuring the UAE/creatinine ratio (UAER) to control for urine dilution. Timed overnight was also used in the past although today it has been replaced by the spot urine [7].

The time for collection should also be taken into account since a circadian variability of UAE excretion and exercise can modify the values. Then, the first voiding urine in the morning is the most used to reduce intraindividual variability.

14.2.2 Method

Dipsticks for both P and UAE are available nowadays. Their use as a screening test provides a rapid assessment but quantification is necessary if the result is positive. A dipstick for UAE also provides creatinine urine concentration at the same time, which gives a rapid assessment of UAER. Considering the large intraindividual variability of UAE excretion, it is recommended to assess two separate samples, obtained on different days.

Quantification of total protein excretion can be performed using different methods, turbidimetry or dye binding, and this depends on the preferences of the different laboratories, although the capacity to detect different molecules differs. For UAE, after the initial radioimmunoassays, immunological methods by enzyme immune assay (ELISA) have the most widespread use [8].

14.2.3 Definitions

Proteinuria is defined when the total protein excretion is >300 mg/dl, is given clinical relevance in values >1 g/24 h, and receives the name of nephrotic range in >3 g/24 h [9].

Microalbuminuria is defined as UAE from 30 to 300 mg/24 h or equivalent amounts of UAER using spot urine samples in mg/g (mg of albumin and g of creatinine). Taking into account the differences by sex, the threshold for women is higher than for men, ≥31 mg/g and ≥22 mg/g, respectively. The definition comes from studies, which have established its value as a marker of risk to develop nephropathy in diabetic subjects. However, when the potential prognostic value of microalbuminuria in cardiovascular disease is being assessed, the threshold value pointing to an increment of risk is largely below the UAE values outlined, regardless of the population included: adult or elderly population, postmenopausal women, or high-cardiovascular-risk subjects. A potential consideration used by the KDIGO is to subdivide the UAER below 30 mg/g into two: normal 0–15 mg/g and high normal 15–30 mg/g.

14.3 Prevalence

Prevalence of both proteinuria and microalbuminuria depends on the population being studied. It is obvious that the prevalence is higher in hypertensive subjects and even higher in diabetics since in the absence of a renal disease, both P and UAE increase by BP elevation and abnormalities in the glucose metabolism. In hypertension, the prevalence of proteinuria is about 3–5 %, while for microalbuminuria it is around 15 %, being a little bit higher in women as compared to men. The prevalence of P and UAE in diabetes is practically twice that observed in hypertensives with the same BP values. In Fig. 14.1, factors that influence the prevalence of microalbuminuria are displayed. In the absence of insulin resistance, prevalence of microalbuminuria is mainly

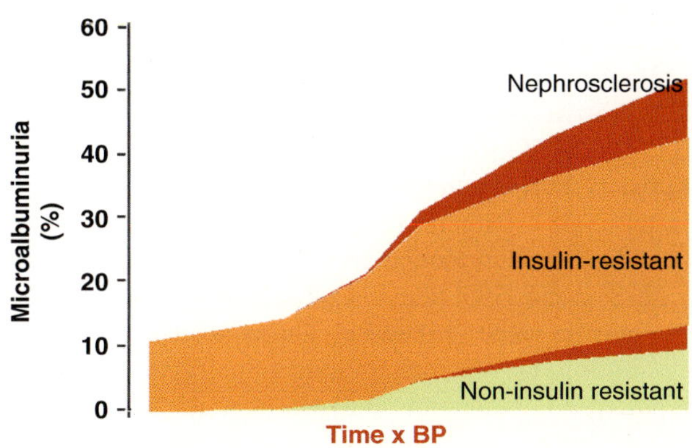

Fig. 14.1 Factors related to the prevalence of microalbuminuria in hypertension (see text for explanation)

dependent on the BP values and the time duration of hypertension: the higher the values and the longer the duration, the higher the prevalence. However, if insulin resistance exists, with or without diabetes, microalbuminuria is present even around normal BP values. Once nephrosclerosis develops, the increment is frequently observed.

14.4 Change with Treatment

Considering the large intraindividual variability of UAE excretion, assessment of significant changes should be performed carefully. One recommended way to evaluate changes over time is to define regression when UAE drops more than 50 % from the initial values, along with a reduction of UAE to <30 mg/24 h for microalbuminurics and <300 mg/24 h for proteinurics.

Despite their relevance as a marker of developing organ damage and cardiovascular risk, changes in UAE over time, other than short-term ones induced by antihypertensive treatment, have received little attention. One study has analyzed factors related to the occurrence of new microalbuminuria during antihypertensive treatment [10]. In mild hypertensives, development of microalbuminuria was linked to insufficient BP control and to a progressive increment of glucose values. However there is less information about the long-term changes in initially increased UAE. According to our data, antihypertensive treatment is able to normalize microalbuminuria in half of the patients, although 10 % progress to overt proteinuria despite treatment. Glomerular filtration rate lower than 60 mL/min/1.73 m^2 decreases the probability to reduce UAE [11].

14.5 Prognostic Value of Change

A significant reduction in proteinuria is a marker of treatment success and is followed by a reduction in the risk to develop end-stage renal disease and cardiovascular events. Whether or not changes in UAE overtime have prognostic value and can be used as an intermediate objective, it is a matter of discussion. Post hoc analyses from the Losartan Intervention for Endpoint Reduction in Hypertension (LIFE) [12], Action in Diabetes and Vascular Disease (ADVANCE) [13–15], Ongoing Telmisartan Alone and in Combination with Ramipril Global Endpoint Trial (ONTARGET), and Telmisartan Randomized Assessment Study In ACE-Intolerant Subjects with Cardiovascular Disease (TRASCEND) have reported positive results in terms of a reduction in UAE being followed by risk reduction [16]. However, Avoiding Cardiovascular Events through Combination Therapy in Patients Living with Systolic Hypertension (ACCOMPLISH) [17] does not confirm the potential prognostic value. Likewise, a prospective study, Olmesartan for the Delay or Prevention of Microalbuminuria in Type 2 Diabetes (ROADMAP) [18], also reported no association between changes in microalbuminuria and cardiovascular events during the double-blind period, although an observational follow-up concluded that the development of microalbuminuria was a marker of cardiovascular events [19]. These studies, which were heterogeneous in terms of patients and analysis of data, did not contribute to the clarification of the potential role of microalbuminuria during antihypertensive treatment. A recent study [20] carried out in a hypertensive clinic demonstrated for first time that, in hypertension, an increment of UAE at any time is a marker of cardiovascular risk. The study also confirms previous observations regarding the prognostic value of microalbuminuria in the risk to develop cardiovascular events and the worse prognosis of persistent or progression to microalbuminuria during treatment.

Bibliography

1. Currie G, Delles C. Proteinuria and its relation to cardiovascular disease. Int J Nephrol Renovasc Dis. 2013;7:13–24.
2. Viazzi F, Pontremoli R. Blood pressure, albuminuria and renal dysfunction: the ‘chicken or egg’ dilemma. Nephrol Dial Transplant. 2014;29:1453–5.
3. Lv J, Ehteshami P, Sarnak MJ, Tighiouart H, Jun M, Ninomiya T, Foote C, Rodgers A, Zhang H, Wang H, Strippoli GF, Perkovic V. Effects of intensive blood pressure lowering on the progression of chronic kidney disease: a systematic review and meta-analysis. CMAJ. 2013;185:949–57.
4. Cravedi P, Remuzzi G. Pathophysiology of proteinuria and its value as an outcome measure in chronic kidney disease. Br J Clin Pharmacol. 2013;76:516–23.
5. Garg P, Rabelink T. Glomerular proteinuria: a complex interplay between unique players. Adv Chronic Kidney Dis. 2011;18:233–42.
6. Parikh CR, Lu JC, Coca SG, Devarajan P. Tubular proteinuria in acute kidney injury: a critical evaluation of current status and future promise. Ann Clin Biochem. 2010;47(Pt 4):301–12.
7. Redon J, Pascual JM. Development of microalbuminuria in essential hypertension. Curr Hypertens Rep. 2006;8:171–7.
8. Redon J, Martinez F. Microalbuminuria as surrogate endpoint in therapeutic trials. Curr Hypertens Rep. 2012;14:345–9.
9. Viswanathan G, Upadhyay A. Assessment of proteinuria. Adv Chronic Kidney Dis. 2011;18:243–8.
10. Pascual JM, Rodilla E, González C, Pérez-Hoyos S, Redon J. Long-term impact of systolic blood pressure and glycemia on the development of microalbuminuria in essential hypertension. Hypertension. 2005;45:1125–30.
11. Pascual JM, Rodilla E, Miralles A, González C, Redon J. Determinants of urinary albumin excretion reduction in essential hypertension: a long-term follow-up study. J Hypertens. 2006;24:2277–84.
12. Ibsen H, Olsen MH, Wachtell K, Borch-Johnsen K, Lindholm LH, Mogensen CE, Dahlöf B, Snapinn SM, Wan Y, Lyle PA. Does albuminuria predict cardiovascular outcomes on treatment with losartan versus atenolol in patients with diabetes, hypertension, and left ventricular hypertrophy? The LIFE study. Diabetes Care. 2006;29:595–600.
13. Patel A; ADVANCE Collaborative Group, MacMahon S, Chalmers J, Neal B, Woodward M, Billot L, Harrap S, Poulter N, Marre M, Cooper M, Glasziou P, Grobbee DE, Hamet P, Heller S, Liu LS, Mancia G, Mogensen CE, Pan CY, Rodgers A, Williams B. Effects of a fixed combination of perindopril and indapamide on macrovascular and microvascular outcomes in patients with type 2 diabetes mellitus (the ADVANCE trial): a randomised controlled trial. Lancet. 2007;370:829–40.
14. de Galan BE, Perkovic V, Ninomiya T, Pillai A, Patel A, Cass A, Neal B, Poulter N, Harrap S, Mogensen CE, Cooper M, Marre M, Williams B, Hamet P, Mancia G, Woodward M, Glasziou P, Grobbee DE, MacMahon S, Chalmers J, ADVANCE Collaborative Group. Lowering blood pressure reduces renal events in type 2 diabetes. J Am Soc Nephrol. 2009;20:883–92.

15. Zoungas S, de Galan BE, Ninomiya T, Grobbee D, Hamet P, Heller S, MacMahon S, Marre M, Neal B, Patel A, Woodward M, Chalmers J; ADVANCE Collaborative Group, Cass A, Glasziou P, Harrap S, Lisheng L, Mancia G, Pillai A, Poulter N, Perkovic V, Travert F. Combined effects of routine blood pressure lowering and intensive glucose control on macrovascular and microvascular outcomes in patients with type 2 diabetes: new results from the ADVANCE trial. Diabetes Care. 2009;32:2068–74.
16. Schmieder RE, Mann JF, Schumacher H, Gao P, Mancia G, Weber MA, McQueen M, Koon T, Yusuf S, ONTARGET Investigators. Changes in albuminuria predict mortality and morbidity in patients with vascular disease. J Am Soc Nephrol. 2011;22:1353–64.
17. Bakris GL, Sarafidis PA, Weir MR, Dahlöf B, Pitt B, Jamerson K, Velazquez EJ, Staikos-Byrne L, Kelly RY, Shi V, Chiang YT, Weber MA, ACCOMPLISH Trial investigators. Renal outcomes with different fixed-dose combination therapies in patients with hypertension at high risk for cardiovascular events (ACCOMPLISH): a prespecified secondary analysis of a randomised controlled trial. Lancet. 2010;375:1173–81.
18. Haller H, Ito S, Izzo Jr JL, Januszewicz A, Katayama S, Menne J, Mimran A, Rabelink TJ, Ritz E, Ruilope LM, Rump LC, Viberti G, ROADMAP Trial Investigators. Olmesartan for the delay or prevention of microalbuminuria in type 2 diabetes. N Engl J Med. 2011;364:907–17.
19. Menne J, Ritz E, Ruilope LM, Chatzikyrkou C, Viberti G, Haller H. The Randomized Olmesartan and Diabetes Microalbuminuria Prevention (ROADMAP) observational follow-up study: benefits of RAS blockade with olmesartan treatment are sustained after study discontinuation. J Am Heart Assoc. 2014;3:e000810.
20. Pascual JM, Rodilla E, Costa JA, Garcia-Escrich M, Gonzalez C, Redon J. Prognostic value of microalbuminuria during antihypertensive treatment in essential hypertension. Hypertension. 2014;64:1228–34.

Glomerular Filtration Rate in Renal Damage

15

Josep Redon, Gernot Pichler, and Fernando Martinez

15.1 Introduction

Renal function is mainly represented by the glomerular filtration (GF), which is dependent on the number and function of the nephrons. Glomerular filtration declines progressively after the third decade with a progressive loss of 1 % per year. In addition to diseases producing direct damage in the glomerular structures, high blood pressure values, diabetes, and dyslipidemia are the main factors increasing the rate of GF decline over the years. Other functional parameters of the kidney such as renal plasma flow or tubular functions are not measured in daily practice in hypertension and are not related to risk for cardiovascular disease (CVD).

The relationship between decreased glomerular filtration rate (GFR) and CVD has been examined in numerous studies with the majority of them involving high-risk populations (individuals with hypertension, heart failure, coronary artery disease, acute coronary syndrome, coronary artery bypass surgery, and diabetes or age >65 years) or low-risk populations demonstrating increased CVD risk with decreased GFR [1, 2]. In a study with more than one million subjects, a graded and inverse association was noted between GFR and CVD events, hospitalizations, and mortality. Data was supported by a collaborative meta-analysis that pooled

J. Redon (✉)
Hypertension Unit, Internal Medicine, Hospital Clinico,
INCLIVA Research Institute, University of Valencia, Valencia, Spain

CIBERObn, Health Institute Carlos III, Madrid, Spain

Avda Blasco Ibañez, 17, 46010 Valencia, Spain
e-mail: josep.redon@uv.es

G. Pichler • F. Martinez
Hypertension Unit, Internal Medicine, Hospital Clinico,
INCLIVA Research Institute, University of Valencia, Valencia, Spain
e-mail: gernotpichler@gmx.at; fernandoctor@hotmail.com

E. Agabiti Rosei, G. Mancia (eds.), *Assessment of Preclinical Organ Damage in Hypertension*, DOI 10.1007/978-3-319-15603-3_15

information from 21 general population cohort studies to assess the relationship between CKD measures and CVD mortality [3]. The increased CVD risk associated with CKD may simply reflect a longer duration or severity of traditional CVD risk factors such as hypertension, diabetes, and dyslipidemia, although nontraditional risk factors consequential to chronic kidney disease (CKD) such as anemia, hyperphosphatemia, increased fibroblast growth factor-23 levels, inflammation, and unmeasured uremic factors account for at least some of the excess cardiovascular risks [4].

15.2 How to Assess

Assessment of glomerular filtration was initially performed by the measurement in serum of an endogenous substance which is filtered in the glomerulus, creatinine. Indirect glomerular filtration can be measured by assessing the clearance of substances that are free filtered in the glomerulus and are not reabsorbed in the tubules. This is the case of endogenous creatinine or administered inulin, ^{51}Cr-EDTA or iodo-thalamate. The former has been used for many years as the routine method despite limitations, and the latter is used for research. The use of creatinine not only has potential for inaccuracies derived from muscle mass, protein intake, exercise, and some drugs (cimetidine, fibrates) but is also misleading (Fig. 15.1). In the range of normal values, small changes in creatinine are related to large changes in GFR. However, in lower values, large changes in creatinine imply small modifications of GFR [5].

Recently, serum levels of cystatin C, a free housekeeping protein ubiquitous in many cellular systems, seem to be superior in reflecting not only the GF but also the CVD risk, mainly in the elderly [6]. Its utility in estimating kidney function derives from the fact that after being freely filtered in the glomerulus, it is then absorbed in

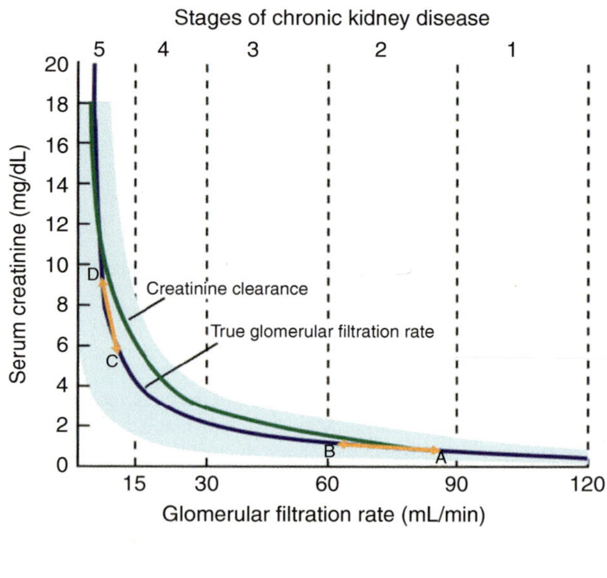

Fig. 15.1 Relationship between serum creatinine, glomerular filtration rate, creatinine clearance, and stages of CKD

the kidney tubules where it is fully degraded locally. There is no active tubular secretion or significant extrarenal elimination, making it an excellent marker of GFR. Cystatin C may also be superior to creatinine as a better predictor of cardiovascular mortality while providing a more accurate estimation of GFR. The serum cystatin C concentration is independent of muscle mass, nutritional status, and sex, although it may be altered in patients with derangements in thyroid function and certain cancers and with glucocorticoid therapy.

The widespread use of equations to calculate GFR has enabled the influence of renal function in cardiovascular risk to be assessed. The calculation was initially performed by the Cockcroft-Gault formula, which includes data on serum creatinine, age, sex, and weight, providing an estimation of creatinine clearance. The MDRD formula, which only needs serum creatinine, age, and sex, estimates the GFR. Both methods provide GF referred to mL/min/1.73 m^2. Several studies have examined the difference between these methods compared to the corresponding gold standard – i.e., GFR calculated by isotopic techniques. In the range of normal values, with true GFR >60 ml/min, the GFR may be underestimated by up to 28 % when applying the formula [7]. As true glomerular filtration decreases, the differences between the methods become smaller – reaching an underestimation of 6 % when the true GFR is <30 ml/min [7]. The original equation to estimate GFR, which was published in 1996, has been constantly refined to improve its use in the general population. A recent updated equation, the CKD-EPI equation, corrects for much of the overestimation of CKD especially among those with GFRs between 60 and 89 mL/min/1.73 m^2, mainly in female and black populations. The formula has also been adapted for other ethnicities, in particular of Asian origin (formulas and automatic calculators are available at www.kidney.org/professionals/kdoqi/gfr_calculator.cfm). It is worthy to remember that these equations should not be used in situations in which renal function is changing rapidly, such as in acute kidney injury. Likewise, they should be used with caution in subjects with extreme body mass since they underestimate in vey muscular patients and overestimate in very small patients.

15.2.1 Definitions

According to the estimated GFR (eGFR), five different stages of chronic kidney disease (CKD) have been defined (see Fig. 15.2) [8]. Stages 3 and higher are those in which CV risk is most pronounced, and within that stage, the risk is particularly elevated in those patients with stage 3b, i.e., eGFR<45 mL/min/1.73 m^2. This fact does not impede the recognition that in less advanced degrees of CKD, an elevated CV mortality has been described. Potential sources of bias include ascertainment problems, intra-patient variation in renal function, single eGFR which is likely to overestimate prevalence, and intra-laboratory variation: the use of raw creatinine to calculate eGFR does not take into account calibration issues between labs.

It is worthy to remember that in evaluating CVD using renal parameters, GFR should be assessed simultaneously with urinary albumin excretion (UAE). The presence of eGFR stage 3 or more and the presence of or an increase in urinary

		UAE	A1	A1	A2	A3	A3
		mg/g	Optimal <15	High normal 15-29	High 30-299	Very high 300-1999	Nefrotic >2000
GFR stage	Description	(ml/min/ 1.73 m²)					
G1	High	>105					
G1	Optimal	90-104					
G2	Mild	60-89					
G3a	Mild to moderate	45-59					
G3b	Moderate to severe	30-44					
G4	Severe	15-29					
G5	Kidney failure	<15					

Fig. 15.2 Cardiovascular and renal risk based on eGFR and UAE

albumin or protein excretion are criteria for CKD. Chronic kidney disease (CKD) is frequently observed in arterial hypertension and is accompanied by a significant enhancement in CV risk that reinforces the need for simultaneous protection of both the renal and the CV system.

15.3 Prevalence

Prevalence of eGFR in levels of 60 or lower is frequent, but it is difficult to estimate since age is an important determinant, as well as sex, hypertension, obesity, and abnormalities in the glucose metabolism. In the general population, several studies have found that around 5 % of the subjects have GFR <60 ml/min/1.73 m^2. In hypertension, one study conducted by our group including 6,227 hypertensive subjects from primary care and using the MDRD equation, renal insufficiency (GFR <60 ml/min/1.73 m^2) was present in 21.8 % of the subjects, and 4.8 % subjects had a GFR ≤ 45 ml/min/1.73 m^2 [9]. Subjects with the lowest GFR were more frequently older patients, women, and diabetics [10].

15.4 Change with Treatment (Criteria for Significant Change, Incidence During Treatment)

Changes in GFR can result from loss of nephrons, which is not reversible and is usually progressive, or from rapid functional changes induced by clinical events, such as acute heart failure and physiological phenomena, or more frequently from drugs used in the treatment of CVD diseases. It is well recognized that at the beginning of antihypertensive treatment, BP reduction can induce a drop in the GFR, which is more evident if drugs that block the renin-angiotensin-aldosterone system (RAAS) are used. The initial reduction induced by the treatment reflects the degree of RAAS activation, and it has been hypothesized that it produces long-term protection. What is demonstrated is that drug withdrawal restores the previous GFR. An important point is the following: when does the change in GFR become clinically significant? Usually a 10 % drop is considered relevant, although a reduction close to or higher than 25 % is a strong recommendation to withdraw treatment.

In the absence of acute events or pharmacological treatment, GFR declines slowly. In the worst cases, in which a diabetic nephropathy exists, the yearly decline is around 10 ml/min/1.73 m^2. Therefore the utility of GFR in the follow-up of hypertensive subjects is limited by the slow rate of changes [11].

15.5 Prognostic Value of Change

Some studies have demonstrated that development of CKD in the hypertensive population is followed by an increase in cardiovascular risk. However, studies looking at the changes in GFR and the prognostic value in hypertension are scarce. In fact, despite the wide availability of GFR, there are few clinical trials for development of chronic kidney disease or for the impact on CV disease of the changes in renal function. This may be because changes in GFR are slow, and the most used criterion, doubling of serum creatinine, corresponds to a 57 % change in GFR, which is a late event requiring long follow-up periods and large sample size. Shorter time changes even in 1 year have been strongly related to risk of ESRD in one study, and some others have estimated the risk for CV events, a situation much more common than ESRD.

Recently a large cooperative study analyzed the impact of GFR changes at 1, 2, and 3 years on the risk to develop ESRD and mortality. Using a CKD-EPI equation, a decrease in estimated GFR smaller than a doubling of serum creatinine occurred more commonly and was consistently associated with the risk of ESRD and mortality, supporting the consideration of lesser declines in estimated GFR as an alternative end point for CKD progression. Although there is a continuous relationship between reduction in GFR and risk, a 30 % reduction over 2 years could be used as a reliable outcome in future trials, since it also predicts long-term mortality [12].

References

1. Chronic Kidney Disease Prognosis Consortium, Matsushita K, van der Velde M, et al. Association of estimated glomerular filtration rate and albuminuria with all-cause and cardiovascular mortality in general population cohorts: a collaborative meta-analysis. Lancet. 2010;375:2073–81.
2. National Kidney Foundation. K/DOQI clinical practice guidelines for chronic kidney disease: evaluation, classification and stratification. Am J Kidney Dis. 2002;39:S46–64.

3. Go AS, Chertow GM, Fan D, McCulloch CE, Hsu C. Chronic kidney disease and the risks of death, cardiovascular events, and hospitalisation. N Engl J Med. 2004;351:1296–306.
4. Boubred F, Saint-Faust M, Buffat C, Ligi I, Grandvuillemin I, Simeoni U. Developmental origins of chronic renal disease: an integrative hypothesis. Int J Nephrol. 2013;2013:346067.
5. Levey AS, Inker LA, Coresh J. GFR estimation: from physiology to public health. Am J Kidney Dis. 2014;63:820–34.
6. Shlipak MG, Mattes MD, Peralta CA. Update on cystatin C: incorporation into clinical practice. Am J Kidney Dis. 2013;62:595–603.
7. Earley A, Miskulin D, Lamb EJ, Levey AS, Uhlig K. Estimating equations for glomerular filtration rate in the era of creatinine standardization: a systematic review. Ann Intern Med. 2012;156:785–95.
8. Levey AS, de Jong PE, Coresh J, El Nahas M, Astor BC, Matsushita K, Gansevoort RT, Kasiske BL, Eckardt KU. The definition, classification, and prognosis of chronic kidney disease: a KDIGO Controversies Conference report. Kidney Int. 2011;80:17–28.
9. Cea-Calvo L, Redón J, Martí-Canales JC, Lozano JV, Llisterri JL, Fernández-Pérez C, Aznar J, González-Esteban J. Prevalence of low glomerular filtration rate in the elderly population of Spain. The PREV-ICTUS study. Med Clin (Barc). 2007;129:681–7.
10. Redon J, Morales-Olivas F, Galgo A, Brito MA, Mediavilla J, Marín R, Rodríguez P, Tranche S, Lozano JV, Filozof C, MAGAL Group. Urinary albumin excretion and glomerular filtration rate across the spectrum of glucose abnormalities in essential hypertension. J Am Soc Nephrol. 2006;17:S236–45.
11. Glassock RJ, Winearls C. Ageing and the glomerular filtration rate: truths and consequences. Trans Am Clin Climatol Assoc. 2009;120:419–28.
12. Coresh J, Turin TC, Matsushita K, Sang Y, Ballew SH, Appel LJ, Arima H, Chadban SJ, Cirillo M, Djurdjev O, Green JA, Heine GH, Inker LA, Irie F, Ishani A, Ix JH, Kovesdy CP, Marks A, Ohkubo T, Shalev V, Shankar A, Wen CP, de Jong PE, Iseki K, Stengel B, Gansevoort RT, Levey AS, CKD Prognosis Consortium. Decline in estimated glomerular filtration rate and subsequent risk of end-stage renal disease and mortality. JAMA. 2014;311:2518–31.

Other Methods to Assess Renal Damage 16

Josep Redon, Gernot Pichler, and Fernando Martinez

16.1 Introduction

Although glomerular filtration rate (GFR) and proteinuria remain gold standard in the evaluation of renal target organ damage, imaging techniques and image-derived parameters allow for both assessment of renal function and estimation of cardiovascular risk. Enhancement in digital image processing permits dynamic measurement of renal vascular and intraparenchymal processes in real time. The most relevant in terms of clinical use to assess hypertension-induced organ damage are the renal resistive index (RRI), renal calcium score, and functional magnetic resonance imaging.

16.2 Ultrasound and Doppler-Derived Renal Resistive Index

Ultrasound and Doppler-derived indexes of renal blood flow are standard procedures in the evaluation of acute and chronic kidney disease (CKD), regardless of the underlying cause. Doppler ultrasonography allows for detection of both macrovascular and microvascular abnormalities, together with structural or functional changes of the renal parenchyma, deduced from vascular impedance patterns [1].

The ESH recommends performing renal ultrasound and renal duplex Doppler ultrasonography in hypertensives when a secondary form of hypertension is

J. Redon (✉)
Hypertension Unit, Internal Medicine, Hospital Clinico, INCLIVA Research Institute, University of Valencia, Valencia, Spain

CIBERObn, Health Institute Carlos III, Madrid, Spain
e-mail: josep.redon@uv.es

G. Pichler • F. Martinez
Hypertension Unit, Internal Medicine, Hospital Clinico, INCLIVA Research Institute, University of Valencia, Valencia, Spain
e-mail: gernotpichler@gmx.at; fernandoctor@hotmail.com

E. Agabiti Rosei, G. Mancia (eds.), *Assessment of Preclinical Organ Damage in Hypertension*, DOI 10.1007/978-3-319-15603-3_16

suspected. However, current evidence suggests that ultrasound Doppler-derived RRI might be a good predictor of subclinical renal, vascular, and target organ damage as well as cardiovascular risk [2, 3].

The RRI is calculated by dividing the difference of the peak systolic velocity and the end diastolic velocity by the peak systolic velocity derived from intrarenal arteries, considering a range of 0.47–0.7, with a difference between the two kidneys of <8 % as normal in the adult population. Vascular compliance and resistance are the main determinants of RRI, and its usefulness has been demonstrated in a broad clinical spectrum, including renal artery stenosis, obstructive renal disease, chronic renal allograft rejection, and prediction of progression risk in CKD and critically ill patients, among others [4].

In the hypertensive population, the relationship between RRI and kidney injury is well established. Alteration of the vascular resistance at the renal parenchymal level is associated with a decline in glomerular filtration rate. Furthermore, RRI has shown to maintain a positive direct relationship with the quantity of UAE, reflecting its potential as a marker of cardiovascular risk. The interaction between renal impedance and vascular hemodynamics in the presence of hypertension has been further investigated. RRI is associated with age, blood pressure including abnormal circadian patterns, pulse pressure, and arterial stiffness. Taking the current evidence together, RRI may be considered as a monitor of the hemodynamic properties in hypertensive subjects [5–8].

Hypertension-induced target organ damage in other territories is also closely related to renal vascular patterns. Patients with a RRI beyond the threshold of 0.7 have higher pulse wave velocity, left ventricular mass, coronary artery calcification, and intima-media thickness than subjects with normal values of RRI. Interestingly, these observations are independent of the degree of renal functional impairment and therefore permit the usage of RRI in both hypertensives without apparent target organ damage and subjects with high cardiovascular risk [9, 10].

Renal impedance expressed by RRI is closely related to central and peripheral hemodynamics. In addition, RRI has shown to be a predictor of the development of diabetes mellitus and hyperuricemia in the hypertensive population. These findings suggest that RRI might be a useful tool for the prediction of cardiovascular events. Up to now, only a few prospective studies have addressed this question. However, recent evidence shows that high RRI values independently predict all-cause mortality and cardiovascular events (ischemic cardiomyopathy, congestive heart failure, stroke, and transient ischemic attack) in hypertensive subjects [11, 12].

The impact of treatment reducing RRI and consecutive changes on the prognosis of cardiovascular events remains uncertain. Blood pressure-lowering treatment has shown to reduce RRI and parallel urine albumin excretion, but long-term studies are necessary to determine whether the decline in RRI is followed by a significant reduction of cardiovascular risk [13, 14].

16.3 Computed Tomography and Renal Artery Calcium

Multidetector computed tomography has gained importance in vascular medicine due to its ability to measure arterial wall properties and to detect vessel alterations. The presence of vascular calcium in coronary and peripheral arteries has shown to maintain a direct relationship with systemic atherosclerosis. Among others, coronary artery calcium is a well-established marker of asymptomatic organ damage and has been validated as a predictor of cardiovascular disease.

Renal artery calcium (RAC) can be assessed noninvasively using the multidetector or the electron beam computed tomography. To determine and quantify the arterial calcium, regions of interest are identified as having a density of more than 130 Hounsfield units (HU) in an area larger than or equal to 1 mm^2. Detectable RAC is commonly classified with the Agatston scoring method adjusted by slice thickness. The established threshold for the presence of RAC is defined as a density of more than 130HU in a given vascular area [15].

The prevalence of RAC differs among the reported data and depends on the studied subpopulation. While RAC is identified in about one third of the general population, the prevalence rises up to 80 % in diabetic patients [16]. However, the presence of RAC is closely related to hypertension, cardiovascular risk factors, systemic atherosclerosis, and end-organ damage of the kidney. Recent evident shows that the presence of RAC results in twofold higher odds of microalbuminuria and hypertension compared to subjects without renal artery alterations. The risk of progression to end-stage renal disease is greater in patients with RAC, independent of other risk factors, favoring the role as a prognostic tool of CKD. Also, RAC has shown to be associated with coronary artery calcium and, more importantly, an increased risk of cardiovascular mortality. Interestingly, there is no independent association between RAC and patients with diabetes mellitus, despite the greater burden of vascular calcium in this subpopulation group. Therefore, the detection of RAC in diabetics might serve as a predictor of systemic vascular calcium [17–20].

Despite the promising properties of RAC in the assessment of cardiovascular disease, there are currently no studies available considering RAC as a treatment target. The question of whether specific treatment is able to reduce RAC and consecutively the cardiovascular risk remains unanswered.

16.4 Functional Magnetic Resonance Imaging

Functional magnetic resonance imaging (MRI) of the kidneys has gained ground in the past several years. MRI permits in vivo measurement of renal perfusion, filtration, diffusion, and oxygenation and provides several benefits compared to other (imaging) techniques to assess renal function: no exposure to ionizing radiation, avoidance of iodinated contrast agents, noninvasiveness, and ability to determine renal function for each kidney separately [21].

There is a lack of current evidence on long-term prospective studies to assess the impact of cardiovascular risk factors and the corresponding treatment on MRI-based determination of renal function. However, various techniques available to assess GFR are described as followed.

16.4.1 Dynamic Contrast-Enhanced MRI

Dynamic contrast-enhanced (DCE) MRI, also termed MR renography, is based on the acquisition of dynamic images before, during, and after administration of gadolinium chelate. The signal intensity of the renal tissue is converted to gadolinium concentration and plotted versus the time to generate various functional parameter curves. With this method, it is possible to resolve the renal cortex from the medulla and collecting system, and it offers the potential to measure renal properties in vivo that previously could only be assessed by biopsy. Current applications of DCE MRI include estimation of GFR as well as diagnostics of renovascular hypertension, functional urinary obstruction, and renal allograft dysfunction [22–24].

16.4.2 Diffusion-Weighted MRI

Diffusion-weighted MRI (DWI) detects random motion, or diffusion, of water molecules in tissue. As renal function decreases, physiologic water reabsorption in the kidneys decreases and reduces diffusion. DWI allows for the calculation of the so-called apparent diffusion coefficient (ADC), which can be used for in vivo quantification of the combined effects of capillary perfusion and diffusion. DWI has shown good linear correlation with serum creatinine both in acute and chronic renal failure and is currently applied to the evaluation of renal fibrosis, renovascular hypertension, and allograft dysfunction [25–27].

16.4.3 Blood-Oxygen-Level-Dependent MRI

Blood-oxygen-level-dependent (BOLD) MRI is a tool for indirect assessment of renal oxygenation. The renal medulla physiologically functions in a state of hypoxia due to low oxygen delivery (low vascular density) and high oxygen consumption (active transcellular transport mechanisms). BOLD MRI is based on the perturbance of the magnetic field caused by the paramagnetic effect of deoxyhemoglobin, which depends on local oxygen concentration.

The high sensitivity of BOLD MRI to subtle changes of oxygen concentration converts this method into a promising tool to detect renal impairment in an early stage. Current applications include evaluation of diabetic nephropathy, renovascular hypertension, unilateral ureteral obstruction, and allograft dysfunction [28–30].

References

1. Calabia J, Torguet P, Garcia I, Martin N, Mate G, Marin A, Molina C, Valles M. The relationship between renal resistive index, arterial stiffness, and atherosclerotic burden: the link between macrocirculation and microcirculation. J Clin Hypertens. 2014;16:186–91.
2. Tublin ME, Bude RO, Platt JF. The resistive index in renal Doppler sonography: where do we stand? AJR Am J Roentgenol. 2003;180:885–92.
3. Lubas A, Kade G, Niemczyk S. Renal resistive index as a marker of vascular damage in cardiovascular diseases. Int Urol Nephrol. 2014;46:395–402.
4. Viazzi F, Leoncini G, Derchi LE, Pontremoli R. Ultrasound Doppler renal resistive index: a useful tool for the management of the hypertensive patient. J Hypertens. 2014;32:149–53.
5. Hashimoto J, Ito S. Central pulse pressure and aortic stiffness determine renal hemodynamics: pathophysiological implication for microalbuminuria in hypertension. Hypertension. 2011;58:839–46.
6. Derchi LE, Leoncini G, Parodi D, Viazzi F, Martinoli C, Ratto E, Vettoretti S, Vaccaro V, Falqui V, Tomolillo C, Deferrari G, Pontremoli R. Mild renal dysfunction and renal vascular resistance in primary hypertension. Am J Hypertens. 2005;18:966–71.
7. Ratto E, Leoncini G, Viazzi F, Vaccaro V, Falqui V, Parodi A, Conti N, Tomolillo C, Deferrari G, Pontremoli R. Ambulatory arterial stiffness index and renal abnormalities in primary hypertension. J Hypertens. 2006;24:2033–8.
8. Afsar B, Ozdemir NF, Elsurer R, Sezer S. Renal resistive index and nocturnal non-dipping: is there an association in essential hypertension? Int Urol Nephrol. 2009;41:383–91.
9. Florczak E, Januszewicz M, Januszewicz A, Prejbisz A, Kaczmarska M, Michałowska I, Kabat M, Rywik T, Rynkun D, Zieliński T, Kuśmierczyk-Droszcz B, Pregowska-Chwała B, Kowalewski G, Hoffman P. Relationship between renal resistive index and early target organ damage in patients with never-treated essential hypertension. Blood Press. 2009;18:55–61.
10. Raff U, Schmidt BM, Schwab J, Schwarz TK, Achenbach S, Bär I, Schmieder RE. Renal resistive index in addition to low-grade albuminuria complements screening for target organ damage in therapy-resistant hypertension. J Hypertens. 2010;28:608–14.
11. Doi Y, Iwashima Y, Yoshihara F, Kamide K, Hayashi S, Kubota Y, Nakamura S, Horio T, Kawano Y. Renal resistive index and cardiovascular and renal outcomes in essential hypertension. Hypertension. 2012;60:770–7.
12. Viazzi F, Leoncini G, Derchi LE, Baratto E, Storace G, Vercelli M, Deferrari G, Pontremoli R. Subclinical functional and structural renal abnormalities predict new onset type 2 diabetes in patients with primary hypertension. J Hum Hypertens. 2013;27:95–9.
13. Leoncini G, Martinoli C, Viazzi F, Ravera M, Parodi D, Ratto E, Vettoretti S, Tomolillo C, Derchi LE, Deferrari G, Pontremoli R. Changes in renal resistive index and urinary albumin excretion in hypertensive patients under long-term treatment with lisinopril or nifedipine GITS. Nephron. 2002;90:169–73.
14. Lubas A, Zelichowski G, Próchnicka A, Wiśniewska M, Saracyn M, Wańkowicz Z. Renal vascular response to angiotensin II inhibition in intensive antihypertensive treatment of essential hypertension. Arch Med Sci. 2010;6:533–8.
15. Agatston AS, Janowitz WR, Hildner FJ, Zusmer NR, Viamonte M, Detrano R. Quantification of coronary artery calcium using ultrafast computed tomography. J Am Coll Cardiol. 1990;15:827–32.
16. Roseman DA, Hwang SJ, Manders ES, O'Donnell CJ, Upadhyay A, Hoffmann U, Fox CS. Renal artery calcium, cardiovascular risk factors, and indexes of renal function. Am J Cardiol. 2014;113:156–61.
17. Allison MA, Lillie EO, DiTomasso D, Wright CM, Criqui MH. Renal artery calcium is independently associated with hypertension. J Am Coll Cardiol. 2007;50:1578–83.
18. Chiu Y-W, Adler S, Budoff M, Takasu J, Ashai J, Mehrotra R. Prevalence and prognostic significance of renal artery calcification in patients with diabetes and proteinuria. Clin J Am Soc Nephrol. 2010;5:2093–100.

19. Rifkin DE, Ix JH, Wassel CL, Criqui MH, Allison MA. Renal artery calcification and mortality among clinically asymptomatic adults. J Am Coll Cardiol. 2012;60:1079–85.
20. Allison MA, DiTomasso D, Criqui MH, Langer RD, Wright CM. Renal artery calcium: relationship to systemic calcified atherosclerosis. Vasc Med Lond Engl. 2006;11:232–8.
21. Zhang JL, Morrell G, Rusinek H, Sigmund EE, Chandarana H, Lerman LO, Prasad PV, Niles D, Artz N, Fain S, Vivier PH, Cheung AK, Lee VS. New magnetic resonance imaging methods in nephrology. Kidney Int. 2014;85:768–78.
22. Huang AJ, Lee VS, Rusinek H. Functional renal MR imaging. Magn Reson Imaging Clin N Am. 2004;12:469–86.
23. Bokacheva L, Rusinek H, Zhang JL, Lee VS. Assessment of renal function with dynamic contrast-enhanced MR imaging. Magn Reson Imaging Clin N Am. 2008;16:597–611.
24. Lee VS, Rusinek H, Bokacheva L, Huang AJ, Oesingmann N, Chen Q, Kaur M, Prince K, Song T, Kramer EL, Leonard EF. Renal function measurements from MR renography and a simplified multicompartmental model. Am J Physiol Renal Physiol. 2007;292:F1548–59.
25. Thoeny HC, De Keyzer F, Oyen RH, Peeters RR. Diffusion-weighted MR imaging of kidneys in healthy volunteers and patients with parenchymal diseases: initial experience. Radiology. 2005;235:911–7.
26. Xu Y, Wang X, Jiang X. Relationship between the renal apparent diffusion coefficient and glomerular filtration rate: preliminary experience. J Magn Reson Imaging. 2007;26:678–81.
27. Carbone SF, Gaggioli E, Ricci V, Mazzei F, Mazzei MA, Volterrani L. Diffusion-weighted magnetic resonance imaging in the evaluation of renal function: a preliminary study. Radiol Med (Torino). 2007;112:1201–10.
28. Prasad PV, Edelman RR, Epstein FH. Noninvasive evaluation of intrarenal oxygenation with BOLD MRI. Circulation. 1996;94:3271–5.
29. Simon-Zoula SC, Hofmann L, Giger A, Vogt B, Vock P, Frey FJ, Boesch C. Non-invasive monitoring of renal oxygenation using BOLD-MRI: a reproducibility study. NMR Biomed. 2006;19:84–9.
30. Dos Santos EA, Li L-P, Ji L, Prasad PV. Early changes with diabetes in renal medullary hemodynamics as evaluated by fiberoptic probes and BOLD magnetic resonance imaging. Invest Radiol. 2007;42:157–62.

Part V

Brain

MRI/CT: Evaluation of Brain Damage in Hypertension

17

Peter Wohlfahrt and Renata Cifkova

Hypertension is the main modifiable risk factor for ischemic and hemorrhagic stroke and vascular brain injury (VBI). Brain imaging in hypertension may be used to detect VBI, which is considered a sign of cerebral small vessel disease (SVD) and an important mediator of the relationship between hypertension and brain aging. SVD leads to substantial cognitive, psychiatric, and physical disabilities; contributes to about a fifth of all strokes, more than doubles the future risk of stroke, and contributes up to 45 % of dementias. VBI can be found in 44 % of middle-aged hypertensive patients without a history of cardiovascular and cerebrovascular disease [1]. Identifying hypertensive subjects with VBI could be helpful in preventive strategies. However, performing brain imaging in all hypertensive patients is unrealistic for economic and practical reasons. Thus, only a selected group of hypertensive patients at high risk of accelerated brain aging may be considered for VBI screening. In the future, screening tools for selection of patients who may profit from VBI screening will have to be developed.

17.1 Types of Vascular Brain Injury

The terminology and definitions used to describe VBI on conventional MRI (magnetic resonance imaging) vary substantially between studies. This precludes comparison between studies and hampers progress in identifying the mechanisms leading to VBI. To overcome this problem, STandards for ReportIng Vascular

P. Wohlfahrt • R. Cifkova (✉)
Center for Cardiovascular Prevention, Charles University in Prague,
First Faculty of Medicine and Thomayer Hospital, Videnska 800,
Prague 140 59, Czech Republic
e-mail: wohlfp@gmail.com; renata.cifkova@ftn.cz

E. Agabiti Rosei, G. Mancia (eds.), *Assessment of Preclinical Organ Damage in Hypertension*, DOI 10.1007/978-3-319-15603-3_17

Table 17.1 MRI terminology and findings of lesions related to vascular brain injury as recommended by STRIVE (STandards for ReportIng Vascular changes on nEuroimaging)

	White matter hyperintensity	Cerebral microbleeds	Recent small subcortical infarct	Lacunes	Dilated perivascular space
Usual diameter	Variable	≤10 mm	≤20 mm	3–15 mm	≤2 mm
Comment	Located in the white matter	Detected on GRE, round or ovoid, blooming	Best identified on DWI	Usually hyperintense rim	Mostly linear without hyperintense rim
DWI	↔	↔	↑	↔/(↓)	↔
FLAIR	↑	↔	↑	↓	↓
T2	↑	↔	↑	↑	↑
T1	↔/(↓)	↔	↓	↓	↓
T2-weighted GRE	↑	↓↓	↔	↔/↓ if hemorrhage	↔

DWI diffusion-weighted imaging, *FLAIR* fluid-attenuated inversion recovery, *SWI* susceptibility-weighted imaging, *GRE* gradient-recalled echo
↑ increased signal, ↓ decreased signal, ↔ isointense signal

changes on nEuroimaging (STRIVE) were recently published [2]. These standards should be used in research studies and in the clinical setting in order to standardize image interpretation, acquisition, and reporting. The following signs of VBI can be recognized on brain imaging: white matter hyperintensity (WMH), cerebral microbleeds (MBs), recent small subcortical infarct (SSI), lacunes, dilated perivascular space, and atrophy. MRI terminology and findings of lesions related to VBI as recommended by STRIVE are summarized in Table 17.1.

17.1.1 White Matter Hyperintensity

17.1.1.1 Definition

WMHs of presumed vascular origin are bilateral, mostly symmetrical hyperintense lesions on T2-weighted sequences of variable size in the white matter. On T1 sequences, WMH can appear as isointense or hypointense (Fig. 17.1, panel a). Lesions in the subcortical gray matter or brainstem are not included in this category. When using CT, white matter hypoattenuation or white matter hypodensities can be detected. CT and MRI rating scales for WMH have been suggested [3].

17.1.1.2 Epidemiology

Among all subtypes of VBI, WMHs are the most prevalent lesions in the general population, and both the frequency and size increase substantially with age. In subjects in their 40s, 50 % have WMH [4], while more than 90 % of individuals aged >80 years have WMH [5].

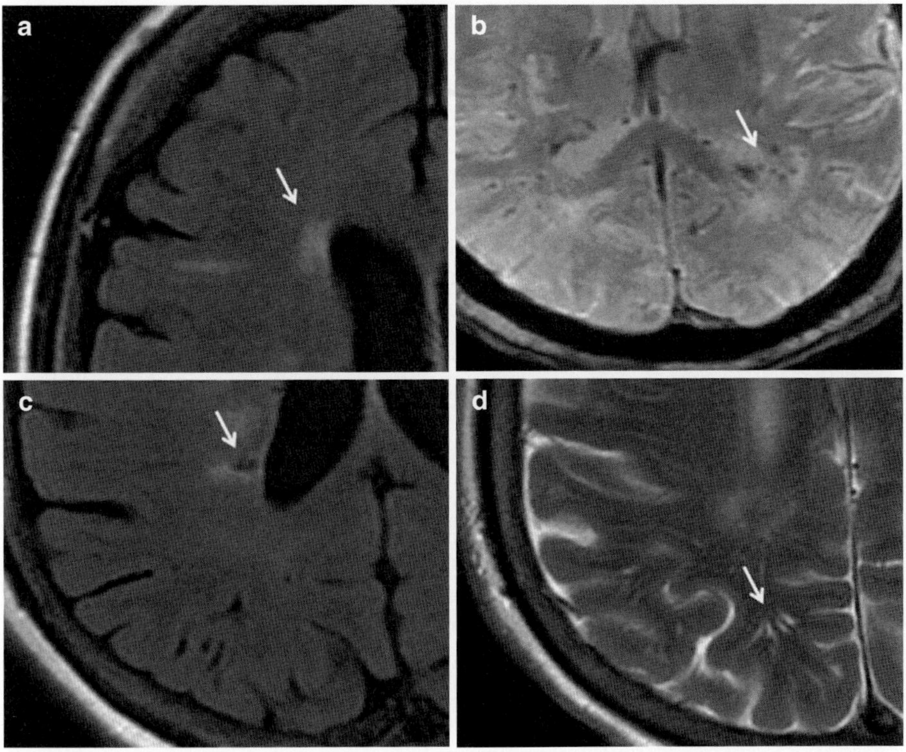

Fig. 17.1 Panel (**a**) Periventricular white matter hyperintensity – fluid-attenuated inversion recovery (FLAIR) MRI. Panel (**b**) Microbleeds – susceptibility-weighted imaging (SWI) MRI. Panel (**c**) Lacunes – fluid-attenuated inversion recovery (FLAIR) MRI. Panel (**d**) Perivascular space – T2-weighted turbo spin-echo MRI. Lesions are shown by *arrows* (MRI scans are courtesy of Dr. Zuzana Ryznarova, Dept of Radiology, Thomayer Hospital, Prague, Czech Republic)

17.1.1.3 Association with Hypertension

Hypertension is currently considered the most important modifiable risk factor for WMH volume and progression [6]. Midlife BP and cumulative systolic blood pressure (BP) and cumulative systolic BP measured over a period of several years seem to be better predictors of WMH than single late-life measurements. Hypertension or a history of hypertension has been associated with a greater WMH volume in the frontal lobe, indicating greater susceptibility of the frontal lobe to the hypertension-related white matter degradation. An association between systolic BP and injury to the white matter microstructure was described already in young adults in their 30s, suggesting that these lesions develop insidiously during life [7].

There is mounting evidence that BP control may reduce the course of WMH progression. In the 3C-Dijon MRI study, baseline BP and BP control over a 4-year follow-up were strong predictors of WMH volume progression [8]. However, the association with BP was only present for total and periventricular WMH. In the PROGRESS MRI substudy, a combination of perindopril plus indapamide was able to reduce WMH progression over a period of 3 years as compared to placebo [9]. The rate of WMH progression is lower in controlled treated hypertensives than in uncontrolled treated or untreated hypertensives [10].

17.1.1.4 Prognostic Value

According to a meta-analysis of 22 longitudinal studies, WMH is an independent indicator of future risk, which triples the risk of stroke and doubles the risk of dementia and death [5]. Extensive WMHs predispose to both ischemic (especially SSI) and hemorrhagic strokes. Moreover, WMHs are associated with covert neurological and cognitive symptoms and physical difficulties such as gait disturbance [11].

17.1.2 Cerebral Microbleeds (MBs)

17.1.2.1 Definition

Cerebral MBs are small (generally 2–5 mm but, occasionally, up to 10 mm in diameter) areas of signal void with associated blooming seen on T2* gradient-recalled echo (GRE) and susceptibility-weighted (SWI) MRI sequences and correspond to areas of hemosiderin breakdown from prior microscopic hemorrhage (Fig. 17.1, panel b). These are commonly caused by hypertensive vasculopathy or cerebral amyloid angiopathy. MRI is able to detect bleeding from vessels as small as 200 μm in diameter. The patterns of MB distribution differ by etiology. MBs in deep subcortical or infratentorial areas are usually associated with the presence of hypertension or vascular risk factors, with lipohyalinosis being the predominant finding. MBs in lobar and cortico-subcortical areas are associated with apolipoprotein E carrier status (ε4), β-amyloid burden, and evidence of cerebral amyloid angiopathy. Low total cholesterol and statin use have been found to be associated with increased risk of lobar MBs. Lacunes and WMH are associated with the deep or infratentorial MBs, but not with those in a lobar region.

17.1.2.2 Epidemiology

MB prevalence gradually increases with age, from 6.5 % in persons aged 45–50 years to 36 % in individuals ≥80 years of age [12]. In patients after stroke, MBs are present more often in patients with hemorrhagic stroke as compared with ischemic stroke. Of ischemic stroke subtypes, MBs occur more often in SSI than in other stroke subtypes. MBs are also more prevalent in subjects with mild cognitive impairment, Alzheimer's disease, and vascular dementia, as compared with subjects with cognitive normal controls. Lovelock et al. demonstrated an excess of MB in warfarin users compared with no antithrombotic users and in warfarin-related intracranial hemorrhage versus spontaneous intracranial hemorrhage, suggesting that MB may increase the risk of warfarin-associated intracranial hemorrhage [13].

17.1.2.3 Association with Hypertension

Hypertension is independently associated with cerebral MBs both in otherwise healthy adults and in adults with cerebrovascular diseases [14]. Among patients with hypertension, 24-h systolic, diastolic, and pulse pressure are independent predictors of MB progression. In subjects after lacunar stroke, higher BP is associated with the development of a new MB; however, a decrease in BP during follow-up does not halt MB progression [15]. Thus, it is not clear whether optimal BP control can slow down progression of MB.

17.1.2.4 Prognostic Value

The presence of MBs is associated with increased risk of incident intracerebral hemorrhage, particularly in patients on anticoagulation therapy. Among patients after ischemic stroke, the presence of MBs significantly increases the risk of recurrent hemorrhagic and ischemic stroke [16]. In the PROSPER study over 7-year follow-up, MBs were associated with a sixfold increased risk of stroke-related death. Those with non-lobar MBs had double the risk of cardiovascular disease-related death independently of other vascular risk factors, whereas those with lobar MBs had a sevenfold increase in the risk of stroke-related death, but not cardiovascular death [17]. In the Rotterdam study, the presence of MBs, and particularly deep or infratentorial MBs, was independently associated with an increased risk of all-cause and cardiovascular mortality [18].

17.1.3 Recent Small Subcortical Infarct

17.1.3.1 Definition

Recent small subcortical infarct (SSI) is defined as a neuroimaging evidence of recent infarction in the territory of one perforating arteriole, with imaging features or clinical symptoms consistent with a lesion occurring in the previous few weeks. The size of the lesion should be ≤20 mm in its maximal diameter in the axial plane. Acute lesions can shrink to leave lacunes, WMH, or completely disappear. A recent study has shown 97 % cavitation of SSI at 90 days [19]. Historically, SSI is commonly called as lacunar stroke or lacunar syndrome. This nomenclature is derived from the French expression for a small fluid-filled cavity (lacuna) that was thought to mark the healed stage of an SSI. Thus, the pre-cavitary stage became the lacunar infarct. As noted above, not all SSIs transform into lacunes, making the term lacunar stroke inaccurate. That is why STRIVE recommend to use the term SSI instead.

The primary location of SSI in the primary motor or sensory pathways explains why these lesions are clinically symptomatic despite their size, while other VBI lesions accumulate silently. An incidentally asymptomatic SSI can be found by chance and is referred to as a silent cerebral infarction.

17.1.3.2 Epidemiology

Clinically evident recent SSI is responsible for about 25 % of all ischemic strokes. Only about 50 % of recent SSIs are visible on CT, while at least 70 % can be found on DWI MRI. The incidence of lacunar strokes increases with age.

17.1.3.3 Association with Hypertension

Hypertension is the most prevalent risk factor for stroke, particularly for SSI. The prevalence of hypertension in patients with SSIs is higher as compared with other ischemic stroke subtypes [20, 21]. However, the mechanisms by which hypertension leads to SSI and other forms of cerebral SVD are largely unknown. Increased pressure pulsatility, impaired autoregulation of cerebral blood flow, and pulse wave encephalopathy (all of which emphasize the central hemodynamic role of aortic stiffness) have been suggested as possible mechanisms. Ischemic SSIs are caused mostly by cerebral arteriolar occlusive disease (e.g., arteriolosclerosis, lipohyalinosis, fibrinoid necrosis, and arteritis), while, in approximately 10 % of cases, occlusion of the perforating arteriole is caused by an embolus from a proximal source. A minority of SSIs are caused by hemorrhage due to amyloid angiopathy, fibrinoid necrosis, and arteritis.

Many clinical trials and meta-analyses have confirmed that BP lowering reduces the risk of stroke in primary and secondary prevention [22]. In the PROGRESS trial with patients after a previous cerebrovascular event, antihypertensive treatment reduced the risk of lacunar stroke by 23 %. In the recent SPS3 trial [23], lowering of systolic BP to a target of <130 mmHg in patients with a recent SSI resulted in nonsignificant reductions in all stroke, disabling or fatal stroke, and major vascular events and a significant reduction in intracerebral stroke, as compared with the treatment target of systolic BP 130–140 mmHg. This suggests that patients after SSI may benefit from lower BP targets.

17.1.3.4 Prognostic Value

Due to its size, SSI is commonly perceived to be associated with lower risk as compared with other ischemic stroke subtypes. While the early mortality and stroke recurrence risk are higher among patients with other stroke subtypes, the long-term risks and the risks of cardiac outcomes are similar [24]. This may be explained by the associated VBI. Furthermore, SSI is associated with increased risk of cognitive impairment and dementia. In a recent meta-analysis, approximately 30 % of patients were cognitively impaired at 4 years following an SSI, a similar proportion to non-SSI stroke.

17.1.4 Lacunes of Presumed Vascular Origin

17.1.4.1 Definition

A lacuna of presumed vascular origin is a round or ovoid, subcortical, fluid-filled cavity of between 3 and 15 mm in diameter. On fluid-attenuated inversion recovery (FLAIR) images, lacunes have a central cerebrospinal fluidlike hypointensity with a surrounding rim of hyperintensity (Fig. 17.1, panel c). However, the rim is not always present. Lacunes can be caused by a previous SSI (symptomatic), silent brain infarction (asymptomatic), or hemorrhage in the territory of one perforating arteriole. Old striato-capsular strokes, which are caused by atherosclerotic or embolic occlusion of several penetrating arteries and are >20 mm in the acute phase, can shrink to form a lacunar-like cavity. This may preclude discrimination of the etiology of old lesions.

As SSIs are described above, silent brain infarction (SBI) will be further discussed. While SBIs are by definition asymptomatic, these infarcts are often accompanied by subtle focal neurological and cognitive deficits, such as a decrease in reaction time and executive deficits. Some authors propose to replace the designation silent with the term covert.

17.1.4.2 Epidemiology

The incidence of SBI is five times that of symptomatic stroke. The prevalence of SBI in the general population ranges from 10 to 20 %, with a higher prevalence in the older age groups and groups with a higher cardiovascular risk profile [25]. The annual incidence of SBI is 3–4 %. According to the population-based Rotterdam Scan Study, 90 % of SBIs are lacunes in the basal ganglia (74 %) or subcortical lacunes (15 %), while only 10 % are cortical, cerebellar, or brainstem infarcts. However, not all SBIs form lacunes, with 30–80 % of infarcts remaining as T2 hyper/T1 hypointense lesions. Recently, criteria to standardize SBI definitions were published [26].

17.1.4.3 Association with Hypertension

In cross-sectional studies, hypertension has consistently been implicated as a risk factor for SBI. It increases the risk of SBI two- to threefold. In the Rotterdam study, associations between BP and incident lacunes on MRI were strongest in the youngest age stratum (60–69 years) and in people without severe WMH at baseline, while, in the oldest people and in those with severe WMH or lacunes at baseline, increased BP was not associated with lesion progression [27]. This may be so because, in the stage of impaired brain autoregulation, increased BP may be essential to maintain adequate cerebral perfusion. This warrants early BP control to prevent changes in brain microcirculation and autoregulation. There are limited longitudinal data assessing the association between BP control and SBI. In a small Japanese study, BP control reduced the risk of incident SBI in hypertensive patients [28]. In the PROGRESS CT substudy, antihypertensive treatment decreased the risk of incident SBI as compared with placebo only in subjects with large artery ischemic stroke, but not in the overall study sample [29].

17.1.4.4 Prognostic Value

Among subjects without stroke, SBI increases the risk of the first-ever stroke four- to fivefold, and the annual risk of stroke is as high as 10 %. Among subjects after stroke, the presence of multiple SBIs increases the risk of recurrent stroke 2.5 times. Elderly people with SBIs are at an increased risk of dementia and show a steeper decline in cognitive function. Also, the odds of death are increased three to four times among those with SBI.

17.1.5 Dilated Perivascular Space (dPVS)

17.1.5.1 Definition

Perivascular space, also known as the Virchow-Robin space, is a fluid-filled space that follows the typical course of a vessel as it goes through the gray or white matter.

The space has signal intensity similar to cerebrospinal fluid on all sequences. As it follows the course of penetrating vessels, it appears linear when imaged parallel to the course of the vessel and round or ovoid, with a diameter generally smaller than 3 mm, when imaged perpendicular to the course of the vessel (Fig. 17.1, panel d). A rating scale for perivascular space was described [30].

17.1.5.2 Epidemiology

The presence and severity of dPVS increase with age. In a population-based study, dPVS in the basal ganglia and white matter was found in all elderly individuals, while 46 % had dPVS within the hippocampus. Status cribrosum can be found in 1.3 % of elderly subjects. dPVS is also found in children, in whom their presence has been associated with behavioral and neurological symptoms. Nonetheless, the etiology of dPVS in children with neuropsychiatric abnormalities is most likely of an etiology different from those of middle-aged and older individuals with cardiovascular risk factors.

17.1.5.3 Association with Hypertension

Hypertension is associated with dPVS in the white matter and basal ganglia, although the association with basal ganglia dPVS seems stronger. Although some risk factors are shared, it is suggested the mechanisms underlying the development of dPVS may differ in different areas of the brain. The presence of dPVS is associated with other forms of VBI such as WMH and lacunes. In the Northern Manhattan Study, antihypertensive therapy was associated with a lower dPVS score; however, longitudinal data on the effect of antihypertensive therapy on dPVS progression are lacking.

17.1.5.4 Prognostic Value

Data assessing the predictive value of dPVS in cardiovascular risk prediction are lacking.

17.1.6 Brain Atrophy

17.1.6.1 Definition

Brain atrophy is defined as a lower brain volume that is not relevant to a specific macroscopic focal injury such as trauma or infarction.

17.1.6.2 Epidemiology

Aging has a significant, but disparate, effect on volume change in brain structure. The volume of the precentral and postcentral cortices decreases linearly with aging, while that of the temporal and occipital cortices and subcortical structures (thalamus, caudate, pallidum, and amygdala) decreases exponentially with aging, with accelerated changes after 60 years of age. Volume reduction in men has steeper trajectories than those of women, especially after age 60 years [31].

17.1.6.3 Association with Hypertension

High BP leads to global and regional brain volume reduction, specifically in the hippocampus and prefrontal cortex [32]. However, the association between BP and brain volume is inconsistent across studies. Most studies have shown an association between higher BP/hypertension and regional brain volume reduction, while other studies reported an association between lower BP and brain volume reduction. These differences may be explained by a confounding effect of age, cerebral blood flow, and differences in methodology. In support of this superposition is the observation that low BP by itself is not sufficient to induce brain atrophy; however, lower BP in combination with lower cerebral blood flow does increase the risk for cortical atrophy [33].

The effect of pharmacological treatment of hypertension on brain volume in longitudinal follow-up is complex and dependent on the timing of treatment initiation and magnitude of BP reduction [34]. Higher diastolic BP in midlife predicts more brain volume loss late in life when antihypertensive therapy is not used. However, when antihypertensive therapy is initiated late in life, it is associated with more profound brain volume loss, particularly when there is a steep decrease in diastolic BP.

17.1.6.4 Prognostic Value

A smaller total brain volume is an independent predictor of total mortality, cardiovascular mortality, and ischemic stroke among patients with manifest cardiovascular disease [35]. Among the elderly, brain atrophy increases the risk of total mortality [36, 37]. Furthermore, brain atrophy is a strong predictor of cognitive decline, dementia, and function disabilities.

Acknowledgment Development of this chapter was supported by grant NT 12102–4 awarded by the Internal Grant Agency of the Ministry of Health of the Czech Republic.

References

1. Henskens LH, van Oostenbrugge RJ, Kroon AA, Hofman PA, Lodder J, de Leeuw PW. Detection of silent cerebrovascular disease refines risk stratification of hypertensive patients. J Hypertens. 2009;27(4):846–53.
2. Wardlaw JM, Smith EE, Biessels GJ, Cordonnier C, Fazekas F, Frayne R, Lindley RI, O'Brien JT, Barkhof F, Benavente OR, Black SE, Brayne C, Breteler M, Chabriat H, Decarli C, de Leeuw FE, Doubal F, Duering M, Fox NC, Greenberg S, Hachinski V, Kilimann I, Mok V, Oostenbrugge R, Pantoni L, Speck O, Stephan BC, Teipel S, Viswanathan A, Werring D, Chen C, Smith C, van Buchem M, Norrving B, Gorelick PB, Dichgans M. Neuroimaging standards for research into small vessel disease and its contribution to ageing and neurodegeneration. Lancet Neurol. 2013;12(8):822–38.
3. Wahlund LO, Barkhof F, Fazekas F, Bronge L, Augustin M, Sjogren M, Wallin A, Ader H, Leys D, Pantoni L, Pasquier F, Erkinjuntti T, Scheltens P. A new rating scale for age-related white matter changes applicable to MRI and CT. Stroke. 2001;32(6):1318–22.
4. Wen W, Sachdev PS, Li JJ, Chen X, Anstey KJ. White matter hyperintensities in the forties: their prevalence and topography in an epidemiological sample aged 44–48. Hum Brain Mapp. 2009;30(4):1155–67.

5. Debette S, Markus HS. The clinical importance of white matter hyperintensities on brain magnetic resonance imaging: systematic review and meta-analysis. BMJ (Clinical Research ed). 2010;341:c3666. doi:10.1136/bmj.c3666.
6. Debette S, Seshadri S, Beiser A, Au R, Himali JJ, Palumbo C, Wolf PA, DeCarli C. Midlife vascular risk factor exposure accelerates structural brain aging and cognitive decline. Neurology. 2011;77(5):461–8.
7. Maillard P, Seshadri S, Beiser A, Himali JJ, Au R, Fletcher E, Carmichael O, Wolf PA, DeCarli C. Effects of systolic blood pressure on white-matter integrity in young adults in the Framingham Heart Study: a cross-sectional study. Lancet Neurol. 2012;11(12):1039–47.
8. Godin O, Tzourio C, Maillard P, Mazoyer B, Dufouil C. Antihypertensive treatment and change in blood pressure are associated with the progression of white matter lesion volumes: the Three-City (3C)-Dijon Magnetic Resonance Imaging Study. Circulation. 2011;123(3): 266–73.
9. Dufouil C, Chalmers J, Coskun O, Besancon V, Bousser MG, Guillon P, MacMahon S, Mazoyer B, Neal B, Woodward M, Tzourio-Mazoyer N, Tzourio C. Effects of blood pressure lowering on cerebral white matter hyperintensities in patients with stroke: the PROGRESS (Perindopril Protection Against Recurrent Stroke Study) Magnetic Resonance Imaging Substudy. Circulation. 2005;112(11):1644–50.
10. Verhaaren BF, Vernooij MW, de Boer R, Hofman A, Niessen WJ, van der Lugt A, Ikram MA. High blood pressure and cerebral white matter lesion progression in the general population. Hypertension. 2013;61(6):1354–9.
11. Inzitari D, Pracucci G, Poggesi A, Carlucci G, Barkhof F, Chabriat H, Erkinjuntti T, Fazekas F, Ferro JM, Hennerici M, Langhorne P, O'Brien J, Scheltens P, Visser MC, Wahlund LO, Waldemar G, Wallin A, Pantoni L. Changes in white matter as determinant of global functional decline in older independent outpatients: three year follow-up of LADIS (leukoaraiosis and disability) study cohort. BMJ (Clinical research ed). 2009;339:b2477. doi:10.1136/bmj.b2477.
12. Poels MM, Vernooij MW, Ikram MA, Hofman A, Krestin GP, van der Lugt A, Breteler MM. Prevalence and risk factors of cerebral microbleeds: an update of the Rotterdam scan study. Stroke. 2010;41(10 Suppl):S103–6.
13. Lovelock CE, Cordonnier C, Naka H, Al-Shahi Salman R, Sudlow CL, Sorimachi T, Werring DJ, Gregoire SM, Imaizumi T, Lee SH, Briley D, Rothwell PM. Antithrombotic drug use, cerebral microbleeds, and intracerebral hemorrhage: a systematic review of published and unpublished studies. Stroke. 2010;41(6):1222–8.
14. Cordonnier C, Al-Shahi Salman R, Wardlaw J. Spontaneous brain microbleeds: systematic review, subgroup analyses and standards for study design and reporting. Brain. 2007;130(Pt 8):1988–2003.
15. Klarenbeek P, van Oostenbrugge RJ, Rouhl RP, Knottnerus IL, Staals J. Higher ambulatory blood pressure relates to new cerebral microbleeds: 2-year follow-up study in lacunar stroke patients. Stroke. 2013;44(4):978–83.
16. Charidimou A, Kakar P, Fox Z, Werring DJ. Cerebral microbleeds and recurrent stroke risk: systematic review and meta-analysis of prospective ischemic stroke and transient ischemic attack cohorts. Stroke. 2013;44(4):995–1001.
17. Altmann-Schneider I, Trompet S, de Craen AJ, van Es AC, Jukema JW, Stott DJ, Sattar N, Westendorp RG, van Buchem MA, van der Grond J. Cerebral microbleeds are predictive of mortality in the elderly. Stroke. 2011;42(3):638–44.
18. Akoudad S, Ikram MA, Koudstaal PJ, Hofman A, van der Lugt A, Vernooij MW. Cerebral microbleeds and the risk of mortality in the general population. Eur J Epidemiol. 2013;28(10): 815–21.
19. Moreau F, Patel S, Lauzon ML, McCreary CR, Goyal M, Frayne R, Demchuk AM, Coutts SB, Smith EE. Cavitation after acute symptomatic lacunar stroke depends on time, location, and MRI sequence. Stroke. 2012;43(7):1837–42.
20. Vemmos KN, Takis CE, Georgilis K, Zakopoulos NA, Lekakis JP, Papamichael CM, Zis VP, Stamatelopoulos S. The Athens stroke registry: results of a five-year hospital-based study. Cerebrovasc Dis. 2000;10(2):133–41.

21. Marti-Vilalta JL, Arboix A. The Barcelona Stroke Registry. Eur Neurol. 1999;41(3):135–42.
22. Law MR, Morris JK, Wald NJ. Use of blood pressure lowering drugs in the prevention of cardiovascular disease: meta-analysis of 147 randomised trials in the context of expectations from prospective epidemiological studies. BMJ (Clinical research ed). 2009;338:b1665.
23. SPS3 Study Group, Benavente OR, Coffey CS, Conwit R, Hart RG, McClure LA, Pearce LA, Pergola PE, Szychowski JM. Blood-pressure targets in patients with recent lacunar stroke: the SPS3 randomised trial. Lancet. 2013;382(9891):507–15.
24. Jackson C, Sudlow C. Comparing risks of death and recurrent vascular events between lacunar and non-lacunar infarction. Brain. 2005;128(Pt 11):2507–17.
25. Fanning JP, Wong AA, Fraser JF. The epidemiology of silent brain infarction: a systematic review of population-based cohorts. BMC Med. 2014;12(1):119.
26. Fanning JP, Wesley AJ, Wong AA, Fraser JF. Emerging spectra of silent brain infarction. Stroke. 2014;45(11):3461–71.
27. van Dijk EJ, Prins ND, Vrooman HA, Hofman A, Koudstaal PJ, Breteler MM. Progression of cerebral small vessel disease in relation to risk factors and cognitive consequences: Rotterdam Scan study. Stroke. 2008;39(10):2712–9.
28. Sugiyama T, Lee JD, Shimizu H, Abe S, Ueda T. Influence of treated blood pressure on progression of silent cerebral infarction. J Hypertens. 1999;17(5):679–84.
29. Hasegawa Y, Yamaguchi T, Omae T, Woodward M, Chalmers J. Effects of perindopril-based blood pressure lowering and of patient characteristics on the progression of silent brain infarct: the Perindopril Protection against Recurrent Stroke Study (PROGRESS) CT Substudy in Japan. Hypertens Res. 2004;27(3):147–56.
30. Adams HH, Cavalieri M, Verhaaren BF, Bos D, van der Lugt A, Enzinger C, Vernooij MW, Schmidt R, Ikram MA. Rating method for dilated Virchow-Robin spaces on magnetic resonance imaging. Stroke. 2013;44(6):1732–5.
31. Pfefferbaum A, Rohlfing T, Rosenbloom MJ, Chu W, Colrain IM, Sullivan EV. Variation in longitudinal trajectories of regional brain volumes of healthy men and women (ages 10 to 85 years) measured with atlas-based parcellation of MRI. Neuroimage. 2013;65:176–93.
32. Beauchet O, Celle S, Roche F, Bartha R, Montero-Odasso M, Allali G, Annweiler C. Blood pressure levels and brain volume reduction: a systematic review and meta-analysis. J Hypertens. 2013;31(8):1502–16.
33. Muller M, van der Graaf Y, Visseren FL, Vlek AL, Mali WP, Geerlings MI. Blood pressure, cerebral blood flow, and brain volumes. The SMART-MR study. J Hypertens. 2010;28(7):1498–505.
34. Friedman JI, Tang CY, de Haas HJ, Changchien L, Goliasch G, Dabas P, Wang V, Fayad ZA, Fuster V, Narula J. Brain imaging changes associated with risk factors for cardiovascular and cerebrovascular disease in asymptomatic patients. JACC Cardiovasc Imaging. 2014;7(10):1039–53.
35. van der Veen PH, Muller M, Vincken KL, Mali WP, van der Graaf Y, Geerlings MI. Brain volumes and risk of cardiovascular events and mortality. The SMART-MR study. Neurobiol Aging. 2014;35(7):1624–31. doi:10.1016/j.neurobiolaging.2014.02.003.
36. Ikram MA, Vernooij MW, Vrooman HA, Hofman A, Breteler MM. Brain tissue volumes and small vessel disease in relation to the risk of mortality. Neurobiol Aging. 2009;30(3):450–6.
37. Kuller LH, Arnold AM, Longstreth Jr WT, Manolio TA, O'Leary DH, Burke GL, Fried LP, Newman AB. White matter grade and ventricular volume on brain MRI as markers of longevity in the cardiovascular health study. Neurobiol Aging. 2007;28(9):1307–15.

Questionnaires for Cognitive Function Evaluation

18

Mónica Doménech, Cristina Sierra, and Antonio Coca

Microvascular brain damage may be the result of age-associated alterations in the large arteries (primarily arterial stiffening) and the progressive mismatch of their cross talk with the small cerebral arteries. The limited, but growing, literature indicates that microvascular brain damage is a potent risk factor for cognitive decline in older individuals and for the onset of dementia [1]. Therefore, neuropsychological evaluation and neuroimaging are required for assessment of the clinical consequences. Clinicians should be aware of the high prevalence of microvascular brain damage and make efforts to screen for cognitive function and follow-up for cognitive deterioration.

Patients with hypertension should be asked during the routine clinical examination whether they have recently experienced changes in memory or mood, speed of thinking and acting, or slowness or unsteadiness during walking [1]. European Guidelines do not recommend any standardized cognitive assessment instrument as routine for hypertensive patients, but it seems reasonable that in people at high risk for vascular cognition impairment (VCI) or for those who have suspected cognitive impairment based on clinician observation, self- (or informant) reported concerns, the use of instruments designed to assess cognitive impairment should be part of the routine examination [2]. The most common screening instruments used to detect mild cognitive impairment (MCI) are, from most to least common, the Mini-Mental State Examination (MMSE) (studies = 15; n = 5,758); the Informant Questionnaire on Cognitive Decline in the Elderly (IQCODE) (studies = 4; n = 975); the Clock Drawing test (CDT) (studies = 4; n = 4,191), the Mini-Cog (studies = 3; n = 1,092), the Telephone Interview for Cognitive Status (TICS) (studies = 3; n = 568), and the Montreal Cognitive Assessment (MoCA) (studies = 2; n = 251) [2].

M. Doménech • C. Sierra • A. Coca (✉)
Hypertension and Vascular Risk Unit, Department of Internal Medicine, Hospital Clínic, University of Barcelona, Villarroel 170, Barcelona 08036, Spain
e-mail: mdomen@clinic.ub.es; csierra@clinic.ub.es; acoca@clinic.ub.es

E. Agabiti Rosei, G. Mancia (eds.), *Assessment of Preclinical Organ Damage in Hypertension*, DOI 10.1007/978-3-319-15603-3_18

The most widely used cognitive screening test is the MMSE, developed by Folstein et al. [3]. It includes five sections: orientation (10 points), registration (3 points), attention and calculation (5 points), recall (3 points), and language (9 points), for a total of 30 points. However, there are a number of limitations, including advanced age, limited education, foreign culture, and sensory impairment, which may easily lead to false-positives. In a limited subset of studies that reported sensitivity and specificity, a cut point of 27 or 28 had a low (and wide ranging) sensitivity to detect MCI, and a cut point of 23 or 24 appears to have a better sensitivity and specificity to detect MCI and dementia than most other screening instruments, albeit still less than optimal [2]. Therefore, even though the MMSE is the most widely used cognitive assessment test, it is being used less and less.

It has been hypothesized that microvascular brain damage electively and predominantly affects executive function, with slower information processing, impairments in the ability to shift from one task to another, and deficits in the ability to hold and manipulate information (i.e., working memory) [4–6]. Executive functions cannot be explored by the MMSE, and it has a low sensitivity for VCI. The National Institute of Neurological Disorders and Stroke-Canadian Stroke Network harmonization standard has proposed the use of the Montreal Cognitive Assessment (MoCA) [7]. This newly designed screening test incorporates subtests assessing executive functions and psychomotor speed [7], which are frequently impaired in VCI. Ideally, neuropsychological evaluation should include tests exploring multiple cognitive domains, particularly in middle-aged patients with hypertension: executive function and activation, language, visuospatial ability, and memory (Fig. 18.1). The MoCA was specifically designed to detect MCI. One fair-quality [8] and one good-quality study [9] assessed the test performance of the MoCA in detecting MCI (excluding people with dementia). Both studies used the Petersen criteria for MCI. One study was conducted in South Korea, with a mean age of 70 years, and found a prevalence of MCI of 24 %. The other study was conducted in an older population (mean age, 76 years) in the United Kingdom and found a prevalence of MCI of 20 %. Using a cut-off point of 25/26, sensitivity and specificity ranged from 80 to 100 % (95 % CI, 56.3–100) and 50 to 76 % (95 % CI, 41–84.9), respectively [2].

The MoCA test showed excellent sensitivity and specificity in identifying VCI and MCI compared to the MMSE (90 % vs 18 %) [10]. It is recommended that patients who present cognitive complaints and functional decline should first be screened with the MMSE and, if this is normal (>25), with the MoCA test [10]. For patients with cognitive complaints without functional impairment, the MoCA should be administered first, as these patients are either normal or have MCI and may not be identified by the MMSE. A recent study in patients with acute transient ischemic attack and minor stroke found that the MoCA is more sensitive than the MMSE in detecting cognitive impairment at 7, 30 and 90 days after the cerebrovascular event, even when other neurological deficits were not evident [11].

The Clock Drawing Test (CDT) is another cognitive screening instrument which requires a wide range of intellectual and perceptual skills and provides a wide net in capturing cognitive dysfunction [11]. The cognitive domain includes comprehension, planning, visual memory, visuospatial ability, motor programming and

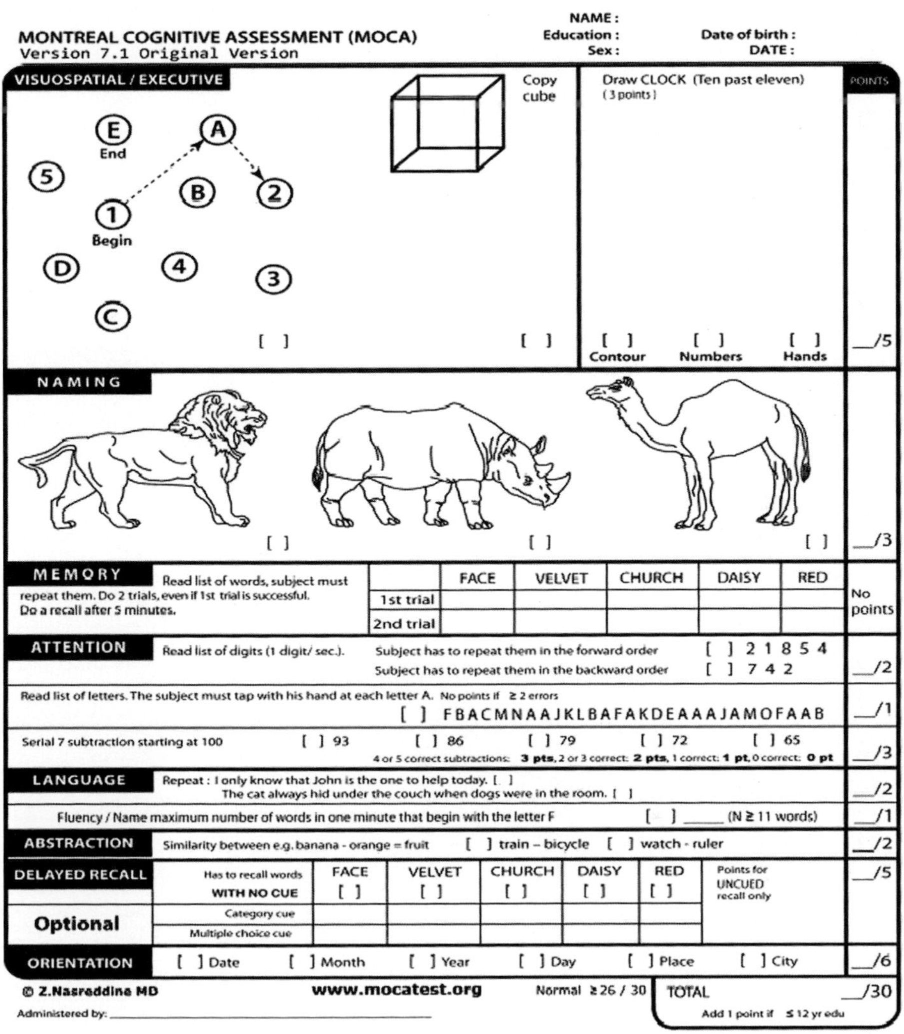

MONTREAL COGNITIVE ASSESSMENT (MOCA)
Version 7.1 Original Version

NAME :
Education : Date of birth :
Sex : DATE :

VISUOSPATIAL / EXECUTIVE — POINTS

E End, A, 5, B, 2, 1 Begin, D, 4, 3, C [ ]

Copy cube [ ]

Draw CLOCK (Ten past eleven) (3 points)

[ ] Contour [ ] Numbers [ ] Hands ___/5

NAMING

[ ] [ ] [ ] ___/3

MEMORY Read list of words, subject must repeat them. Do 2 trials, even if 1st trial is successful. Do a recall after 5 minutes.

	FACE	VELVET	CHURCH	DAISY	RED	
1st trial						No points
2nd trial						

ATTENTION Read list of digits (1 digit/ sec.). Subject has to repeat them in the forward order [ ] 2 1 8 5 4
Subject has to repeat them in the backward order [ ] 7 4 2 ___/2

Read list of letters. The subject must tap with his hand at each letter A. No points if ≥ 2 errors
[ ] FBACMNAAJKLBAFAKDEAAAJAMOFAAB ___/1

Serial 7 subtraction starting at 100 [ ] 93 [ ] 86 [ ] 79 [ ] 72 [ ] 65
4 or 5 correct subtractions: **3 pts**, 2 or 3 correct: **2 pts**, 1 correct: **1 pt**, 0 correct: **0 pt** ___/3

LANGUAGE Repeat : I only know that John is the one to help today. [ ]
The cat always hid under the couch when dogs were in the room. [ ] ___/2

Fluency / Name maximum number of words in one minute that begin with the letter F [ ] ___ (N ≥ 11 words) ___/1

ABSTRACTION Similarity between e.g. banana - orange = fruit [ ] train – bicycle [ ] watch - ruler ___/2

DELAYED RECALL	Has to recall words WITH NO CUE	FACE [ ]	VELVET [ ]	CHURCH [ ]	DAISY [ ]	RED [ ]	Points for UNCUED recall only	___/5
Optional	Category cue							
	Multiple choice cue							

ORIENTATION [ ] Date [ ] Month [ ] Year [ ] Day [ ] Place [ ] City ___/6

© Z.Nasreddine MD www.mocatest.org Normal ≥ 26 / 30 TOTAL ___/30
Administered by: ___ Add 1 point if ≤ 12 yr edu

Fig. 18.1 Montreal Cognitive Assessment (MoCA) (Copyright Z. Nasreddine MD. Reproduced with permission. Copies are available at www.mocatest.org)

execution, abstraction, concentration, and response inhibition [11]. The CDT provides a user-friendly visual record of cognitive function and takes less than 1 min to conduct, which is ideal for busy clinicians. Therefore, the CDT could be used as a complement to the widely used and validated MMSE and should provide a significance advance in the early detection of dementia and in monitoring cognitive change in a few minutes [12] (Fig. 18.2).

A recent study evaluating the cognitive executive function in adult treated hypertensive patients has shown that poor BP control, confirmed by ambulatory blood pressure monitoring, is associated to impaired global cognitive function and

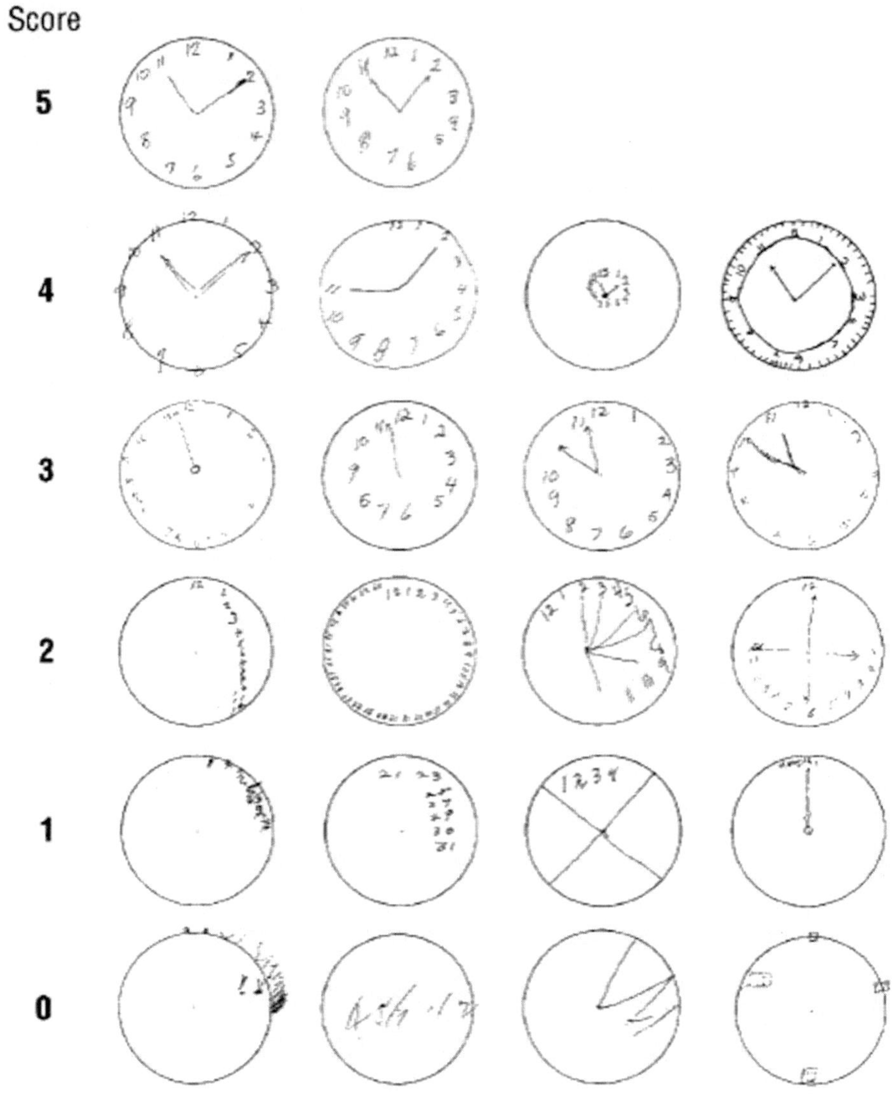

Fig. 18.2 Clock Drawing Test. Example of severity scores progressing from 5 (minimum) to 0

especially executive/attention functions [13]. Prose Memory Immediate and Delayed Recall (DR) [14] and Digit Span (DS) Forwards [15] tests were used to investigate verbal long-term memory and verbal short-term memory, respectively. The cognitive domains of attention and executive functions were measured by the DS Backwards test that examines verbal working memory [15], specially affected in patients with white coat effect. This study showed accelerated deterioration of cognitive performances in adult treated hypertensive with an insufficient BP control, mainly in the functions regulated by frontal-subcortical circuits and DR and DS seems to be more specific test in these situations.

In conclusion, screening tests in all or targeted older adults may help identify patients with dementia or MCI who are otherwise missed. Early identification of cognitive impairment would ideally allow patients and their families to receive care at an earlier stage in the disease process, leading to improved prognosis and decreased morbidity. Knowledge of the patient's cognitive status is important for the management of comorbid conditions, especially in older hypertensive patients, a population in which further specific research is necessary.

18.1 Summary

Microvascular brain damage is a potent risk factor for cognitive decline in elderly hypertensive individuals and for the onset of dementia [1]. In addition to elderly patients, cognitive decline has also been detected in asymptomatic middle-aged hypertensive patients. Therefore, neuropsychological evaluation and neuroimaging are required to assess silent brain damage induced by hypertension and the associated cardiovascular risk factors. With respect to cognitive decline, clinicians should be aware of the high prevalence of microvascular brain damage and make an effort to screen for cognitive function very early in the natural history of the disease and follow-up for cognitive deterioration. Patients with hypertension should be asked during the routine clinical examination whether they have recently experienced changes in memory or mood, speed of thinking and acting, or slowness or unsteadiness during walking. The use of some of the different instruments designed to assess cognitive function and impairment, such as the Mini-Mental State Examination (MMSE), the Informant Questionnaire on Cognitive Decline in the Elderly (IQCODE), the Clock Drawing test (CDT), the Mini-Cog, the Telephone Interview for Cognitive Status (TICS), the Montreal Cognitive Assessment (MoCA), and the more sensitive Prose Memory Immediate and Delayed Recall (DR) and Digit Span (DS) Forwards tests, should be part of the routine clinical examination in hypertension.

References

1. Scuteri A, Nilsson PM, Tzourio C, et al. Microvascular brain damage with aging and hypertension: pathophysiological consideration and clinical implications. J Hypertens. 2011;29: 1469–77. Brief but complete review of microvascular brain damage and hypertension that considers what should be done to improve understanding.
2. Screening for cognitive impairment in older adults: an evidence update for the U.S. Preventive Services Task Force. 2013. www.ahrq.gov.
3. Folstein M, Folstein S, McHugh P. Mini mental state. A practical method for grading the cognitive state of patients for the clinician. J Psychiatr Res. 1975;12:189–98.
4. Garrett KD, Browndyke JN, Whelihan W, Paul RH, DiCarlo M, Moser DJ, et al. The neuropsychological profile of vascular cognitive impairment – no dementia: comparisons to patients

at risk for cerebrovascular disease and vascular dementia. Arch Clin Neuropsychol. 2004;19:745–57.
5. Nyenhuis DL, Gorelick PB, Geenen EJ, Smith CA, Gencheva E, Freels S, DeToledo-Morrell L. The pattern of neuropsychological deficits in vascular cognitive impairment-no dementia (vascular CIND). Clin Neuropsychol. 2004;18:41–9.
6. Troyer AK, Moscovitch M, Winocur G, Alexander MP, Stuss D. Clustering and switching on verbal fluency: the effects of focal frontal- and temporal lobe lesions. Neuropsychologia. 1998;36:499–504.
7. Hachinski V, Iadecola C, Petersen RC, et al. National Institute of Neurological Disorders and Stroke-Canadian Stroke Network vascular cognitive impairment harmonization standards. Stroke. 2006;37:2220–41.
8. Lee JY, Dong WL, Cho SJ, et al. Brief screening for mild cognitive impairment in elderly outpatient clinic: validation of the Korean version of the montreal cognitive assessment. J Geriatr Psychiatry Neurol. 2008;21(2):104–10. PMID: 18474719.
9. Markwick A, Zamboni G, de Jager CA. Profiles of cognitive subtest impairment in the Montreal Cognitive Assessment (MoCA) in a research cohort with normal Mini-Mental State Examination (MMSE) scores. J Clin Exp Neuropsychol. 2012;34(7):750–7. PMID: 22468719.
10. Zahinoor I, Rajji TK, Shulman KI. Brief cognitive screening instruments: an update. Int J Geriatr Psychiatry. 2010;25:111–20.
11. Sivakumar L, Kate M, Jeerakathil T, Camicioli R, Buck B, Butcher K. Serial montreal cognitive assessments demonstrate reversible cognitive impairment in patients with acute transient ischemic attack and minor stroke. Stroke. 2014;45:1709–15.
12. Shulman KI. Clock-drawing: is it the ideal cognitive screening test? Int J Geriatr Psychiatry. 2000;15(6):548–61.
13. Spinelli C, De Caro MF, Schirosi G, Mezzapesa D, De Benedittis L, Chiapparino C, Serio G, Federico F, Nazzaro P. Impaired cognitive executive dysfunction in adult treated hypertensives with a confirmed diagnosis of poorly controlled blood pressure. Int J Med Sci. 2014; 11(8):771–8.
14. Bianchi A, Prà Dai M. Twenty years after Spinnler and Tognoni: new instruments in the Italian neuropsychologist's toolbox. Neurol Sci. 2008;29:209–17.
15. Orsini A, Grossi D, Capitani E, et al. Verbal and spatial immediate memory span: normative data from 1355 adults and 1112 children. Ital J Neurol Sci. 1987;8:539–48.

Other Techniques for Neurological Damage Evaluation

19

Cristina Sierra, Mónica Doménech, and Antonio Coca

It is known that high blood pressure (BP) is a major risk factor for ischemic and hemorrhagic stroke in men and women [1] and for small vessel disease predisposing to lacunar infarction, white matter lesions (WML), and cerebral microbleeds, which are frequently silent [1, 2]. Functional and structural abnormalities due to hypertension may be detected in neurologically asymptomatic individuals by computerized tomography (CT), magnetic resonance imaging (MRI), transcranial Doppler (TCD) ultrasound, positron emission tomography (PET), and single-photon emission computed tomography (SPECT). Neuropsychological tests may also provide useful information, as mentioned in the previous chapter.

However, availability and cost considerations do not allow the widespread use of MRI in the evaluation of middle-aged and elderly hypertensives in order to search for asymptomatic structural organ damage. Likewise, availability, cost, and radiation hazards are disadvantages of techniques investigating hemodynamic abnormalities (PET, SPECT). TCD ultrasound may be useful in investigating cerebral hemodynamics in hypertensive individuals, although its predictive value has not been evaluated in longitudinal studies.

19.1 Cerebral Autoregulation and High Blood Pressure

Autoregulation of the cerebral circulation system enables the cerebral blood flow (CBF) to remain constant despite changes in arterial BP. Under normal conditions, autoregulation is effective between 60 and 150 mmHg. High BP influences the cerebral circulation, causing adaptive vascular changes. Thus, hypertension

C. Sierra • M. Doménech • A. Coca (✉)
Hypertension and Vascular Risk Unit, Department of Internal Medicine, Hospital Clínic, University of Barcelona, Villarroel 170, Barcelona 08036, Spain
e-mail: csierra@clinic.ub.es; mdomen@clinic.ub.es; acoca@clinic.ub.es

E. Agabiti Rosei, G. Mancia (eds.), *Assessment of Preclinical Organ Damage in Hypertension*, DOI 10.1007/978-3-319-15603-3_19

influences the autoregulation of CBF by shifting both the lower and upper limits of autoregulatory capacity toward higher BP. For this reason, hypertensive patients may be especially vulnerable to episodes of hypotension [3], which may play a role in the development of silent cerebrovascular damage. Increased cerebral vascular resistance may be due to narrowing of the small vessels by lipohyalinosis and microatherosclerosis. The effect of high BP on small vessels is known, with vascular remodeling occurring in cerebral blood vessels during chronic hypertension. It has been suggested that this structural alteration impairs autoregulation, exposing the white matter to fluctuations in BP. For this reason, it has been hypothesized that changes in cerebral hemodynamics may play a role in the development of WML [3].

The perfusion pressure of the brain cannot be measured directly in humans. Parameters indirectly reflecting cerebral perfusion pressure are (a) the regional CBF/regional cerebral blood volume ratio, evaluated by PET or SPECT and (b) the reactivity of the cerebral vasculature to various vasodilating stimuli (CO_2, acetazolamide), evaluated by regional CBF techniques or TCD.

19.2 Transcranial Doppler and Cerebral Hemodynamics

TCD has been used extensively in various clinical situations and in the last two decades has established a role in the management of patients with cerebrovascular disease and stroke. Based on the Doppler principle, it uses ultrasound waves to insonate the blood vessels supplying the brain in order to obtain hemodynamic information. Anatomic abnormalities due to vascular occlusion, stenosis, and spasm can be indirectly detected. TCD ultrasonography is noninvasive and relatively inexpensive, can be performed at the bedside, and is simpler than other complex methods (SPECT, PET, xenon-computed tomography) for the investigation of cerebral hemodynamics.

The Doppler principle, in physics, is a wave theory that describes the relationship between the velocity of objects and transmitted or received wave frequencies. TCD provides continuous recordings of the instantaneous flow velocity in cerebral arteries and veins. The human brain receives blood through defined cerebral artery systems; each system consists of a cerebral artery with its branches extending down to the capillaries. When investigating the cerebral circulation, we thus examine the behavior of the blood flow at certain points along these transmission lines. TCD records blood velocities in the precerebral neck arteries and in the basal cerebral arteries and their branches. Velocity recordings from the mainstem middle cerebral artery (MCA) are the first choice (insonating through the temporal bone) in order to relate cerebral artery blood velocity to hemispheric blood flow.

The mechanics of flow in a vascular bed are usually simplified in three concepts: (a) perfusion pressure, the pressure differential between the inflow side and the outflow side, (b) the resistance to flow, and (c) the resultant flow volume.

The pulsatility index measured by TCD is postulated to reflect the degree of downstream vascular resistance [4]. An increase in cerebral vascular resistance could be due to narrowing of the small vessels by lipohyalinosis and microatherosclerosis.

An association has been found between the presence of silent WML and the pulsatility index, assessed by TCD ultrasonography, in middle-aged patients with uncomplicated, never-treated, essential hypertension [5].

TCD has become widely used to assess cerebral vasomotor reactivity, which provides information on cerebral autoregulation and collateral circulation. Cerebral vasomotor reactivity is defined as a shift between cerebral blood flow and cerebral blood velocity before and after administration of a potent vasodilatory stimulus test. Three such tests are currently used for this purpose: the apnea test (breath-holding index), CO_2 inhalation, and the Diamox test (i.v. acetazolamide), all of which are based on the dilatatory response of cerebral blood flow to hypercapnia. Certain advantages of the Diamox test have been described, but each of the three tests has advantages and disadvantages.

Early investigators of cerebrovascular reactivity used CO_2 as the cerebral vasodilating stimuli. However, patients with chronic lung disease or those with coronary heart disease and congestive heart failure cannot undergo this test. In contrast, acetazolamide testing is influenced less by the patient's cooperation. Acetazolamide is a selective inhibitor of carbonic anhydrase. One gram of this drug given intravenously increases CBF by more than 50 % in 10–20 min. Both techniques are comparable in their potential to identify patients with severely reduced cerebral perfusion pressure.

The cerebral vasomotor reactivity (VMR) (or vasodilatory capacity or cerebrovascular reserve capacity) of cerebral vessels is usually evaluated 10 min after the intravenous injection of 1 g of acetazolamide (Diamox test), and the response is calculated using the following formula:

$$\mathrm{VMR} = \left[\left(\mathrm{MCA\ velocity}_{\mathrm{acetazolamide}} - \mathrm{MCA\ velocity}_{\mathrm{baseline}}\right) / \mathrm{MCA\ velocity}_{\mathrm{baseline}}\right] \times 100.$$

The measurement of VMR by TCD has been shown to be a valuable noninvasive instrument for both practical clinical work and pathophysiological research in the field of stroke and cerebrovascular disease. Cerebral VMR reflects the compensatory dilatory capacity of cerebral arterioles to a dilatory stimulus. In the absence of major stenosis, an impaired cerebral VMR may reflect increased rigidity of the arteriolar walls. Decreased cerebral VMR has been observed in patients with hypertension and those with insulin-dependent diabetes mellitus [6]. Moreover, impaired cerebral VMR in young hypertensive subjects appears to improve after the initiation of antihypertensive treatment, suggesting that hypertensive microangiopathic changes could be, at least initially, reversible [7].

Tzourio et al. [8] using TCD in 628 individuals (39 % treated hypertensives) found that the degree of WML was associated with a reduction in CBF velocity.

However, until now, most studies have been performed in elderly people or have included treated hypertensive patients or patients with a history of cardiovascular disease, carotid stenosis, previous stroke, or diabetes, which could act as confounding factors. In order to establish cutoff values for cerebral hemodynamic parameters to define silent cerebral organ damage, longitudinal studies in homogeneous samples of middle-aged hypertensive patients will be necessary.

19.3 Cerebral SPECT

Cerebral SPECT with ^{99m}Tc-HMPAO allows semiquantitative evaluation of brain perfusion in humans. HMPAO (hexamethyl-propylene amine oxime) is a lipophilic molecule that crosses the blood–brain barrier and is converted within the brain cell into a hydrophilic form that remains stable for many hours and displays areas of increased or decreased perfusion. The striatum and thalamus are the brain areas most susceptible to lacunar thrombotic infarction, particularly in hypertensive patients, due to the vessel anatomy and vascular supply in these areas. Cerebral blood flow in hypertensive patients is maintained at the same level as in normotensive individuals by cerebral autoregulation, until significant arteriosclerosis and hypertensive vascular disease develop [9].

Cerebral SPECT is an accurate examination for the evaluation of regional CBF. The disadvantages are radiation hazard (not optimal for screening), poor spatial resolution, and the fact that the technique does not permit continuous registration.

The possible relationship between CBF and the existence of target organ damage at other levels in essential hypertensive patients is unclear. A relationship between left ventricular hypertrophy and a reduction in regional CBF–SPECT, especially in the striatum region, has been shown in asymptomatic middle-aged untreated essential hypertensive patients [10].

19.4 Summary

It remains unclear whether early functional cerebral alterations in hypertension are related to a higher risk of stroke or not. Optimal techniques for the detection of early silent brain damage should (a) be simple, relatively cheap, noninvasive, and easy to perform; (b) have excellent topographical resolution for the detection of regional abnormalities; and (c) have the capacity to assess therapeutic efficacy. The measurement of VMR by transcranial Doppler is a valuable noninvasive examination for both practical clinical work and pathophysiological research in the field of stroke and cerebrovascular disease. Cerebral VMR reflects increased rigidity of the arteriolar walls, and this abnormality has been observed in patients with hypertension. In addition, impaired cerebral VMR in young hypertensive subjects improves with antihypertensive treatment, suggesting that hypertensive microangiopathic changes could be, at least initially, reversible. Cerebral SPECT is an excellent technique for the evaluation of regional CBF, but the radiation hazard and poor spatial resolution means it is not recommended for the detection of early silent cerebral damage in hypertension in routine clinical practice.

References

1. Goldstein LB, Bushnell CD, Adams RJ, Appel LJ, Braun LT, Chaturvedi S, et al. Guidelines for the primary prevention of stroke: a guideline for healthcare professionals from the American Heart Association/American Stroke Association. Stroke. 2011;42:517–84.
2. The task force for the management of arterial hypertension of the European Society of Hypertension (ESH) and of the European Society of Cardiology (ESC). 2013 ESH/ESC Guidelines for the management of arterial hypertension. J Hypertens 2013;31:1281–357.
3. Pantoni L. Cerebral small vessel disease: from pathogenesis and clinical characteristics to therapeutic challenges. Lancet Neurol. 2010;9:689–701.
4. Lindegaard KF. Indices of pulsatility. In: Newell DW, Aaslid R, editors. Transcranial Doppler. New York: Raven Press; 1992. p. 67–81.
5. Sierra C, de la Sierra A, Chamorro A, Larrousse M, Domenech M, Coca A. Cerebral hemodynamics and silent cerebral white matter lesions in middle-aged essential hypertensive patients. Blood Press. 2004;13:304–9.
6. Troisi E, Attanasio A, Matteis M, Bragoni M, Monaldo BC, Caltagirone C, et al. Cerebral hemodynamics in young hypertensive subjects and effects of atenolol treatment. J Neurol Sci. 1998;159:115–9.
7. Sierra C. Essential hypertension, cerebrovascular reactivity and risk of stroke. In: Yim PJ, editor. Vascular hemodynamics bioengineering and clinical perspectives. Hoboken: Wiley Publishers; 2008. p. 299–314.
8. Tzourio C, Levy C, Dufouil C, Touboul PJ, Ducimetiere P, Alperovitch A. Low cerebral blood flow velocity and risk of white matter hyperintensities. Ann Neurol. 2001;49:411–4.
9. Strandgaard S, Paulson OB. Cerebral blood flow and its pathophysiology in hypertension. Am J Hypertens. 1989;2:486–92.
10. Sierra C, de la Sierra A, Lomeña F, Paré JC, Larrousse M, Coca A. Relation of left ventricular hypertrophy to regional cerebral blood flow: single photon emission computed tomography abnormalities in essential hypertension. J Clin Hypertens (Greenwich). 2006;8:700–5.

Part VI

Relationships Between Target Organ Damage and Blood Pressure Changes

Organ Damage and Blood Pressure in Untreated and Treated Hypertensives

20

Giuseppe Mancia, Cesare Cuspidi, and Sverre E. Kjeldsen

20.1 Introduction

A large number of studies in experimental animals and man show that angiotensin II, catecholamines and many other substances with cardiovascular and/or metabolic effects can favour alterations of organ function and structure independently on their ability to modify blood pressure (BP). There is, however, also a large body of evidence that these alterations are related to BP levels "per se" both in untreated and treated hypertensive patients. This chapter will offer some examples of this relationship mainly based on past work by the authors. The examples will largely focus on organ damages of more common assessment in clinical practice as well as of a more clear prognostic value, i.e. left ventricular hypertrophy, increased urinary protein excretion or reduction of glomerular filtration rate and carotid intima-media thickening or plaques. However, other types of organ damage will be also mentioned, albeit more briefly.

G. Mancia (✉)
University of Milano Bicocca–IRCCS Istituto Auxologico, Italiano, Milan Italy

C. Cuspidi
University of Milano-Bicocca - Dept. of Health Sciences-IRCCS Istituto Auxologico Italiano Centro Ricerche Cliniche, Italiano, Milan Italy

S.E. Kjeldsen
University of Oslo, Faculty of Medicine, Ullevaal Hospital, Department of Cardiology, Oslo, Norway

University of Michigan Health System, Division of Cardiovascular Medicine, Ann Arbor, Michigan, Norway

E. Agabiti Rosei, G. Mancia (eds.), *Assessment of Preclinical Organ Damage in Hypertension*, DOI 10.1007/978-3-319-15603-3_20

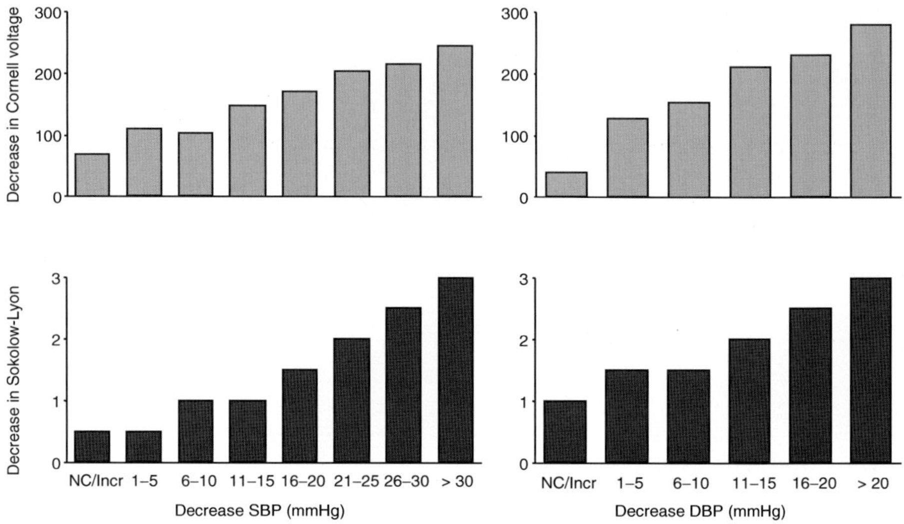

Fig. 20.1 Reduction in the incidence of left ventricular hypertension as a function of the treatment-induced reduction of systolic (*S*) and diastolic (*D*) blood pressure (*BP*) in the patients of the LIFE study. Left ventricular hypertrophy was assessed by electrocardiographic criteria, and the graphs show average values after 12 months of treatment (Kjeldsen)

20.1.1 BP and Cardiac Damage

20.1.1.1 Left Ventricular Hypertrophy (LVH)

Both when assessed by echocardiography and when determined by electrocardiographic criteria, the prevalence of LVH increases progressively with the increase in office systolic or diastolic BP [1–4]. Evidence is also available that in hypertensive patients a BP reduction is associated with LVH regression regardless of the drug used to obtain BP-lowering effect [5], a greater BP fall being accompanied by a greater and more spread-out reduction in the markers of the abnormally elevated values of left ventricular volume, thickness and mass [6]. This is exemplified in Fig. 20.1, which refers to the large number of hypertensive patients recruited for the Losartan Intervention For Endpoint reduction (LIFE) trial. Both when the increase of left ventricular mass was assessed by Cornell voltage and when it was assessed by Sokolow-Lyon electrocardiographic criteria, the percentage of patients undergoing a LVH regression 12 months into the study became progressively greater as the treatment-reduced systolic or diastolic BP fall increased. Similar observations have been made for echocardiographic estimations of LVH regression and for treatments different from those (losartan or atenolol) used in the LIFE trial [7].

20.1.1.2 Other Measures of Cardiac Damage

Although many more studies have focused on LVH, evidence is also available that other measures of cardiac damage exhibit a relationship with BP. One, observational studies have consistently shown that the diameter of the left atrium, the prevalence and the severity of systolic left ventricular dysfunction and the prevalence or the severity of diastolic dysfunction are both related to BP values [8, 9]. Furthermore, a

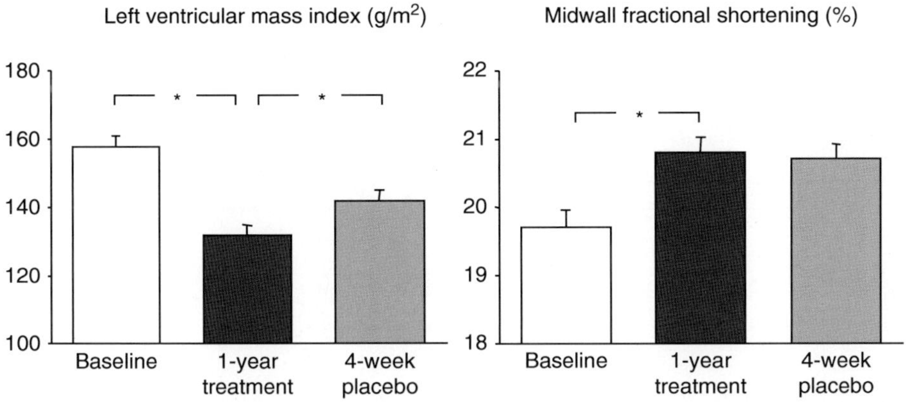

Fig. 20.2 Regression of left ventricular hypertrophy and improvement of left ventricular systolic function (midwall fractional shortening) with 24 h BP reduction over 1 year antihypertensive treatment in patients with hypertension and left ventricular hypertrophy. The left ventricular systolic function improvement was maintained when BP increased towards the initial baseline values after a final month of administration of placebo. From left to right histograms show baseline, 1 year treatment and final placebo data, respectively (From [14], with permission)

treatment-induced BP reduction has been repeatedly shown to improve these measures of cardiac damage, irrespectively of the antihypertensive drugs used and independently on the concomitant modifications of other biomarkers with potential cardiac effects [10, 11]. A pertinent example is offered by the Study on Ambulatory Monitoring of Pressure and Lisinopril Evaluation (SAMPLE), in which hypertensive patients with echocardiographic LVH exhibited not only a LVH regression but also a distinct improvement of LV contractile performance, assessed by a sensitive marker such as fractional midwall shortening [12], after 1 year reduction of office and out-of-office BP reduction by treatment (Fig. 20.2) [13]. Interestingly, the improvement was entirely maintained after BP returned to the initially elevated values over a final month of placebo administration, indicating that the contractile function had not improved because of the favourable effect of a reduced afterload on cardiac performance but it had a persistent structural and/or functional basis (Fig. 20.2) [14].

20.1.2 BP and Renal Damage

20.1.2.1 Microalbuminuria and Proteinuria

A huge number of studies have provided conclusive evidence that the prevalence of microalbuminuria or proteinuria is closely related to BP values, this being the case both in the general population and in diabetic or hypertensive nondiabetic patients [15, 16]. The evidence is also conclusive that a BP reduction by treatment is accompanied by a reduction of urinary protein excretion, regardless of the type of treatment employed, including that based on drug classes which also have a BP-independent antiproteinuric effect [17]. This is shown in Fig. 20.3 which refers to patients under treatment with drugs capable or not capable (irbesartan and amlodipine, respectively) to lower urinary protein excretion independently on BP

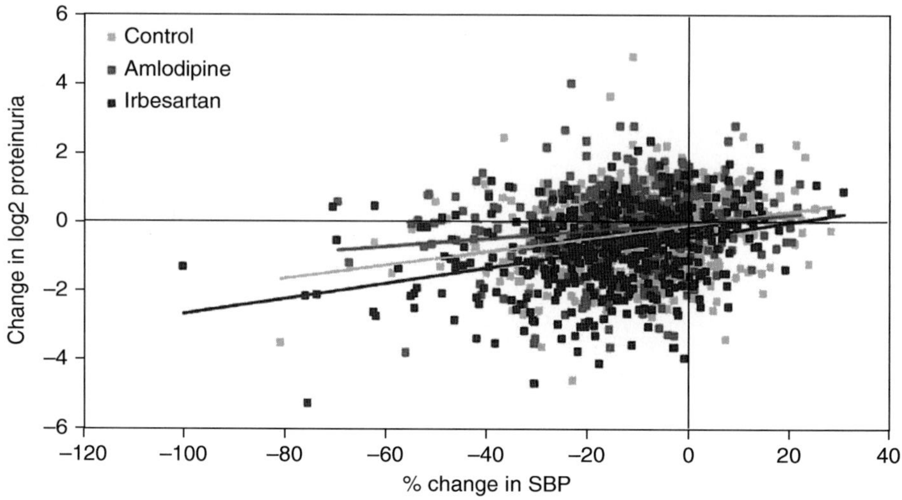

Fig. 20.3 Change in proteinuria associated with change of systolic BP after 1 year treatment in control patients as well as in patients treated with irbesartan or amlodipine. Regression lines between changes in proteinuria and BP are also shown (From [18], with permission)

changes. In both instances, the amount of urinary protein decreased progressively with the BP decrease, a similar phenomenon being apparent in the control group [18]. A further example is provided by the patients of the Ongoing Telmisartan Alone and in Combination with Ramipril Global Endpoint Trial (ONTARGET) in whom treatment consisted of an ACE inhibitor, an angiotensin receptor antagonist or a combination of the two drugs. In the patients pooled, the incidence of new-onset microalbuminuria or proteinuria was closely related to systolic BP down to very low on-treatment values, whose achievement was conversely associated with a more frequent return to normo-albuminuria in patients in whom an increased urinary protein excretion was detected at baseline (Fig. 20.4) [19].

20.1.2.2 Reduction of Glomerular Filtration Rate

Observational studies have shown that in the general population, in diabetic patients and in patients with chronic kidney disease, glomerular filtration rate (GFR) as estimated (e) by conventional formulae [20] becomes progressively less as BP progressively increases [21]. It has further been shown that although the reduction of renal perfusion pressure may raise serum creatinine in the first few weeks after initiation of antihypertensive treatment, in the long term lower on-treatment BP values favour preservation of renal function and delay progression to end-stage renal disease in hypertensive patients with or without chronic nephropathy. This is again shown in Fig. 20.4 again for the normotensive and hypertensive patients recruited for the ONTARGET trial [19]. It has further been documented for the patients with hypertension and diabetic nephropathy addressed in a variety of studies in which the time-related loss of eGFR was plotted vs the achieved BP values [22]. As shown in Fig. 20.5, the lower was the on-treatment BP, the lesser was the decline of renal function as assessed by a reduction in GFR,

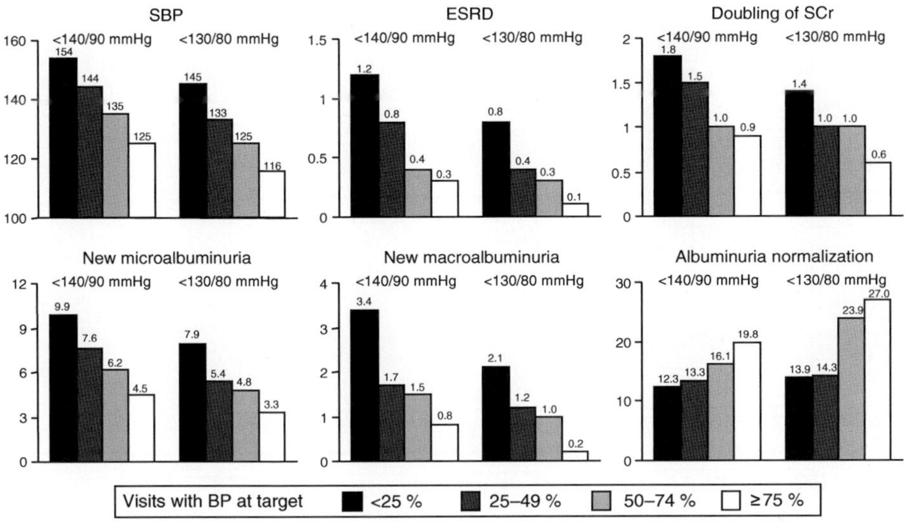

Fig. 20.4 Incidence of renal endpoints according to the % of on-treatment visits before the renal event in which BP was reduced to < 140/90 mmHg or < 130/80 mmHg. The greater the % of visits with BP at target, the lower the mean SBP over the treatment period (upper right panel). *SBP* systolic blood pressure, *ESRD* end-stage renal disease, *SCr* serum creatinine (Modified from [19], with permission)

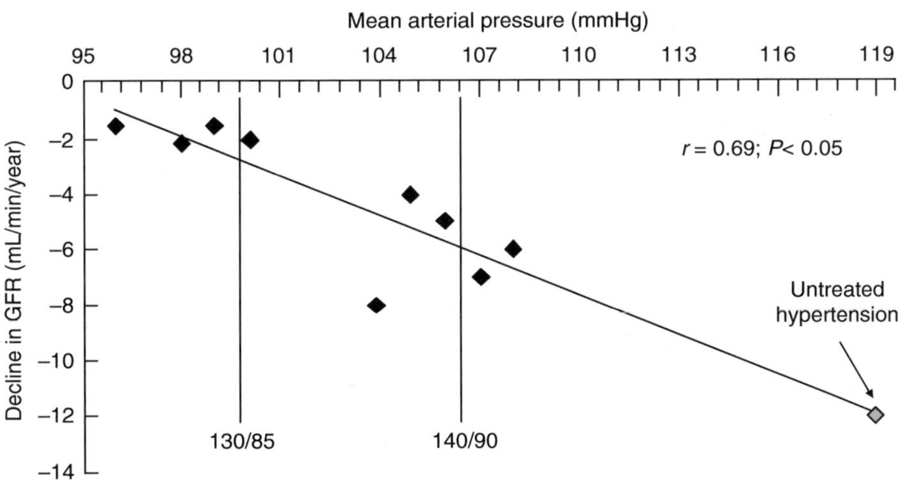

Fig. 20.5 Decline in glomerular filtration rate (*GFR*) according to on-treatment mean arterial pressure values in studies on diabetic nephropathy. Compared to untreated hypertension, antihypertensive treatment was associated with lower degrees of GFR decline. The smallest decline occurred at on-treatment mean arterial BP around 100 mg (From [22], with permission)

the most effective renal protection being observed for mean arterial pressures (diastolic + one third of systolic) of about 100 mmHg, i.e. a value approximately corresponding to 120 mmHg systolic and 75 mmHg diastolic BP.

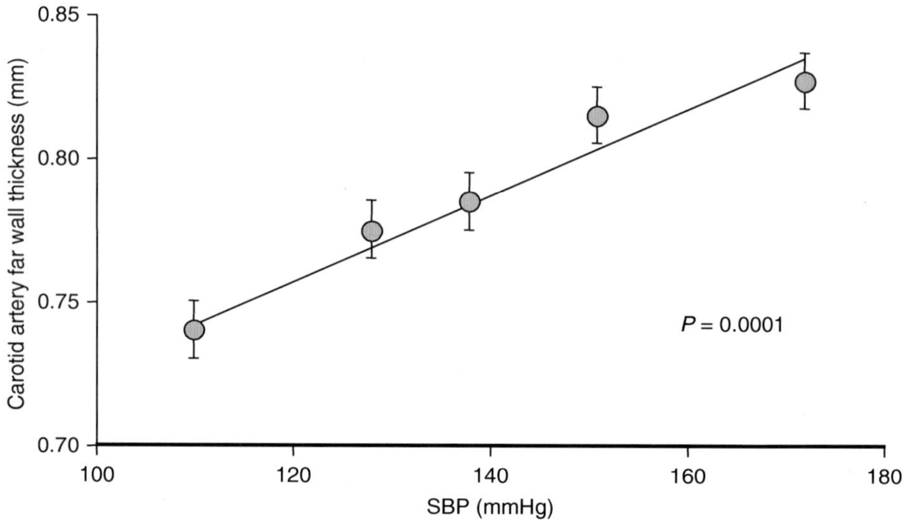

Fig. 20.6 Relationship between carotid artery far wall thickness and systolic blood pressure (*SBP*) in 1006 normotensive and hypertensive subjects (From [23] with permission)

20.1.3 BP and Vascular Damage

20.1.3.1 Carotid Intima-Media Thickness

As exemplified in Fig. 20.6, thickening of the common or internal carotid artery walls increases progressively as BP increases [23]. Furthermore, evidence has been obtained that when BP is reduced by treatment, the progressive increase of carotid wall thickness that occurs with ageing and type 2 diabetes can be delayed and that some reduction may sometimes occur [24, 25]. Although the amount of evidence is not comparable with that available for LVH and renal damage, this justifies the conclusion that vascular structural alterations that reflect atherosclerosis are also in direct relationship with BP values. This is strengthened by the evidence obtained with the use of more direct measures of atherosclerotic lesions such as that obtainable by intravascular quantification of the volume of an atherosclerotic plaque (IVUS). The intravascular measured coronary plaque volume showed a continuous relationship with the BP changes induced by antihypertensive treatment supporting the notion of a direct antiatherogenic effect of BP-lowering interventions [26].

20.2 Office or Out-of-Office BP?

Several studies have shown that in hypertensive patients cardiac, renal and vascular damages are more closely related to ambulatory than to office BP values. To quote some examples, both the prevalence of LVH and the echocardiographic left ventricular mass index value have been repeatedly found to have a higher correlation coefficient with the 24 h mean BP than with office BP values (Table 20.1) [27].

Table 20.1 Relationship of left ventricular mass index with office (or clinic) and 24 h mean systolic blood pressure (SBP)

Study	*N*	Clinic SBP	24 h SBP
Rowlands	50	0.45	0.60
Drayer	12	0.55	0.81
Devereux	100	0.24	0.38
Lattuada	50	0.07	0.40
Palatini	42	0.52	0.62
Gosse	61	0.40	0.49
White	30	0.13	0.54
Gosse	23	0.60	0.72[a]
Prisant	55	0.33	0.50
Verdecchia	150	0.44	0.57
Ravogli[b]	45	0.38	0.47

From Mancia et al. [27]
Data refer to coefficients of variation
[a]Daytime mean
[b]N with familiar H

The prevalence of microalbuminuria and proteinuria has been reported to have a better association with 24 h mean than to office BP [28, 29], the correlation being closer for the night than for the daytime values [30]. Closer relationships with ambulatory than office BP values have finally been reported for carotid intima-media thickness [31, 32], the superior organ damage-ambulatory BP association extending in other studies to additional types of vascular-dependant organ damage, including those reflecting (1) small-artery functional or structural abnormalities [33] and (2) functional or structural brain alterations such as decline of cognitive function or white matter lesions [34, 35].

Its closer association with organ damage has strongly contributed to the current notion that ambulatory BP is prognostically superior to the BP derived from measurement in the physician's office, presumably because ambulatory values reflect more accurately the BP regimen existing in daily life. Limited information exists, however, on the ability of out-of-office BP to predict progression or regression of organ damage over long-term longitudinal studies, although the available data also speak in favour of a greater ability of out-of-office BP, or of the treatment-induced out-of-office BP changes, to predict patients' cardiovascular risk. In the hypertensive patients of the SAMPLE study, for example, the regression of LVH that occurred over 1 year antihypertensive treatment was more closely related to the reduction of 24 h mean than to office BP, the home BP reduction lying approximately in between (Fig. 20.7) [13]. Similarly, in the hypertensive patients of the European Lacidipine Study on Atherosclerosis (ELSA) and the Plaque Hypertension Lipid-Lowering Italian Study (PHYLLIS), the changes in left ventricular mass and carotid intima-media thickness, respectively, were significantly predicted by changes in ambulatory but not by changes in office BP [36, 37]. Finally, in the type I diabetic patients studied by the Valencia group, not only was the presence of proteinuria associated with a higher ambulatory BP value (Fig. 20.8), but a higher ambulatory BP value predicted the progression to microalbuminuria and

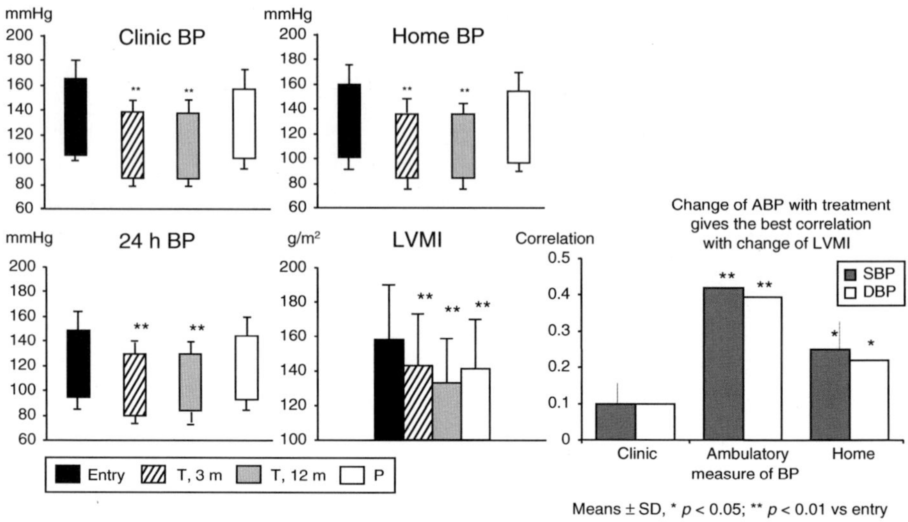

Fig. 20.7 Reduction from entry values of clinic (or office) self-measured home and 24 h (h) mean systolic blood pressure as well as of echocardiographic left ventricular mass index (*LVMI*) after 3 and 12 months of antihypertensive treatment in hypertensive patients with left ventricular hypertrophy. Data are also shown after a final month of placebo (*P*). Correlations between different BP and LVMI changes are shown at right *BP* blood pressure; *A* ambulatory (From [13] with permission)

nephropathy in individuals who did not have renal abnormalities at the start, independently on the office BP values [38].

20.3 Organ Damage and BP Phenomena Other than Mean Values

In the last few years, attention has been reserved also to the clinical importance of BP phenomena that occur within the 24 h, in particular the morning BP rise and the BP variations that characterize the day- and to a lesser extent the night-time. While recent studies have not confirmed [39, 40] the initial suggestion that morning arousal has an independent prognostic value [41], evidence is available that 24 h BP variability may adversely affect patients' prognosis over and above the role played by 24 h mean BP values. Many years ago evidence was obtained that for any given 24 h mean BP elevation (1), BP variability, as quantified by the standard deviation of the mean, was associated with an increased prevalence of a comprehensive score of organ damage [42] and (2) over several years of follow-up, hypertensive patients exhibited a greater increase of echocardiographic left ventricular mass as well as a more frequent progression to LVH if 24 h BP variability was greater [43]. There have also been several cross-sectional reports of an independent association between 24 h BP variability and other types of organ damage, including brain lesions and carotid intima-media thickness (Fig. 20.9) [32]. Finally, the regression of echocardiographic left ventricular hypertrophy seen after 1 year of successful

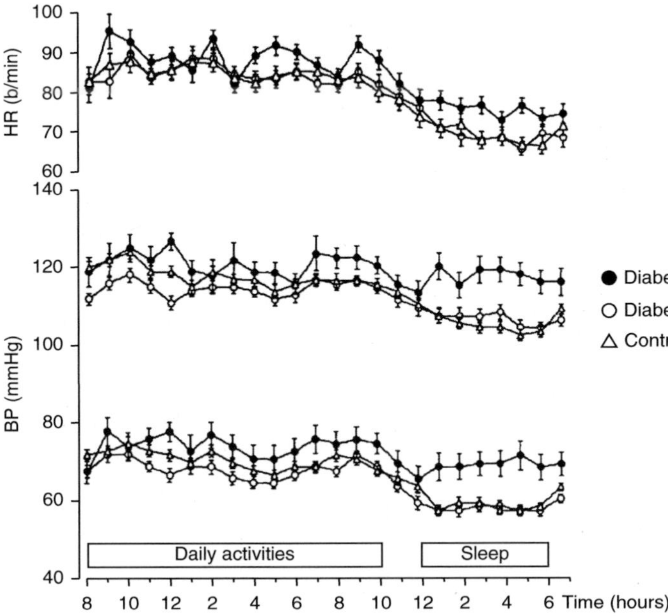

Fig. 20.8 24 h circadian blood pressure (*BP*) profile in control subjects, diabetic patients with an increased urinary albumin excretion (*UAE*) and normoproteinuric diabetics (Modified from [38] with permission)

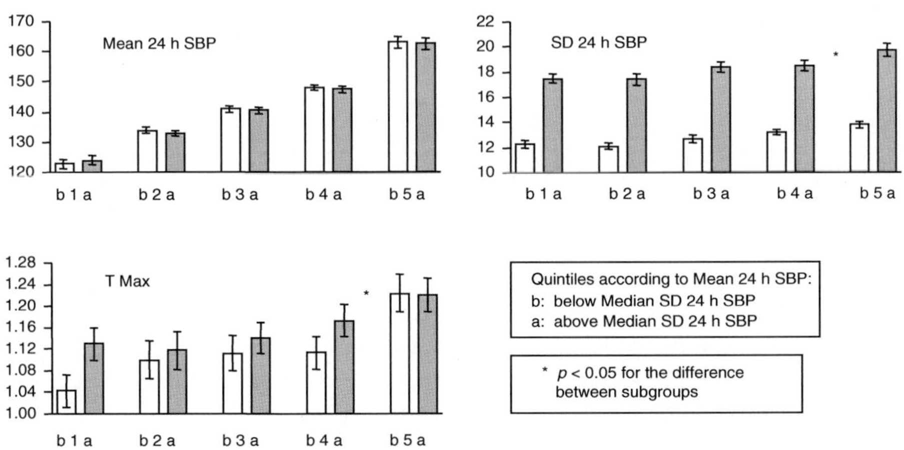

Fig. 20.9 Increase of carotid intima-media thickness (*T max*) according to quintiles of mean 24 h (h) systolic blood pressure (*SBP*) and, within each quintile, to the 24 h SBP standard deviation (*SD*) above and below the median value. Baseline data from the ELSA trial (From [32], with permission)

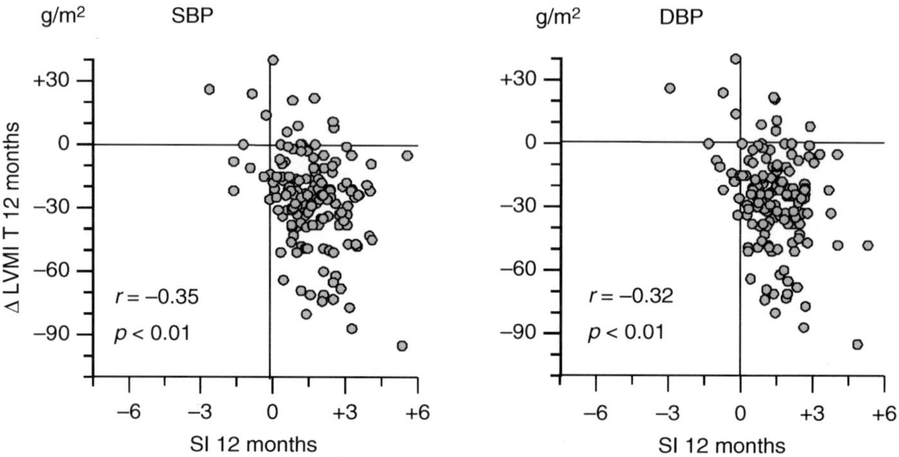

Fig. 20.10 Relationship changes in left ventricular mean index (*LVMI*) and the smoothness index (*SI*) of systolic and diastolic blood pressure (*SBP* and *DBP*) 12 months of treatment (From [44] with permission)

antihypertensive treatment has been shown to relate to the smoothness index (Fig. 20.10), i.e. a measure of the "homogeneity" of the BP reduction induced by treatment between different day and night hours that reflects the magnitude of on-treatment BP variations [44]. This favours the conclusion that BP variability may have a causative role in the development of organ damage, for which it serves as a long-term independent predictor, in line with the observation that greater 24 h BP variations independently predict cardiovascular and all cause mortality [45].

BP undergoes marked variations not only within the 24 h but also between days, weeks, months and seasons [46, 47]. Day-to-day BP variability has been related to cardiovascular risk in one study [48], and an adverse prognostic role has been repeatedly ascribed to the BP variations that occur between visits spaced by several months. In post hoc analyses of trials on hypertensive patients at high cardiovascular risk, visit-to-visit BP variability has been related to cardiovascular or renal outcomes, independently on the mean BP levels achieved over the same period [49, 50]. However, although similar evidence has been reported for the general population [51] (suggesting an adverse role of long-term BP variations not only at high but also at normal BP values) [51, 52], it is still not clear whether an inconsistent BP control between visits may have the same adverse consequences in individuals with a mild hypertensive condition, and an overall low added risk in which lack of control may mean BP values only few mmHg above target. In the patients with mild hypertension and a low-to-moderate risk of the ELSA trial, cardiovascular events were predicted by on-treatment mean but not by visit-to-visit variability [53]. As shown in Fig. 20.11, this was the case also for the end-of-treatment carotid intima-media thickness value which increased progressively from the quartile with the lowest to that with the highest on-treatment office systolic BP, while showing no relationship with the quartile values of on-treatment office systolic BP coefficient of variation,

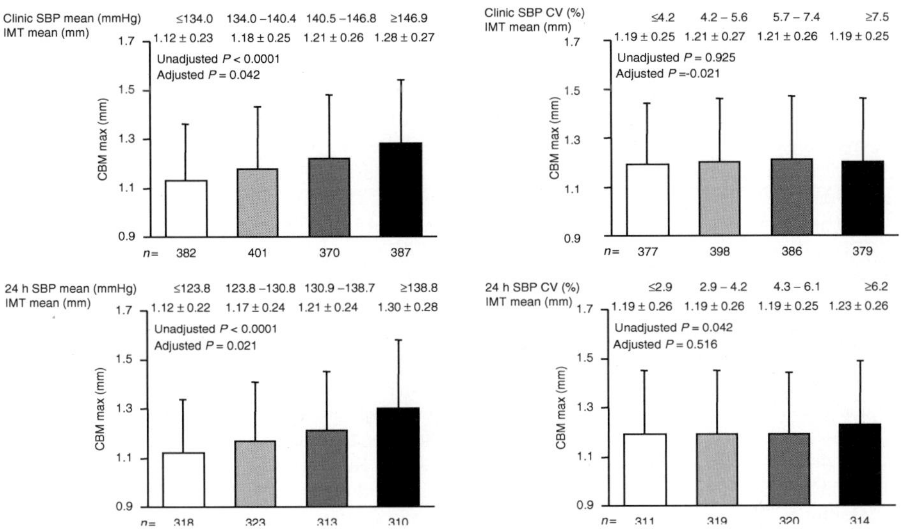

Fig. 20.11 Relationship between end-of-treatment carotid intima-media thickness (*IMT*) and on-treatment clinic (or office) or 24 h (h) systolic blood pressure (*SBP*) mean or between visit variability. Between-visit variability is shown as coefficient of variation (*CV*) of mean on-treatment values. Data are shown as quintiles. Adjustments were made for baseline confounders and for SBP CV (quintiles of mean SBP) or SBP mean (quintiles of visit-to-visit SBP CV) (From [53], with permission)

i.e. a measure of visit-to-visit BP variability independent on the mean BP value. The same was true for the visit-to-visit variability of 24 h mean systolic BP vs the 24 h average on-treatment value, strengthening the conclusion that under this circumstance BP variation may matter less than the achieved mean.

References

1. Mancia G, Carugo S, Grassi G, Lanzarotti A, Schiavina R, Cesana G, Sega R. Prevalence of left ventricular hypertrophy in hypertensive patients without and with blood pressure control : data from the PAMELA population. Pressioni Monitorate E Loro Associazioni. Hypertension. 2002;39:744–9.
2. Cuspidi C, Sala C, Negri F, Mancia G, Morganti A. Prevalence of left ventricular hypertrophy in hypertension: an updated review of echocardiographic study. J Hum Hypertens. 2012;26:343–9.
3. Cuspidi C, Rescaldani M, Sala C, Negri F, Grassi G, Mancia G. Prevalence of electrocardiographic left ventricular hypertrophy in human hypertension: an updated review. J Hypertens. 2012;30:2066–73.
4. Cuspidi C, Meani S, Sala C, Valerio C, Negri F, Mancia G. Age-related prevalence of severe left ventricular hypertrophy in essential hypertension. Echocardiographic findings of the ETODH study. Blood Press. 2012;21:139–45.
5. Fagard R, Celis H, Thijs L, Woulters S. Regression of left ventricular mass by antihypertensive treatment : a meta-analysis of randomized comparative trials. Hypertension. 2009;54:1084–91.
6. Solomon SD, Appelbaum E, Manning WJ, Verma A, Berglund T, Lukashevich V, Cherif Papst C, Smith BA, Dahlöf B, Aliskiren in Left Ventricular Hypertrophy (ALLAY) Trial Investigators. Effect of the direct Renin inhibitor aliskiren, the Angiotensin receptor blocker losartan, or both

on left ventricular mass in patients with hypertension and left ventricular hypertrophy. Circulation. 2009;119:530–7.
7. Devereux RB, Palmieri V, Sharpe N, De Quattro V, Bella JN, de Simone G, et al. Effects of once-daily angiotensin-converting enzyme inhibition and calcium channel blockade-based antihypertensive treatment regimens on left ventricular hypertrophy and diastolic filling in hypertension. The Prospective Randomized Enalapril Study Evaluating Regression of Ventricular Enlargement (PRESERVE) Trial. Circulation. 2001;104:1248–54.
8. Solomon SD, Janardhanan R, Verma A, Bourgoun M, Daley WL, Purkayastha D, Lacourcière Y, Hippler SE, Fields H, Naqvi TZ, Mulvagh SL, Arnold JM, Thomas JD, Zile MR, Aurigemma GP, Valsartan in Diastolic Dysfunction (VALIDD) Investigators.. Effect of angiotensin receptor blockade and antihypertensive drugs on diastolic function in patients with hypertension and diastolic dysfunction: a randomised trial. Lancet. 2007;369:2079–87.
9. Bombelli M, Facchetti R, Cuspidi C, Villa P, Dozio D, Brambilla G, Grassi G, Mancia G. Prognostic significance of left atrial enlargement in a general population. Results of the PAMELA study. Hypertension. 2014;64:1205–11.
10. Terpstra WF, May JF, Smit AJ, de Graeff PA, Havinga TK, van den Veur E, et al. Long-term effects of amlodipine and lisinopril on left ventricular mass and diastolic function in elderly, previously untreated hypertensive patients : the ELVERA trial. J Hypertens. 2001;19:303–9.
11. Wachtell K, Palmieri V, Olsen MH, Gerdts E, Papademetriou V, Nieminen MS, Smith G, Dahlöf B, Aurigemma GP, Devereux RB. Change in systolic left ventricular performance after 3 years of antihypertensive treatment: the Losartan Intervention for Endpoint (LIFE) Study. Circulation. 2002;106:227–32.
12. Aurigemma GP, Meyer TE, Sharma M, Sweeney A, Gaasch WH. Evaluation of extent of shortening versus velocity of shortening at the endocardium and midwall in hypertensive heart disease. Am J Cardiol. 1999;83:792–4.
13. Mancia G, Zanchetti A, Agabiti-Rosei E, Benemio G, De Cesaris R, Figari R, Pessina A, Porcellati C, Rappelli A, Salvetti A, Trimarco B. Ambulatory blood pressure is superior to clinic blood pressure in predicting treatment-induced regression of left ventricular hypertrophy. SAMPLE Study Group. Circulation. 1997;95:1464–70.
14. Perlini S, Muiesan ML, Cuspidi C, Sampieri L, Trimarco B, Aurigemma GP, Agabiti-Rosei E, Mancia G. Midwall mechanics are improved after regression of hypertensive left ventricular hypertrophy and normalization of chamber geometry. Circulation. 2001;103:678–83.
15. Bramlage P, Pittrow D, Lehnert H, Hofler M, Kirch W, Ritz E, Wittchen H. Frequency of albuminuria in primary care: a cross-sectional study. Eur J Cardiovasc Prev Rehabil. 2007;14: 107–13.
16. Hara H, Kougami K, Shimokawa K, Nakajima S, Nakajima R, Nakamura R, Hirahata K, Hoshi H, Nakamura M. The prevalence and risk factors of microalbuminuria in hypertensive patients under current medical treatment. Intern Med. 2014;53:1275–81.
17. Ando K, Ueshima K, Tanaka S, Kosugi S, Sato T, Matsuoka H, Nakao K, Fujita T. Comparison of the antialbuminuric effects of L-/N-type and L-type calcium channel blockers in hypertensive patients with diabetes and microalbuminuria: the study of assessment for kidney function by urinary microalbumin in randomized (SAKURA) trial. Int J Med Sci. 2013;10:1209–16.
18. Atkins RC, Briganti EM, Lewis JB, Hunsicker LG, Braden G, Champion de Crespigny PJ, DeFerrari G, Drury P, Locatelli F, Wiegmann TB, Lewis EJ. Proteinuria reduction and progression to renal failure in patients with type 2 diabetes mellitus and overt nephropathy. Am J Kidney Dis. 2005;45:281–7.
19. Mancia G, Schumacher H, Redon J, Verdecchia P, Schmieder R, Jennings G, Yusoff K, Ryden L, Liu GL, Teo K, Sleight P, Yusuf S. Blood pressure targets recommended by guidelines and incidence of cardiovascular and renal events in the Ongoing Telmisartan Alone and in Combination With Ramipril Global Endpoint Trial (ONTARGET). Circulation. 2011;124: 1727–36.
20. Levey A, Stevens LA, Schmid CH, Zhang YL, Castro 3rd AF, Feldman HI, Kusek JW, Eggers P, Van Lente F, Greene T, Coresh J, CKD-EPI (Chronic Kidney Disease Epidemiology Collaboration). A new equation to estimate glomerular filtration rate. Ann Intern Med. 2009;150:604–12.

21. Gansevoort RT, Correa-Rotter R, Hemmelgarn BR, Jafar TH, Heerspink HJ, Mann JF, Matsushita K, Wen CP. Chronic kidney disease and cardiovascular risk: epidemiology, mechanisms, and prevention. Lancet. 2013;382:339–52.
22. Bakris GL, Williams M, Dworkin L, Elliott WJ, Epstein M, Toto R, Tuttle K, Douglas J, Hsueh W, Sowers J. Preserving renal function in adults with hypertension and diabetes: a consensus approach. National Kidney Foundation Hypertension and Diabetes Executive Committees Working Group. Am J Kidney Dis. 2000;36:646–61.
23. Gamble G, MacMahon S, Culpan A, Ciobo C, Whalley G, Sharpe N. Atherosclerosis and left ventricular hypertrophy: persisting problems in treated hypertensive patients. J Hypertens. 1998;16:1389–95.
24. Cuspidi C, Negri F, Giudici V, Capra A, Sala C. Effects of antihypertensive drugs on carotid intima-media thickness: Focus on angiotensin II receptor blockers. A review of randomized, controlled trials. Integr Blood Press Control. 2009;2:1–8.
25. Roman MJ, Howard BV, Howard WJ, Mete M, Fleg JL, Lee ET, Devereux RB. Differential impacts of blood pressure and lipid lowering on regression of ventricular and arterial mass: the Stop Atherosclerosis in Native Diabetics Trial. Hypertension. 2011;58:367–71.
26. Nissen SE, Tuzcu EM, Libby P, Thompson PD, Ghali M, Garza D, Berman L, Shi H, Buebendorf E, Topol EJ, CAMELOT Investigators. Effect of antihypertensive agents on cardiovascular events in patients with coronary disease and normal blood pressure: the CAMELOT study: a randomized controlled trial. JAMA. 2004;292:2217–25.
27. Mancia G, Gamba PL, Omboni S, Paleari F, Parati G, Sega R, Zanchetii A. Ambulatory blood pressure monitoring. J Hypertens 1996;14 Suppl. 2:S61-6.
28. Boulatov VA, Stenehjem A, Os I. Association between albumin:creatinine ratio and 24-hour ambulatory blood pressure in essential hypertension. Am J Hypertens. 2001;14:338–44.
29. Rodilla E, Pascual JM, Costa JA, Martin J, Gonzalez C, Redon J. Regression of left ventricular hypertrophy and microalbuminuria changes during antihypertensive treatment. J Hypertens. 2013;31:1683–91.
30. Oliveras A, Armario P, Martell-Claròs N, Ruilope LM, de la Sierra A, Spanish Society of Hypertension-Resistant Hypertension Registry. Urinary albumin excretion is associated with nocturnal systolic blood pressure in resistant hypertensives. Hypertension. 2011;57:556–60.
31. Zanchetti A, Bond MG, Hennig M, Neiss A, Mancia G, Dal Palu' C, et al. Risk factors associated with alterations in carotid intima-media thickness in hypertension: baseline data from the European Lacidipine Study on Atherosclerosis. J Hypertens. 1998;16:949–61.
32. Mancia G, Parati G, Hennig M, Flatau B, Omboni S, Glavina F, Costa B, Scherz R, Bond G, Zanchetti A. ELSA Investigators. Relation between blood pressure variability and carotid artery damage in hypertension: baseline data from the European Lacidipine Study on Atherosclerosis (ELSA). J Hypertens. 2001;19:1981–9.
33. Rizzoni D, Porteri E, Platto C, Rizzardi N, De Ciuceis C, Boari GE, Muiesan ML, Salvetti M, Zani F, Miclini M, Paiardi S, Castellano M, Rosei EA. Morning rise of blood pressure and subcutaneous small resistance artery structure. J Hypertens. 2007;25:1698–703.
34. Kwon HS, Lim YH, Kim HY, Kim HT, Kwon HM, Lim JS, Lee YJ, Kim JY, Kim YS. Association of ambulatory blood pressure and heart rate with advanced white matter lesions in ischemic stroke patients. Am J Hypertens. 2014;27:177–83.
35. Klarenbeek P, van Oostenbrugge RJ, Rouhl RP, Knottnerus IL, Staals J. Ambulatory blood pressure in patients with lacunar stroke: association with total MRI burden of cerebral small vessel disease. Stroke. 2013;44:2995–9.
36. Agabiti-Rosei E, Trimarco B, Muiesan ML, Reid J, Salvetti A, Tang R, Hennig M, Baurecht H, Parati G, Mancia G, Zanchetti A, ELSA Echocardiographic Substudy Group. Cardiac structural and functional changes during long-term antihypertensive treatment with lacidipine and atenolol in the European Lacidipine Study on Atherosclerosis (ELSA). J Hypertens. 2005;23:1091–8.
37. Zanchetti A, Crepaldi G, Bond MG, Gallus G, Veglia F, Mancia G, Ventura A, Baggio G, Sampieri L, Rubba P, Sperti G, Magni A, PHYLLIS Investigators.. Different effects of antihypertensive regimens based on fosinopril or hydrochlorothiazide with or without lipid lowering

by pravastatin on progression of asymptomatic carotid atherosclerosis: principal results of PHYLLI-- randomized double-blind trial. Stroke. 2004;35:2807–12.
38. Lurbe A, Redón J, Pascual JM, Tacons J, Alvarez V, Batlle DC. Altered blood pressure during sleep in normotensive subjects with type I diabetes. Hypertension. 1993;21:227–35.
39. Verdecchia P, Angeli F, Mazzotta G, Garofoli M, Ramundo E, Gentile G, Ambrosio G, Reboldi G. Day-night dip and early-morning surge in blood pressure in hypertension: prognostic implications. Hypertension. 2012;60:34–42.
40. Bombelli M, Fodri D, Toso E, Macchiarulo M, Cairo M, Facchetti R, Dell'Oro R, Grassi G, Mancia G. Relationship among morning blood pressure surge, 24-hour blood pressure variability, and cardiovascular outcomes in a white population. Hypertension. 2014;64:943–50.
41. Kario K, Pickering TG, Umeda Y, Hoshide S, Hoshide Y, Morinari M, Murata M, Kuroda T, Schwartz JE, Shimada K. Morning surge in blood pressure as a predictor of silent and clinical cerebrovascular disease in elderly hypertensives: a prospective study. Circulation. 2003;107: 1401–6.
42. Parati G, Pomidossi G, Albini F, Malaspina D, Mancia G. Relationship of 24-hour blood pressure mean and variability to severity of target-organ damage in hypertension. J Hypertens. 1987;5:93–8.
43. Frattola A, Parati G, Cuspidi C, Albini F, Mancia G. Prognostic value of 24-hour blood pressure variability. J Hypertens. 1993;11:1133–7.
44. Parati G, Omboni S, Rizzoni D, Agabiti-Rosei E, Mancia G. The smoothness index: a new, reproducible and clinically relevant measure of the homogeneity of the blood pressure reduction with treatment for hypertension. J Hypertens. 1998;16:1685–91.
45. Sega R, Facchetti R, Bombelli M, Cesana G, Corrao G, Grassi G, Mancia G. Prognostic value of ambulatory and home blood pressures compared with office blood pressure in the general population: follow-up results from the Pressioni Arteriose Monitorate E Loro Associazioni (PAMELA) study. Circulation. 2005;111:1777–83.
46. Rose G. Seasonal variation in blood pressure in man. Nature. 1961;189:235.
47. Sega R, Cesana G, Bombelli M, Grassi G, Stella ML, Zanchetti A, Mancia G. Seasonal variations in home and ambulatory blood pressure in the PAMELA population. Pressione Arteriose Monitorate E Loro Associazioni. J Hypertens. 1998;16:1585–92.
48. Kikuya M, Ohkubo T, Metoki H, Asayama K, Hara A, Obara T, Inoue R, Hoshi H, Hashimoto J, Totsune K, Satoh H, Imai Y. Day-by-day variability of blood pressure and heart rate at home as a novel predictor of prognosis: the Ohasama study. Hypertension. 2008;52:1045–50.
49. Rothwell PM, Howard SC, Dolan E, O'Brien E, Dobson JE, Dahlof B, Sever PS, Poulter NR. Prognostic significance of visit-to-visit variability, maximum systolic blood pressure and episodic hypertension. Lancet. 2010;375:895–905.
50. Rothwell PM, Howard SC, Dolan E, O'Brien E, Dobson JE, Dalhof B, Poulter NR, Sever PS, ASCOT-BPLA and MRC Trial Investigators. Effect of-blockers and calcium channel blockers on within-individual variability in blood pressure and risk of stroke. Lancet Neurol. 2010;9:469–80.
51. Diaz KM, Tanner RM, Falzon L, Levitan EB, Reynolds K, Shimbo D, Muntner P. Visit-to-visit variability of blood pressure and cardiovascular disease and all cause mortality; a systematic review and meta-analysis. Hypertension 2014;64:965–82.
52. Sega R, Corrao G, Bombelli M, Beltrame L, Facchetti R, Grassi G, Ferrario M, Mancia G. Blood pressure variability and organ damage in a general population: results from the PAMELA study (Pressioni Arteriose Monitorate E Loro Associazioni). Hypertension. 2002;39:710–4.
53. Mancia G, Facchetti R, Parati G, Zanchetti A. Visit-to-visit blood pressure variability, carotid atherosclerosis, and cardiovascular events in the European Lacidipine Study on Atherosclerosis. Circulation. 2012;126:569–78.

Printed by Printforce, the Netherlands